Handbook of Inpatient Cardiology

Bryan J. Wells • Pablo A. Quintero
Geoffrey Southmayd
Editors

Handbook of Inpatient Cardiology

Springer

Editors
Bryan J. Wells
Division of Cardiology
Emory University School of Medicine
Atlanta, GA
USA

Geoffrey Southmayd
Division of Cardiology
Emory University School of Medicine
Atlanta, GA
USA

Pablo A. Quintero
Division of Cardiology
Beth Israel Deaconess Medical Center
Harvard Medical School
Boston, MA
USA

ISBN 978-3-030-47867-4 ISBN 978-3-030-47868-1 (eBook)
https://doi.org/10.1007/978-3-030-47868-1

This Springer imprint is published by the registered company Springer Nature Switzerland AG
The registered company address is: Gewerbestrasse 11, 6330 Cham, Switzerland

This book is dedicated to students and trainees past, present and future.

Contents

Contributors

Akanksha Agrawal, MD Department of Internal Medicine, Division of Cardiology, Emory University, Atlanta, GA, USA

Talal Khalid Al-Otaibi, MD Department of Medicine, Cardiovascular Institute, Beth Israel Deaconess Medical Center, Boston, MA, USA

Hakeem Ayinde, MD, MS Department of Cardiac Electrophysiology, Emory University, Atlanta, GA, USA

Vasilis C. Babaliaros, MD, FACC Cardiology, Emory University Hospital, Atlanta, GA, USA

Ankit Ajay Bhargava, MD Department of Cardiovascular Medicine, Emory University Hospital School of Medicine, Atlanta, GA, USA

George Black, MD Division of Cardiology, Emory University, Atlanta, GA, USA

Alfred E. Buxton, MD Department of Medicine, Cardiovascular Division, Beth Israel Deaconess Medical Center, Harvard Medical School, Boston, MA, USA

Dandan Chen, MD, PhD Department of Medicine, Division of Cardiology, Emory University, Atlanta, GA, USA

Mohsin Chowdhury, MD Cardiovascular Medicine, Beth Israel Deaconess Medical Center/Harvard Medical School, Boston, MA, USA

Devinder S. Dhindsa, MD Emory Clinical Cardiovascular Research Institute, Division of Cardiology, Department of Medicine, Emory University School of Medicine, Atlanta, GA, USA

Allen L. Dollar, MD, FACC, FACP Department of Cardiovascular Medicine, Emory University Hospital School of Medicine, Atlanta, GA, USA

Logan Eberly, MD Department of Medicine, Division of Cardiology, Emory University, Atlanta, GA, USA

Mikhael El Chami, MD Medicine, Division of Cardiology, Emory University Hospital-Midtown, Atlanta, GA, USA

Mariana Garcia, MD Division of Cardiovascular Disease, Emory University School of Medicine, Atlanta, GA, USA

Michael C. Gavin, MD, MPH Department of Medicine, Beth Israel Deaconess Medical Center, Boston, MA, USA

Eli V. Gelfand, MD, FACC Department of Cardiology, Beth Israel Deaconess Medical Center, Harvard Medical School, Boston, MA, USA

C. Michael Gibson, MD Cardiovascular Division, Department of Medicine, Beth Israel Deaconess Medical Center, Harvard Medical School, Boston, MA, USA

Edward W. Grandin, MD, MPH, MEd Department of Medicine, Beth Israel Deaconess Medical Center, Boston, MA, USA

Thomas H. Hauser, MD, MPH, MMSc Department of Medicine, Cardiovascular Institute, Beth Israel Deaconess Medical Center, Boston, MA, USA

David Hirsh, MD Division of Cardiology, Emory University, Atlanta, GA, USA

Jesse T. Jacob, MD Division of Infectious Diseases, Emory University School of Medicine, Atlanta, GA, USA

Maan Jokhadar, MD Department of Medicine, Division of Cardiology, Emory University, Atlanta, GA, USA

Joseph P. Kannam, MD Division of Cardiology, Beth Israel Deaconess Medical Center/Harvard Medical School, Boston, MA, USA

Vladimir Kaplinskiy, MD Beth Israel Deaconess Medical Center, Harvard Medical School, Boston, MA, USA

Daniel H. Katz, MD Department of Medicine, Beth Israel Deaconess Medical Center, Boston, MA, USA

Cyrus Kholdani, MD Department of Pulmonary, Critical Care and Sleep Medicine, Beth Israel Deaconess Medical Center, Harvard Medical School, Boston, MA, USA

Soroosh Kiani, MD, MS Department of Medicine, Division of Cardiology, Section of Electrophysiology and Pacing, Emory University School of Medicine, Atlanta, GA, USA

Bryan Kindya, MD Department of Medicine, Division of Cardiology, Emory University School of Medicine, Atlanta, GA, USA

Priya Kohli, MD Department of Cardiology, Emory University School of Medicine, Atlanta VA Medical Center, Decatur, GA, USA

Serge Korjian, MD Cardiovascular Division, Department of Medicine, Beth Israel Deaconess Medical Center, Harvard Medical School, Boston, MA, USA

Rebecca LeLeiko, MD, MS Department of Internal Medicine, Division of Cardiology, Emory University Hospital, Atlanta, GA, USA

Bruno B. Lima, MD PhD Emory Clinical Cardiovascular Research Institute, Department of Medicine, Division of Cardiology, Emory University School of Medicine, Atlanta, GA, USA

John C. Lisko, MD, MPH Cardiology, Emory University Hospital, Atlanta, GA, USA

Michael S. Lloyd, MD Department of Medicine, Division of Cardiology, Section of Electrophysiology and Pacing, Emory University School of Medicine, Atlanta, GA, USA

Department of Cardiac Electrophysiology, Emory University, Atlanta, GA, USA

Marvin Louis Roy Lu, MD Cardiovascular Disease, Emory University School of Medicine, Atlanta, GA, USA

Gina Lundberg, MD Division of Cardiovascular Disease, Emory University School of Medicine, Atlanta, GA, USA

Waddah Malas, MD Emory Clinical Cardiovascular Research Institute, Department of Medicine, Division of Cardiology, Emory University School of Medicine, Atlanta, GA, USA

Anant Mandawat, MD Emory Clinical Cardiovascular Research Institute, Division of Cardiology, Department of Medicine, Emory University School of Medicine, Atlanta, GA, USA

Winship Cancer Institute, Department of Hematology and Medical Oncology, Emory University School of Medicine, Atlanta, GA, USA

Michael McDaniel, MD Division of Cardiology, Emory University School of Medicine, Atlanta, GA, USA

Susan McIlvaine, MD Department of Cardiology, Beth Israel Deaconess Medical Center, Boston, MA, USA

Puja K. Mehta, MD Emory Clinical Cardiovascular Research Institute, Department of Medicine, Division of Cardiology, Emory University School of Medicine, Atlanta, GA, USA

Faisal Merchant, MD Division of Cardiology, Emory University, Atlanta, GA, USA

Mistyann-Blue Miller, MD Department of Interventional Cardiology, Beth Israel Deaconess Medical Center/Harvard Medical School, Boston, MA, USA

Appesh Mohandas, MD Department of Cardiology, Emory University School of Medicine, Atlanta, GA, USA

Donya Mohebali, MD Department of Medicine, Division of Cardiology, Beth Israel Deaconess Medical Center, Boston, MA, USA

Debby Ngo, MD Department of Pulmonary, Critical Care and Sleep Medicine, Beth Israel Deaconess Medical Center, Harvard Medical School, Boston, MA, USA

M. Carolina Gongora Nieto, MD Department of Internal Medicine, Division of Cardiology, Emory University, Atlanta, GA, USA

Amole O. Ojo, MD Department of Medicine, Cardiovascular Division, Beth Israel Deaconess Medical Center, Harvard Medical School, Boston, MA, USA

Duane Pinto, MD, MPH Department of Interventional Cardiology, Beth Israel Deaconess Medical Center/Harvard Medical School, Boston, MA, USA

Pablo A. Quintero, MD Cardiovascular Medicine, Beth Israel Deaconess Medical Center/Harvard Medical School, Boston, MA, USA

John Ricketts, MD Division of Cardiovascular Disease, Emory University Hospital, Atlanta, GA, USA

Muhie Dean Sabayon, MD Clinical Cardiac Electrophysiology, Emory University Hospital, Atlanta, GA, USA

Marwa Sabe, MD, MPH Department of Medicine, Division of Cardiology, Beth Israel Deaconess Medical Center, Boston, MA, USA

Nikoloz Shekiladze, MD Department of Cardiology, Emory University School of Medicine, Atlanta, GA, USA

Geoffrey Southmayd, MD Division of Cardiology, Emory University, Atlanta, GA, USA

Dustin Staloch, MD Department of Medicine, Division of Cardiology, Emory University Hospital, Atlanta, GA, USA

Mark K. Tuttle, MD Division of Cardiology, Beth Israel Deaconess Medical Center/Harvard Medical School, Boston, MA, USA

Stephanie Wang, MD Division of Cardiology, Emory University, Atlanta, GA, USA

Bryan J. Wells, MD Department of Medicine, Division of Cardiology, Emory University Hospital Midtown, Atlanta, GA, USA

Byron Robinson Williams III, MD Department of Medicine, Division of Cardiology, Emory University School of Medicine, Atlanta, GA, USA

Shu Yang, MD Department of Medicine, Beth Israel Deaconess Medical Center, Boston, MA, USA

An Young, MD, MPH Division of Cardiovascular Disease, Emory University School of Medicine, Atlanta, GA, USA

Peter Zimetbaum, MD Department of Medicine, Beth Israel Deaconess Medical Center, Boston, MA, USA

Abbreviations

A2C	Apical two chamber
A4C	Apical four chamber
AAS	Acute aortic syndrome
ABI	Ankle-brachial index
ABPM	Ambulatory blood pressure monitoring
ACE	Angiotensin converting enzyme
ACEI	Angiotensin converting enzyme inhibitor
ACLS	Advanced cardiac life support
ACOG	American College of Obstetricians and Gynecologists
ACR	American College of Rheumatology
ACS	Acute Coronary Syndrome
ACT	Activated clotting time
ADHF	Acute decompensated heart failure
AF	Atrial fibrillation
AF-CM	Atrial fibrillation-induced cardiomyopathy
AiCM	Arrhythmia-induced cardiomyopathy
AIDS	Autoimmune deficiency syndrome
AL	Amyloid light chain
ALI	Acute limb ischemia
aPTT	Partial thromboplastin time
AR	Aortic regurgitation
ARB	Angiotensin II Receptor Blocker
ARNIs	Angiotensin Receptor-Neprilysin Inhibitors
AS	Aortic stenosis
ASA	Acetyl salicylic acid (Aspirin)
ASCVD	Atherosclerotic Cardiovascular Disease
ASD	Atrial septal defect

AT	Atrial tachycardia
ATC	Anticoagulation
ATP	Anti-tachycardia pacing
ATTR	Transthyretin
AV	Atrioventricular
AV node	Atrioventricular node
AVA	Aortic valve area
AVNRT	Atrioventricular nodal reentrant tachycardia
AVRT	Atrioventricular reentrant tachycardia
BB	β - blocker
BMPR2	Bone morphogenetic protein receptor 2
BNP	β-type natriuretic peptide / Brain natriuretic peptide
BP	Blood pressure
BPM	Beat per minute
BTT	Bridge to transplant
CABG	Coronary artery bypass graft surgery
CAC	Coronary artery calcium
CAD	Coronary artery disease
CAS	Carotid artery stent
CBC	Complete blood count
CCB	Calcium channel blocker
CCTA	Coronary Computed Tomography Angiography
CDT	Catheter directed thrombolysis
CEA	Carotid endarterectomy
CHB	Complete heart block
CHD	Congenital heart disease
CHF	Congestive heart failure
CI	Cardiac Index
CIED	Cardiac implantable electronic device
CKD	Chronic kidney disease
CLI	Chronic limb ischemia
CM	Cardiomyopathy
CMP	Complete Metabolic Profile
CMR	Cardiac magnetic resonance
CMV	Cytomegalovirus
CO	Cardiac Output
COPD	Chronic obstructive pulmonary disease

CPK	Creatine phosphokinase
CRP	C- Reactive Protein
CRT	Cardiac resynchronization therapy
CRT-D	Cardiac resynchronization therapy- defibrillator
CRT-P	Cardiac resynchronization therapy- pacemaker
CS	Cardiogenic shock
CSM	Carotid sinus massage
CSP	Carotid sinus pressure
CT	Computed tomography
CTA	Computed tomography angiography
CTEPH	Chronic thromboembolic pulmonary hypertension
CTEPH	Chronic thromboembolic pulmonary hypertension
CTI	Cavo-tricuspid isthmus
CTPA	Computed tomography pulmonary angiogram
CV	Cardiovascular
CVA	Cerebrovascular accident
CVD	Cardiovascular disease
CXR	Chest X ray
DAPT	Dual antiplatelet therapy
DASH	Dietary approaches to stop hypertension
DBP	Diastolic blood pressure
DCCV	Direct current cardioversion
DCM	Dilated Cardiomyopathy
DKA	Diabetic ketoacidosis
DM	Diabetes mellitus
DOAC	Direct oral anticoagulant
DTS	Duke treadmill score
DUS	Duplex ultrasound
DVT	Deep vein thrombosis
EBV	Epstein-Barr Virus
ECG	Electrocardiogram
EF	Ejection fraction
ELR	External loop recorder

EMB	Endomyocardial biopsy
EPS	Electrophysiologic study
EROA	Effective regurgitant orifice area
ESC	European society of cardiology
ESD	End systolic diameter
ESR	Erythrocyte sedimentation rate
ETOH	Ethanol
FDA	Food and Drug Administration
FDG	Fluorodeoxyglucose
FFP	Fresh frozen plasma
FFR	Fractional flow reserve
FMD	Fibromuscular dysplasia
GCM	Giant cell myocarditis
GDMT	Guideline directed medical therapy
GERD	Gastroesophageal reflux disease
HACEK	Haemophilus, Aggregatibacter, Cardiobacterium, Eikenella, Kingella
HBPM	Home blood pressure monitoring
HCM	Hypertrophic cardiomyopathy
HCTZ	Hydrochlorothiazide
HCV	Hepatitis C virus
HELLP	Hemolysis, elevated liver enzymes, low platelet count
HF	Heart Failure
HFmrEF	Heart failure with moderately-reduced ejection fraction
HFpEF	Heart Failure with preserved ejection fraction
HFrecEF	Heart failure with recovered ejection fraction
HFrEF	Heart Failure with reduced ejection fraction
HIV	Human immunodeficiency virus
HJR	Hepatojugular reflex
HLD	Hyperlipidemia
HR	Heart rate
HTN	Hypertension
HTN-CM	Hypertension induced cardiomyopathy
IC	Intermittent claudication
ICA	Internal carotid artery
ICD	Implantable cardioverter- defibrillator

ICH	Intracranial hemorrhage
ICM	Ischemic Cardiomyopathy
ICU	Intensive care unit
IDU	Intravenous drug use
IE	Infective endocarditis
IFDVT	Ileofemoral deep vein thrombosis
iFR	Instantaneous Wave-Free Ratio
ILD	Interstitial lung disease
ILR	Implantable loop recorder
IMH	Intramural hematoma
INR	International normalized ratio
IV	Intravenous
IVC	Inferior vena cava
IVUS	Intravascular ultrasound
JT	Junctional tachycardia
JVP	Jugular venous pressure
LAA	Left atrial appendage
LBBB	Left bundle branch block
LDH	Lactate dehydrogenase
LE	Lower extremity
LFTs	Liver function tests
LMCA	Left main coronary artery
LMWH	Low molecular weight heparin
LV	Left ventricle
LVEF	Left ventricular ejection fraction
LVH	Left ventricular hypertrophy
MACE	Major adverse cardiac event
MCOT	Mobile cardiac outpatient telemetry
MCS	Mechanical circulatory support
MET	Metabolic equivalent
MI	Myocardial Infarction
MR	Mitral regurgitation
MRA	Mineralocorticoid receptor antagonist
MRC	Medical research council
MRI	Magnetic Resonance Imaging
MS	Mitral stenosis
NHANES	National health and nutrition examination survey

NOAC	Novel oral anticoagulant
NPV	Negative predictive value
NSAID	Nonsteroidal anti-inflammatory drug
NSTEMI	Non-ST Elevation Myocardial Infarction
NT-proBNP	N-terminal pro-β-type natriuretic peptide
NTG	Nitroglycerin
NYHA	New York Heart Association
OCT	Optical coherence tomography
OSA	Obstructive sleep apnea
PA	Pulmonary artery
PAC	Premature atrial contraction, pulmonary artery catheter
PAD	Peripheral arterial disease
PAN	Poliarteritis nodosa
PAU	Penetrating aortic ulcer
PBMC	Percutaneous balloon mitral commissurotomy
PCC	Prothrombin complex concentrate
PCI	Percutaneous coronary intervention
PCWP	Pulmonary Capillary Wedge Pressure
PE	Pulmonary embolism
PEFR	Peak expiratory flow rate
PET	Positron Emission Tomography
PFO	Patent foramen ovale
PFT	Pulmonary function tests
PHTN	Pulmonary hypertension
PLAX	Parasternal long axis
PMHx	Past medical history
PMT	Pacemaker-mediated tachycardia
PMT	Percutaneous mechanical thrombectomy
PND	Paroxysmal nocturnal dyspnea
PPCM	Peripartum cardiomyopathy
PPM	Patient prosthesis mismatch
PR	Pulmonic regurgitation
PS	Pulmonic stenosis
PSAX	Parasternal short axis
PTCA	Percutaneous coronary angioplasty
PTP	Pretest probability
PVC	Premature ventricular contraction

PVC-CM	Paroxysmal ventricular contraction induced cardiomyopathy
PVL	Paravalvular leak
PVR	Pulmonary vascular resistance
Qp:Qs	Ratio of pulmonary to systemic flow
RA	Rheumatoid arthritis
RAAS	Renin-angiotensin-aldosterone system
RAE	Right atrial enlargement
RCT	Randomized controlled trial
RFA	Radiofrequency ablation
RH	Right heart
RHC	Right heart catheterization
RV	Right ventricle
RVH	Right ventricular hypertrophy
RVR	Rapid ventricular response
SA node	Sinoatrial node
SA node	Sinoatrial node
SAH	Subarachnoid hemorrhage
SAVR	Surgical aortic valve replacement
SBP	Systolic blood pressure
SCAD	Spontaneous coronary artery dissection
SGLT2	Sodium glucose co-transporter 2
SHEP	Systolic hypertension in the elderly program
SIHD	Stable ischemic heart disease
SL	Sub-lingual
SLE	Systemic Lupus Erythematosus
SND	Sinus node dysfunction
SPECT	Single photon Emission Computed Tomography
SPRINT	Systolic pressure intervention trial
STE	ST-elevations
STEMI	ST-Elevation Myocardial Infarction
STS-PROM	Society for Thoracic Surgeons predicted risk of mortality score
SVC	Superior vena cava
SVi	Stroke volume index
SVR	Systemic vascular resistance
SVT	Supraventricular tachycardia

Syst-EUR	Systolic hypertension in Europe
T-CM	Tachycardia mediated cardiomyopathy
TAPSE	Tricuspid annular planar excursion
TAVR	Transcatheter aortic valve replacement
TBI	Toe-branchial index
TD	Thermodilution
TEE	Transesophageal echocardiogram
TIA	Transient ischemic attack
TID	Three times daily
TNF	Tumor necrosis factor
TOF	Tetralogy of Fallot
TPA	Alteplase
TR	Tricuspid regurgitation
TS	Tricuspid stenosis
TSPG	Trans-lesional systolic pressure gradient
TTE	Transthoracic echocardiogram
UA	Unstable angina
UFH	Unfractionated heparin
US	Ultrasound
V/Q Scan	Ventilation/Perfusion Scan
VAD	Ventricular Assist Device
VEGF	Vascular endothelial growth factor
VF	Ventricular fibrillation
VKA	Vitamin K antagonist
VM	Valsalva maneuver
VRE	Vancomycin resistant enterococcus
VSD	Ventricular septal defect
VT	Ventricular Tachycardia
VTE	Venous thromboembolism
WHO	World Health Organization
WMA	Wall Motion Abnormality

… the practice of medicine is predominantly a humanistic act. Physicians must care about their patients, and they must constantly improve their scientific knowledge about disease. To care and not know is dangerous. To know and not care is even worse. Caring and knowing must be combined to succeed in doctoring.

–J. Willis Hurst, MD

Introduction

The initial inspiration for this book was to create a handbook style reference of common cardiac conditions primarily for hospitalists. Throughout the writing process, it became evident that many providers will benefit from this text—ranging from internists to cardiologists including physicians, affiliate providers, and all levels of trainees in the medical field.

This book provides a concise overview of cardiac care for the hospitalized patient. Topics range from acute coronary syndrome to congestive heart failure to arrhythmias, and much more. Each chapter includes a summary of the presentation, diagnosis, and management of each condition. In addition, we provide a clinical approach to common cardiac chief complaints, as well as an overview of commonly encountered cardiac imaging and procedures. The chapters are formatted in an easy-to-read bullet format that includes "clinical pearls" and "key learning points" along with figures to illustrate the salient content.

We would like to thank all of the authors who contributed to the writing of this important book, which includes cardiology fellows and faculty from Emory University and Beth Israel Deaconess Medical Center. We are forever grateful for their time and expertise.

We hope that this book serves as a practical, reliable reference for anyone who cares for cardiac patients in the hospital setting.

Part I
Cardiac Pathology

Chapter 1
Acute Coronary Syndrome

Mark K. Tuttle and Joseph P. Kannam

Abbreviations

ACE	Angiotensin converting enzyme
ACS	Acute coronary syndrome
ARB	Angiotensin receptor blocker
ASA	Aspirin
CABG	Coronary artery bypass graft
ECG	Electrocardiogram
LVEF	Left ventricular ejection fraction
MI	Myocardial infarction
NSTEMI	Non-ST-elevation myocardial infarction
NTG	Nitroglycerin
PCI	Percutaneous coronary intervention
SL	Sublingual
STE	ST elevation
STEMI	ST-elevation myocardial infarction
UA	Unstable angina

M. K. Tuttle (✉) · J. P. Kannam
Division of Cardiology, Beth Israel Deaconess Medical Center/
Harvard Medical School, Boston, MA, USA
e-mail: mtuttle1@bidmc.harvard.edu; jkannam@bidmc.harvard.edu

B. J. Wells et al. (eds.), *Handbook of Inpatient Cardiology*,
https://doi.org/10.1007/978-3-030-47868-1_1

Clinical Pearls

- In ACS, supplemental oxygen should be given to hypoxemic patients only. Hyperoxia can lead to coronary vasospasm.
- While ST elevations can be used to localize a culprit coronary lesion, ST depressions perform poorly in this regard and should not be relied upon for localization.
- Known prior coronary lesions do not reliably predict the culprit lesion in a subsequent acute coronary syndrome.

Definitions (Table 1.1)

- *Acute myocardial infarction* [1]
  - Detection of a rise and/or fall of troponin (see Table 1.2) with at least one value above the 99th percentile WITH ≥1 of the following:
    - Symptoms of ischemia
    - New ischemic ECG changes (Figs. 1.1 and 1.2)
    - Development of pathological Q waves on ECG
    - Imaging evidence of new loss of viable myocardium (e.g., echo regional wall motion abnormality or perfusion defect on nuclear study)

TABLE 1.1 Acute coronary syndrome, a spectrum of disease

	Unstable angina (UA)	**Non-ST-elevation myocardial infarction (NSTEMI)**	**ST-elevation myocardial infarction (STEMI)**
Characteristics	Ischemic symptoms ECG +/– changes Negative biomarkers	Ischemic symptoms ECG +/– changes Positive biomarkers	Ischemic symptoms ECG with 1 mm STE in two contiguous leads (2 mm STE in V2-V3)

ECG Electrocardiogram, *ASA* aspirin, *STE* ST-elevation, *MI* Myocardial infarction

TABLE 1.2 Characteristics of Cardiac Biomarkers [3–5]

Biomarker	Peak	Return to normal	Sensitivity for MI at presentation	Sensitivity for MI at subsequent measurement
CK-MB (no longer recommended in guidelines)	24 h	48–72 h	66%	81% (at 6 h)
Troponin	24–48 h	5–14 d	79%	89% (at 6 h)
High-sensitivity troponin	24–48 h	–	97%	98.4% (at 1 h)

CK-MB Creatine kinase-MB isoform, *MI* Myocardial infarction

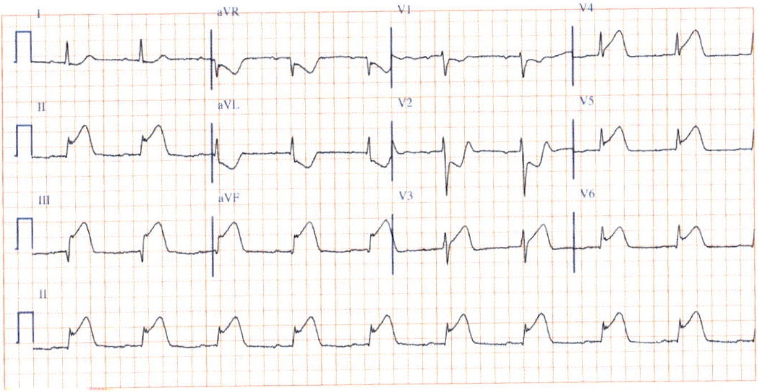

FIGURE 1.1 ST-elevation myocardial infarction. Note the ST elevations in the inferior leads and lateral precordial leads. Also note in V1-V2, the ST depressions with R waves and upright T waves suggest concurrent posterior wall involvement. This patient was found to have an occluded right coronary artery which was revascularized with primary percutaneous coronary intervention

Identification of an intracoronary thrombus by angiography or autopsy

- *Unstable angina*: New onset angina at rest, with minimal exertion, or crescendo angina [2] without elevation in cardiac biomarkers

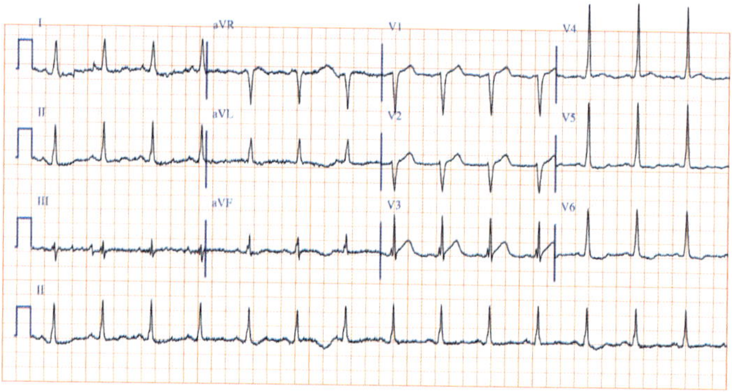

FIGURE 1.2 Non-ST-elevation myocardial infarction. This tracing demonstrates ST depressions in lateral leads suggestive of coronary ischemia, but ST depressions are not useful for localizing culprit coronary lesion. This patient was found to have mid-right coronary artery lesion on coronary angiography [6]

Pathophysiology

- In NSTEMI/unstable angina, likely from embolization and endothelial dysfunction rather than epicardial occlusion (as is seen in STEMI)
  - Single culprit lesion identified just 49% of the time. Complete occlusion in 36% [7].
  - Even in absence of occlusion, cath shows impaired tissue perfusion (↓blush), which predicts ↑ troponin
- Location of stable coronary artery disease is a poor predictor of future location of plaque rupture/occlusion
  - No correlation between severity of prior stenosis and new culprit lesion ($r^2 = 0.0005$, p = NS) [8]

Clinical Pearl
Known prior coronary lesions do not reliably predict the culprit lesion in a subsequent acute coronary syndrome.

Prognosis

- *STEMI*: 5.5% in-hospital mortality, 11% major bleeding [9], 11% 30-day case fatality rate, 8% 1-year CFR [10]
- *NSTEMI*: 3.9% in-hospital mortality, 9% major bleeding [9], 14% 30-day case fatality rate, 18% 1-year CFR [10]

Classification

- *Type I NSTEMI:* Spontaneous MI
  - *Atherosclerotic coronary artery disease*

    Reduced myocardial perfusion from coronary artery narrowing caused by a nonocclusive thrombus formed on a disrupted atherosclerotic plaque; release of injury markers is thought to result from microembolization of thrombus/plaque debris and blockage of distal blood vessels (most common).

    Fixed severe narrowing from progressive atherosclerosis or stent restenosis
  - *Inflammatory or infectious process* causing arterial narrowing, plaque rupture, and/or thrombogenesis
- *Type II MI: "Demand ischemia"* – Does not represent ACS event. Oxygen supply/demand mismatch where a condition other than coronary artery disease contributes.
  - *Increased myocardial O_2 requirement*: Fever, tachycardia, sepsis
  - *Reduced coronary blood flow*: Hypotension, coronary vasospasm
  - *Reduced myocardial O_2 delivery:* Anemia, hypoxemia
- *Type III:* Sudden cardiac death with suggestive symptoms with presumed new ECG changes but no time to check for biomarker elevation
- *Type IV*: Associated with percutaneous coronary intervention (PCI)
- *Type V*: Associated with coronary artery bypass graft surgery

- *Non-MI Troponin Elevation:* Myocardial injury not due to ischemia. Examples include decompensated heart failure, blunt cardiac injury, or defibrillator shocks.

Initial Management (Fig. 1.3)

- *Rule-out STEMI: Serial* 12-lead ECGs.
  - Repeat at 15–30 min intervals if patient remains symptomatic since NSTEMI can evolve to STEMI

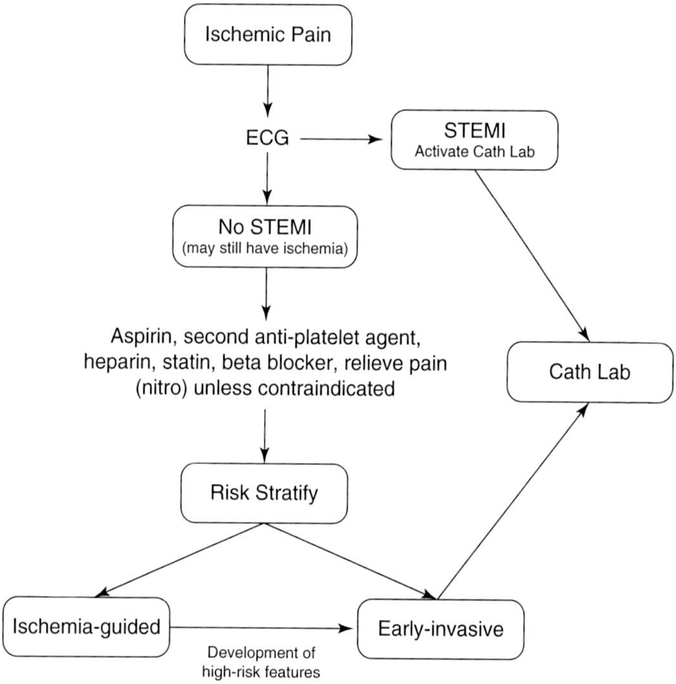

FIGURE 1.3 Management algorithm for acute coronary syndrome

> **Clinical Pearl**
> While ST elevations can be used to localize a culprit coronary lesion, ST depressions perform poorly in this regard and should not be relied upon for localization.

- *Relieve ischemic pain*:
  - *Nitroglycerin:* Titrate to chest pain-free (see below)
  - *Morphine*: Minimize use to avoid masking, rather than treating, ongoing ischemic symptoms.
  - *DON'T USE NSAIDS:* ↑ risk of cardiovascular events (death, MI, heart failure, stroke)
- *Decrease myocardial oxygen demand*: Reduce tachycardia and hypertension
  - *Beta blocker*: Cardioselective is preferred (atenolol or metoprolol)

    Addresses tachycardia, hypertension, and prevents ventricular arrhythmias

    Goal of HR 60–70

    Contraindicated in:
    - Cocaine-induced MI. (Give benzodiazepines instead!) Or labetalol.
    - Hypotension
    - Decompensated heart failure
    - Reactive airway disease
    - PR interval > 0.24 s, or second degree AV block

    Mortality ↓ in patients who receive β-blockers [11].
  - *Nitroglycerin*: Predominantly venodilator (↓ preload), also arteriodilator (↓ afterload)

    May cause reflex tachycardia (↑ myocardial oxygen consumption$_2$) unless concurrent beta-blocker given

    SL NTG (0.4 mg) every 5 min for a total of three doses

    IV NTG for up to 48 h after UA/NSTEMI for ischemia/ongoing chest pain, heart failure, HTN
    - Does not decrease mortality. Should not preclude other mortality-reducing therapy.
    - Development of tachyphylaxis to NTG gtt after ~24 h.

Contraindicated in:

- MI with RV involvement due to risk of hypotension. Consider RV infarct with inferior STEMI, can use right-sided leads to confirm.
- Severe aortic stenosis, since patients are preload-dependent
- Phosphodiesterase inhibitor (e.g. sildenafil) taken within 24 h

- *Increase oxygen delivery to myocardium*
  - Supplemental O_2 for hypoxemic patients only. Hyperoxia can cause coronary vasospasm [12]

- *Antithrombotic therapy (Table 1.3)*
  - *Aspirin:* Aspirin 325 mg chewed immediately, then 81 mg daily in all patients who can tolerate
  - *Second antiplatelet therapy*: This decision should be discussed with a cardiologist.

    Some patients may require *urgent* CABG, and may bleed excessively if given a second anti-platelet agent. But for patients receiving PCI, pre-loading with P2Y12 inhibitor was shown to reduce composite major adverse cardiac events.

    Trials demonstrate anti-ischemic benefits of clopidogrel without an increase in life-threatening bleeding during CABG [13].

Clinical Pearl

In ACS, supplemental oxygen should be given to hypoxemic patients only. Hyperoxia can lead to coronary vasospasm.

- *Anticoagulant therapy*: Heparin or enoxaparin w/aspirin reduced 7-day mortality or MI by 50% in early studies [14], but this data largely comes from the pre-PCI era and its contemporary benefit is likely attenuated.

  Duration: 48 h or until PCI is performed (Class I, LOE B) [15]

Table 1.3 Pharmacology of $P2Y_{12}$ Anti-platelet Agents

Characteristic	**Clopidogrel (Plavix™)**	**Ticagrelor (Brilinta™)**	**Prasugrel (Effient™)**
Loading dose	600 mg	180 mg	60 mg
Maintenance dose	75 mg QD	90 mg BID	10 mg QD
ADP $P2Y_{12}$ inhibition	Irreversible	Reversible	Irreversible
Onset with loading	3–5 h	2 h	1 h (loading dose contraindicated until after diagnostic angiography)
Duration of effect	5–9 days	1–2 days	5–9 days
Side effects	Bleeding, rash, neutropenia (rare)	Bleeding, dyspnea (14%), bradyarrhythmias, ↑uric acid	Bleeding
Clearance	Renal	Hepatic (75%), renal (25%)	Renal
Contraindications	Active bleeding, allergy	History of intracranial hemorrhage, active bleeding, allergy	History of TIA/stroke, active bleeding, allergy

QD once daily, *BID* twice daily, *ADP* Adenosine diphosphate

- *Guard against ventricular arrhythmias*
  - Beta-blocker as above
  - Correct electrolyte abnormalities, replete K^+ to 4 mEq/L and Mg^{2+} to 2 mEq/L [16]
- *Guard against ventricular remodeling/aneurysm formation/rupture*
  - Discontinue NSAIDs and COX-2 inhibitors (other than ASA)
  - Start ACE-inhibitor/ARB if pulmonary congestion or LVEF <40% and no hypotension

Risk Stratification

- *Early invasive (cath within 4–48 h) strategy if:*
  - Unstable: Refractory pain, hemodynamically unstable, electrically unstable (arrhythmia) (*Class I, LOE A*) [15]
  - *Initially stable, but with high-risk features (Class I, LOE B)* [15]:
    - Recurrent angina or ischemia at rest or with low-level activities despite medical therapy
    - PCI within 6 months
    - Prior CABG
    - High risk score: TIMI ≥3, GRACE >140 (see below)
    - Reduced left ventricular function (LVEF less than 40%)
    - Elevated cardiac biomarkers (TnT or TnI)
    - New or presumably new ST-segment depression
    - Signs or symptoms of HF or new or worsening mitral regurgitation
    - High-risk findings from noninvasive testing
- *Risk stratification scoring systems advised by AHA*: TIMI, GRACE
  - *TIMI score*: *ARSERBA* acronym. Predicts mortality, new/recurrent MI, or revascularization at 14 days

    1 point each. Low: 0–2 (5–8% risk), Medium: 3–4 (13–20% risk), High: 5–7 (26–40% risk)
    - *A*ge > = 65 years
    - *R*isk factors (3+) for CHD: HTN, DM, HLD, smoking, or positive family history of early MI
    - *S*tenosis of coronaries > = 50% (known from prior angiography)
    - *E*CG ST segment deviation
    - *R*ecurrent angina (2+ anginal episodes in prior 24 h)
    - *B*iomarkers: Elevated serum cardiac biomarkers
    - *A*SA within 7 days (marker for more severe coronary disease if event occurred despite ASA)

Conservative/Ischemia-Guided Strategy

- If during the conservative strategy, the patient develops high risk features, they should go to angiography
  - *High risk features: recurrent symptoms, heart failure, malignant arrhythmias*
- Echocardiogram to evaluate LVEF: consider angiography if LVEF is newly reduced <40%
- Stress test: Patients without high risk features and free of ischemia for 12–24 h (Class I, LOE B) [15]
  - For intermediate or high risk results: angiography
  - Low risk: can generally be managed with medications alone
- Continue heparin for 48 h or until PCI

Early Invasive Management Strategy

- *Benefits*: ↓ angina, ↓ readmission, ↓ MI risk, ↑ long-term survival in appropriately selected patients.
- *Risks*: AKI (6–13%. Contrast and atheroemboli. No ↑ risk of HD [17]), bleeding
- Selected possible scenarios based on cardiac catheterization
  - Percutaneous coronary intervention
    Continue ASA
    Start/continue second antiplatelet agent as directed by cardiology
    Discontinue anticoagulation following uncomplicated cases
  - Requiring CABG (e.g., 3VD)
    Continue ASA
    Continue heparin until 12–24 h prior to CABG
    Discontinue second anti-platelet agent 5–7 days prior to elective CABG
  - Non-obstructive CAD: Suggestive of non-ACS event, or entity termed MINOCA (Myocardial infarction with nonobstructive coronary arteries) (5% of MIs) [18]

Continue ASA
Continue second antiplatelet agent if ongoing suspicion for ACS
Continue heparin for 48 h
Entertain possible underlying causes (e.g., myocarditis)

Post-ACS Management

- *Medical management of ACS without PCI*
  - ASA 81 mg indefinitely
  - Clopidogrel/ticagrelor for 12 months. (Prasugrel is only FDA approved when PCI is planned.)
- *Bare metal stent*
  - No benefit for bare metal stents in the era of modern drug-eluting stents when anticipated DAPT duration is ≥3 months [19], and the next generation of drug-eluting stents may narrow this margin to 1 month or shorter.
- *Drug-eluting stent*
  - ASA 81 mg daily indefinitely
  - Clopidogrel/prasugrel/ticagrelor for 12 months (ACS), or 6 months (stable CAD). Shorter durations depending on the patient's thrombotic/bleeding risk profile and stent characteristics and should be directed by interventional cardiology
- *Statins:* High intensity statin (Atorvastatin 40–80 mg, Rosuvastatin 20–40 mg) is preferred indefinitely regardless of LDL
  - ↓ death from any cause, myocardial infarction, documented unstable angina requiring rehospitalization, revascularization and the benefit of high intensity statin emerges at 30 days and is persistent [20]
- *Long-term anticoagulation:* for atrial fibrillation or LV thrombus/apical aneurysm
- *ACE-inhibitor/ARB* for anterior MI, EF ≤ 40%, or with clinical heart failure symptoms.
- *Beta blocker*: All patients without contraindications

Key Learning Points

1. The definition of myocardial infarction is not simply troponin elevation, but must also include at least one of the following: symptoms of ischemia, ischemia/infarction on ECG, new regional wall motion abnormality on TTE/nuclear study, or coronary thrombosis at autopsy.
2. Distinguishing acute coronary syndrome (ACS) from other causes of chest pain requires careful evaluation of patient history, ECG, imaging and laboratory data. The primary goal of ACS management is to relieve ischemia, either via medical or invasive therapies.
3. For Type II MI ("demand ischemia") the initial treatment should focus on addressing the underlying cause of increased myocardial oxygen demand, not on invasive coronary evaluation.
4. Clinical risk stratification with the TIMI or GRACE scores can help decide which ACS patients should proceed to cardiac catheterization, and which patients can be treated medically up front.

References

1. Thygesen K, Alpert JS, Jaffe AS, Chaitman BR, Bax JJ, Morrow DA, White HD. Executive Group on behalf of the Joint European Society of Cardiology (ESC)/American College of Cardiology (ACC)/American Heart Association (AHA)/World Heart Federation (WHF) Task Force for the Universal Definition of Myocardial Infarction (2018) Fourth Universal Definition of Myocardial Infarction. J Am Coll Cardiol. 2018;72:2231–64.
2. (2011) NCDR® CathPCI Registry® v4.4 Coder's Data Dictionary. https://www.ncdr.com/WebNCDR/docs/default-source/public-data-collection-documents/cathpci_v4_codersdictionary_4-4.pdf. Accessed 1 Jun 2019
3. Jaffe AS, Babuin L, Apple FS. Biomarkers in acute cardiac disease: the present and the future. J Am Coll Cardiol. 2006;48:1–11.

4. Eggers KM, Oldgren J, Nordenskjöld A, Lindahl B. Diagnostic value of serial measurement of cardiac markers in patients with chest pain: limited value of adding myoglobin to troponin I for exclusion of myocardial infarction. Am Heart J. 2004;148:574–81.
5. Solecki K, Dupuy AM, Kuster N, et al. Kinetics of high-sensitivity cardiac troponin T or troponin I compared to creatine kinase in patients with revascularized acute myocardial infarction. Clin Chem Lab Med. 2015;53:707–14.
6. Abouantoun S, Ahnve S, Savvides M, Witztum K, Jensen D, Froelicher V. Can areas of myocardial ischemia be localized by the exercise electrocardiogram? A correlative study with thallium-201 scintigraphy. Am Heart J. 1984;108:933–41.
7. Kerensky RA, Wade M, Deedwania P, Boden WE, Pepine CJ. Revisiting the culprit lesion in non--Q-wave myocardial infarction: results from the VANQWISH trial angiographic core laboratory. J Am Coll Cardiol. 2002;39:1456–63.
8. Little WC, Constantinescu M, Applegate RJ, Kutcher MA, Burrows MT, Kahl FR, Santamore WP. Can coronary angiography predict the site of a subsequent myocardial infarction in patients with mild-to-moderate coronary artery disease? Circulation. 1988;78:1157–66.
9. Roe MT, Messenger JC, Weintraub WS, et al. Treatments, trends, and outcomes of acute myocardial infarction and percutaneous coronary intervention. J Am Coll Cardiol. 2010;56:254–63.
10. McManus DD, Gore J, Yarzebski J, Spencer F, Lessard D, Goldberg RJ. Recent trends in the incidence, treatment, and outcomes of patients with STEMI and NSTEMI. Am J Med. 2011;124:40–7.
11. Ellis K, Tcheng JE, Sapp S, Topol EJ, Michael Lincoff A. Mortality benefit of beta blockade in patients with acute coronary syndromes undergoing coronary intervention: pooled results from the Epic, Epilog, Epistent, Capture and Rapport Trials. J Interv Cardiol. 2003;16:299–305.
12. Moradkhan R, Sinoway LI. Revisiting the role of oxygen therapy in cardiac patients. J Am Coll Cardiol. 2010;56:1013–6.
13. Fitchett D, Eikelboom J, Fremes S, et al. Dual antiplatelet therapy in patients requiring urgent coronary artery bypass grafting surgery: a position statement of the Canadian Cardiovascular Society. Can J Cardiol. 2009;25:683–9.
14. Eikelboom JW, Anand SS, Malmberg K, Weitz JI, Ginsberg JS, Yusuf S. Unfractionated heparin and low-molecular-weight

heparin in acute coronary syndrome without ST elevation: a meta-analysis. Lancet. 2000;355:1936–42.
15. Amsterdam EA, Wenger NK, Brindis RG, et al. 2014 AHA/ACC guideline for the management of patients with non-ST-elevation acute coronary syndromes: a report of the American College of Cardiology/American Heart Association Task Force on Practice Guidelines. Circulation. 2014;130:e344–426.
16. Goyal A, Spertus JA, Gosch K, Venkitachalam L, Jones PG, Van den Berghe G, Kosiborod M. Serum potassium levels and mortality in acute myocardial infarction. JAMA. 2012;307:157–64.
17. James MT, Tonelli M, Ghali WA, Knudtson ML, Faris P, Manns BJ, Pannu N, Galbraith PD, Hemmelgarn BR, Alberta Provincial Project for Outcome Assessment in Coronary Heart Disease and Alberta Kidney Disease Network Investigators. Renal outcomes associated with invasive versus conservative management of acute coronary syndrome: propensity matched cohort study. BMJ. 2013;347:f4151.
18. Tamis-Holland JE, Jneid H, Reynolds HR, et al. Contemporary diagnosis and management of patients with myocardial infarction in the absence of obstructive coronary artery disease: a scientific statement from the American Heart Association. Circulation. 2019;139:e891–908.
19. Colombo A, Giannini F, Briguori C. Should we still have bare-metal stents available in our catheterization laboratory? J Am Coll Cardiol. 2017;70:607–19.
20. Cannon CP, Braunwald E, McCabe CH, et al. Intensive versus moderate lipid lowering with statins after acute coronary syndromes. N Engl J Med. 2004;350:1495–504.

Chapter 2
Stable Ischemic Heart Disease

Daniel H. Katz and Michael C. Gavin

Abbreviations

ACS	Acute Coronary Syndrome
BNP	Brain Natriuretic Peptide
CAD	Coronary Artery Disease
CBC	Complete Blood Count
CCTA	Coronary Computed Tomography Angiography
CMP	Complete Metabolic Profile
ECG	Electrocardiogram
MI	Myocardial Infarction
MRI	Magnetic Resonance Imaging
PCI	Percutaneous Coronary Intervention
PET	Positron Emission Tomography
SIHD	Stable Ischemic Heart Disease
SPECT	Single Photon Emission Computed Tomography
UA	Unstable Angina

D. H. Katz (✉) · M. C. Gavin
Department of Medicine, Beth Israel Deaconess Medical Center, Boston, MA, USA
e-mail: dkatz@bidmc.harvard.edu; mgavin2@bidmc.harvard.edu

B. J. Wells et al. (eds.), *Handbook of Inpatient Cardiology*,
https://doi.org/10.1007/978-3-030-47868-1_2

Diagnosis

Differentiating CAD, SIHD, and ACS

- Coronary artery disease (CAD) is the presence of atheromatous plaque in the coronary arteries, which may or may not cause symptoms.
- Stable ischemic heart disease (SIHD) is a syndrome marked by *stable* angina: pain or pressure brought on reliably by exertion or emotion and relieved by rest or nitroglycerin. This may or may not be associated with obstructive CAD.
- In contrast, *unstable* angina (UA) describes angina of increasing severity or frequency beyond baseline, sometimes occuring at rest without an apparent trigger and is the clinical manifestation of an acute coronary syndrome (ACS) (see Chap. 1).
- ACS occurs when there is an abrupt reduction in coronary blood flow or a mismatch in myocardial oxygen supply and demand, and includes a spectrum from UA to myocardial infarction (MI).
- *Do not confuse a new diagnosis of SIHD with ACS*; they are separate clinical syndromes as explained above.
  - Patients may present for the first time with the clinical syndrome of SIHD after many months of symptoms, but they do not have UA.

Cardiovascular Risk in Patients Presenting with Chest Pain (Fig. 2.1)

- Begin with baseline risk using the patient's age, sex, and type of angina (Table 2.1).
- *Add in other canonical risk factors* that increase the likelihood of CAD and can shift the likelihood of a given symptomatic patient having obstructive coronary disease significantly [1].
- The American College of Cardiology provides an online calculator to estimate lifetime and 10-year cardiovas-

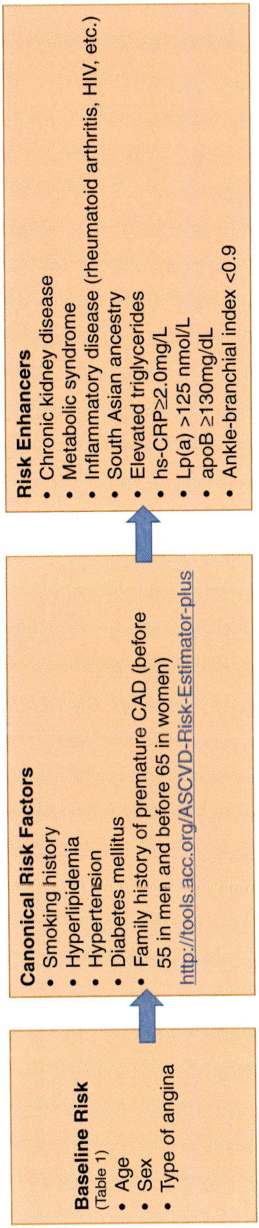

FIGURE 2.1 Approach to CAD risk assessment. Begin with baseline risk and modify using canonical risk factors, utilizing the risk calculator available online. Further risk stratification can be achieved with risk enhancers

Table 2.1 Pretest likelihood of coronary artery disease in symptomatic patients according to age and sex

Age, y	Non-anginal Chest Pain, %		Atypical Angina, %		Typical Angina, %	
	Men	Women	Men	Women	Men	Women
30–39	17.7	5.3	28.9	9.6	59.1	27.5
40–49	24.8	8.0	38.4	14.0	68.9	36.7
50–59	33.6	11.7	48.9	20.0	77.3	47.1
60–69	43.7	16.9	59.4	27.7	83.9	57.7
70-79	54.4	23.8	69.2	37.0	88.9	67.7
>80	64.6	32.3	77.5	47.4	92.5	76.3

Adapted with permission from Ref. [4]

cular risk based on risk factors (http://tools.acc.org/ASCVD-Risk-Estimator-Plus).

- Current guidelines acknowledge that certain *risk enhancers* beyond the factors in the calculator exist [2].

Physical Exam

- The physical examination is often normal or nonspecific in patients with SIHD, but it is useful to look for other associated findings that suggest non-coronary atherosclerotic vascular disease [3].

Preliminary Workup of Suspected SIHD

- *Labs*
  - Lab work in SIHD is not a critical element of diagnosis, but is needed to assess comorbidities and risk.
  - CBC, CMP, lipid panel, HbA1c, BNP, and baseline CK should all be considered especially at initial diagnosis of CAD.

Uninterpretable ECG for Stress

- Left ventricular hypertrophy with associated repolarization abnormalities
- Left bundle branch block
- Ventricular pacing
- Digitalis effect
- Wolf-Parkinson-White
- ≥1mm resting ST segment depression

FIGURE 2.2 Features of an uninterpretable ECG

- *Electrocardiogram*
  - All patients with suspected SIHD should have a resting electrocardiogram (ECG) [1].
  - Most patients with SIHD have a normal resting ECG, but pathologic Q waves indicate a prior myocardial infarction (MI).
  - Also, resting ECG abnormalities help determine which stress test to select for patients who need stress testing (Fig. 2.2).
- *Echocardiography*
  - Rest echocardiography is not always needed.
  - Consider rest echocardiography when patients have:
    - Signs or symptoms suggesting heart failure or cardiac valve disease
    - Known prior MI or a pathologic Q-wave on the ECG suggesting prior infarction
    - ECG findings of complex ventricular arrhythmias, which could suggest underlying cardiomyopathy [1].

Specific Testing in Suspected CAD: Who to Test

- The goal of non-invasive testing is to reliably identify patients with CAD and to estimate prognosis.
- The value of testing symptomatic patients is greatest when the cause of chest pain is truly uncertain (i.e., pretest probability between 20% and 80%).

- Among patients with a very low probability of CAD (Fig. 2.1 and Table 2.1), additional testing is generally not indicated and may result in a false positive test.
- Before testing, consider the pretest probability for CAD in symptomatic patients, the ability to exercise, and any abnormalities on the resting ECG (Fig. 2.3) [4].

Specific Testing in Suspected CAD: Stress Testing (See Table 2.2)

- Stress testing, or functional testing, is the most common form of non-invasive testing.
- The clinician must select both the stressor (exercise or pharmacologic) and the modality to assess ischemia (*ECG, Echocardiography, or Single photon Emission Computed Tomography [SPECT]*, and, less often, *Positron Emission Tomography [PET] or cardiac MRI)*.
- If patients have intermediate risk, can exercise, and have an interpretable ECG (Fig. 2.3), exercise ECG without imaging carries a Class IA indication [1].
- Sensitivity of exercise without imaging is limited at 61% (i.e., 39% false negative rate) and worse for women [1].
- *In practice*, it is often preferred to add imaging to improve sensitivity. Use of imaging for this indication carries a Class IIa indication in the guidelines [1]. It is essential to add imaging if the ECG is uninterpretable.
- Adding any imaging modality – echocardiography, SPECT, or PET – can significantly improve sensitivity. See Chap. 31 for more detail.
- Pharmacologic stress with imaging can be used for patients who cannot exercise or cannot exercise strenuously enough to generate a valid test result.
  - Most commonly, dobutamine is the pharmacologic stress agent of choice for echocardiography
  - Vasodilators (regadenoson or dipyridamole) are the preferred agents for SPECT imaging.

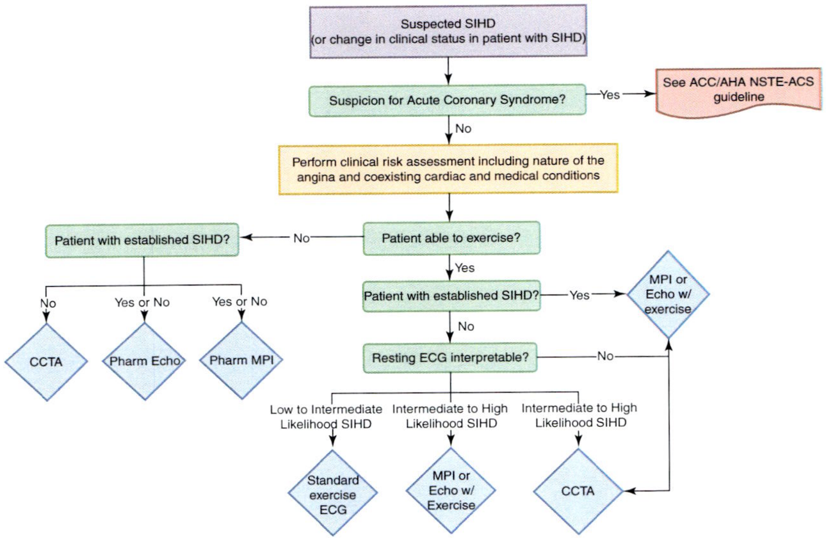

FIGURE 2.3 Choice of non-invasive study for the evaluation of newly suspected SIHD or a change in clinical status in a patient with SIHD. SIHD stable ischemic heart disease; ACC/AHA NSTE-ACS American College of Cardiology/American Heart Association Non-ST segment elevation Acute Coronary Syndrome; MPI myocardial perfusion imaging; Pharm pharmacologic; ECG electrocardiogram; Echo echocardiogram; CCTA Coronary Computed Tomography Angiogram. (Reproduced with permission from Katz and Gavin [29])

TABLE 2.2 Summary of CAD testing options

Test	Preferred Stress Modalities	Pros	Cons
ECG without imaging	Exercise	Low cost	Lowest sensitivity (61%)limited by ECG suitability
Stress Echo	Exercise, Dobutamine	Highly sensitive Also obtain valvular data and filling pressures No radiation	Less interpretable in LBBB or paced hearts Poor image quality can occur in very thin or very obese individuals
SPECT	Exercise, vasodilator (regadenoson, dipyridamole, adenosine)	Highly sensitive Works well in overweight individuals	Radiation More expensive
PET	Vasodilator (regadenoson, dipyridamole, adenosine)	Extremely sensitive Works well in overweight individuals Can provide microvascular dysfunction data	Radiation More expensive Not widely available
MRI	Dobutamine, Vasodilator (regadenoson, dipyridamole, adenosine)	Extremely sensitive Works well in overweight individuals Can provide viability data	Requires breath-holds for quality More expensive Not widely available

TABLE 2.2 (continued)

Test	Preferred Stress Modalities	Pros	Cons
CCTA	N/A	No exercise required Only non-invasive anatomic test, giving data on coronary anomalies Less radiation than SPECT	Requires iodinated contrast Some radiation Images limited in irregular rhythms or high heart rates

ECG electrocardiogram, *LBBB* Left Bundle Branch Block, *Echo* echocardiogram, *CCTA* Coronary Computed Tomography Angiogram, *SPECT* Single-Photon Emission Computed Tomography, *PET* Positron Emission Tomography, *MRI* Magnetic Resonance Imaging

- The sensitivity of SPECT and stress echo for CAD are similar enough that choice of test depends in part on *the resources and technical expertise at a given institution* [1]. These additional factors should also be considered:
  - Echocardiography has no radiation and provides information on valvular function and filling pressures.

Clinical Pearl
In patients with left bundle branch block or ventricular pacing, stress echo is not recommended because the abnormal electrical activation of the heart impairs the interpretation of ischemia in the interventricular septum (LAD territory).

  - SPECT and PET imaging are less susceptible to poor image quality related to body habitus.

Specific Testing in Suspected CAD: Anatomical Testing

- An alternative to functional testing is non-invasive anatomical testing in the form of coronary computed tomography angiography (CCTA).
- Anatomical testing is best in those with contraindication to stress testing or who cannot exercise.
- It also has the advantage of identifying non-obstructive coronary disease and coronary congenital anomalies.
- *CCTA showed no difference in adverse cardiovascular events compared to functional testing when used as the initial diagnostic test among intermediate risk patients with symptomatic SIHD* (PROMISE, NEJM 2015) [5].
- *When added to standard care in SIHD, CCTA lowered rates of combined primary endpoint of death from CHD or non-fatal MI* (SCOT-HEART, NEJM 2018) [6].

Specific Testing in Suspected CAD: Invasive Coronary Angiography

- Often the best initial test in ACS, less useful in SIHD
- In patients with a high likelihood of disease (i.e., >90%) based on symptoms and clinical risk factors (especially when already on anti-anginal medication), non-invasive testing provides little additional information, so invasive testing is required if it will affect therapy.

Specific Testing in Already Known CAD

- For patients who carry a confirmed diagnosis of CAD and are having symptoms on anti-anginal therapy, functional testing with imaging is used to localize and quantify the extent of ischemic myocardium to inform decisions on revascularization [7].
- CCTA is less valuable in this setting.

SIHD Without Obstructive CAD

- Up to 30% of patients presenting with angina have no obstructive CAD.
- Among these patients, 50–65% are believed to have coronary microvascular dysfunction.
- Angina without obstructive coronary disease is more common among women [8].
- MRI and PET protocols have the ability to detect microvascular dysfunction non-invasively [9].
- There is an increased risk of ischemic events in both microvascular disease and non-obstructive epicardial coronary atherosclerosis [10, 11]. Medical therapy is still indicated!

When to Refer to a Cardiologist

- Patients in whom noninvasive testing is contraindicated.
- Patients with a high likelihood of CAD, or uncertain diagnosis after noninvasive testing in whom coronary angiography should be considered [7].
- Patients with suspected microvascular dysfunction or variant (Prinzmetal's) angina.

Guideline-Directed Medical Treatment (GDMT)

Goals of Treatment

- Prevention of ischemic events (cerebral, coronary, and peripheral) (Fig. 2.4).
- Reducing the burden of anginal symptoms.
- Patients with CAD still benefit substantially from treatments that reduce cardiovascular events even if symptoms are minimal or none.

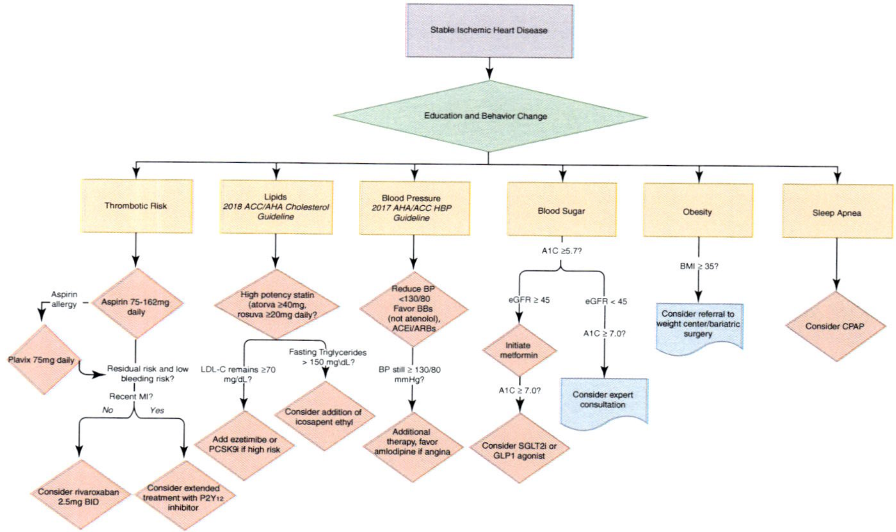

FIGURE 2.4 Guideline-directed medical therapy for patients with stable ischemic heart disease. A1c hemoglobin A1c; ACC American College of Cardiology; ACEi Angiotensin converting enzyme inhibitor; AHA American Heart Association; ARB angiotensin receptor blocker; BBs beta blockers; BID twice daily; BMI body mass index; CPAP continuous positive airway pressure; eGFR estimated glomerular filtration rate; GLP1 glucagon-like peptide 1; HBP high blood pressure; LDL-C low density lipoprotein cholesterol; MI myocardial infarction; SGLT2i sodium-glucose cotransporter 2 inhibitor. (Reproduced with permission from Katz and Gavin [29])

Behavior Modification

- *Smoking cessation:* Smoking increases cardiovascular disease mortality by 50%.
- *Physical activity:* Current guidelines recommend 150 minutes of at least moderate activity per week [22]. Patients with SIHD and those post-MI should participate in a cardiac rehabilitation program [1].
- *Dietary modification:* Emphasize intake of vegetables, fruits, whole grains, legumes, healthy protein sources (low-fat dairy products, low-fat poultry (without the skin), fish/ seafood, and nuts), and non-tropical vegetable oils. The intake of sweets, sugar-sweetened beverages, and red meats should be limited [2].
- *Alcohol Moderation:* No harm and possible cardiovascular benefit for one drink per day with no benefit and likely harm beyond two drinks per day [12]. Bouts of heavy drinking worsen hypertension and precipitate ischemia in SIHD, and should be avoided [13].
- *Psychological well-being:* Interventions to reduce psychological stress may improve clinical outcomes in patients with SIHD [14].

Pharmacologic Therapy for Specific Risk Factors

Lipids

- HMG-COA reductase inhibitors (*statins*) should be used for lipid management, unless contraindicated or adverse events occur.
- In SIHD patients under 75, high-potency statin (atorvastatin 80 mg or rosuvastatin 20–40 mg) is recommended.
- A moderate potency statin can be considered for patients over 75.
- As an update in the 2018 guidelines, adding *ezetimibe and PCKS9 inhibitors in sequence* to reach a low-density lipoprotein cholesterol (LDL-C) goal of <70 mg/dL should be considered for patients at high risk

  - This group includes patients with a history of multiple previous events, or those with one event and multiple risk factors
- *Niacin is no longer recommended* for the lowering of LDL-C [2].
- Low doses of over-the-counter fish oil have not shown consistent benefits, and are not presently recommended [15].
- *However,* icosapent ethyl, *a highly purified and stable EPA ethyl ester, reduced cardiovascular events 25% on top of high-dose statins and aspirin in patients with SIHD and elevated triglycerides (LDL-C between 41 and 100 mg/dL and fasting triglycerides 135–499 mg/dL)* (REDUCE-IT, NEJM 2019) [16].

Hypertension

- Current guidelines recommend a goal BP of <130/80 mmHg in SIHD [17].
- *In patients over 50 with SIHD, achieving a systolic blood pressure of 121 mmHg* versus *136 mmHg with anti-hypertensives decreased major adverse cardiovascular events (MACE) by 31% with a number needed to treat (NNT) of 44* (SPRINT, NEJM 2015) [18].
- Agent of choice depends on other comorbidities (e.g., angina, congestive heart failure, chronic kidney disease, or diabetes)

Diabetes

- Certain SGLT2 inhibitors (*empagliflozin and canagliflozin*) have been shown to reduce cardiovascular events [19].
- Certain GLP-1 receptor agonists (*liraglutide and semaglutide*) have also been shown to reduce ischemic events in patient with SIHD [19].
- It is recommended to add these agents to metformin in SIHD patients not at their glycemic target [19, 20].

Obesity

- Beyond lifestyle change, if BMI > 35, weight loss surgery should be discussed in all patients with SIHD, especially in patients with type 2 diabetes for whom Roux-en-Y gastric bypass has been shown to reduce cardiovascular events [21].

Pharmacologic Therapy to Prevent MI or Death in SIHD Independent of Risk Factors

Antiplatelet Therapy

- All patients with CAD should be treated with low-dose *aspirin*, usually 81 mg.
- When aspirin is contraindicated, patients can be treated with *clopidogrel* 75 mg daily.

Anticoagulation

- *Rivaroxaban* at a very reduced dose of 2.5 mg twice daily likewise demonstrated a reduction in cardiovascular mortality among patients with SIHD at the expense of increased bleeding (COMPASS, NEJM 2017) [22] and may be useful in patients with favorable bleeding profiles.

Other Therapies

- Patients with SIHD should receive an annual influenza vaccine [1, 23].

Medications that Treat Angina

- Short acting nitrates in the form of *sublingual nitroglycerin or nitroglycerin spray* should be used for immediate relief of angina.

  - Patients can administer one dose every 5 minutes for up to three doses.
  - Warn patients about the interaction between nitrates and PDE5 inhibitors leading to hypotension.
- *β-blockers* should be prescribed as initial therapy for prolonged relief of symptoms.

> **Clinical Pearl**
> All beta blockers reduce symptoms, though in patients with peripheral arterial disease, drugs with additional alpha blockade, such as *carvedilol or labetalol*, may prevent vasoconstriction mediated by unopposed alpha agonism [1].

  - In patients with reduced EF, carvedilol, metoprolol succinate, and bisoprolol should be favored per guidelines [24].
- *Calcium channel blockers* or long-acting nitrates (*isosorbide or nitropaste*) can be prescribed when β-blockers are contraindicated (e.g., severe bronchospastic lung disease) or produce unacceptable side effects.
  - Non-dihydropyridine calcium channel blockers (*diltiazem and verapamil*) should be avoided in patients with reduced ejection fraction given their negative inotropic effects; dihydropyridine calcium channel blockers such as *amlodipine* are preferred.
- Ranolazine is an anti-anginal that appears to reduce angina through its effect on the late sodium current.
  - It prolongs QTc and therefore should be used with caution if a patient is on other QT prolonging medications. Side effects are primarily GI upset. Usually a fourth line agent.

Revascularization in SIHD

- Revascularization (either by PCI or CABG) is indicated in patients with ischemic symptoms that are *progressive or*

refractory to maximal medical management (Class 1A recommendation) [1].
- Among patients with a low burden of angina, a sham-controlled trial of up front revascularization plus aggressive medical management did not demonstrate additional angina reduction. (ORBITA, Lancet 2018) Anginal frequency should therefore be taken into consideration when making revascularization decisions.
- In a large randomized control trial of patients with SIHD and moderate-severe ischemia on stress test, routine invasive therapy did not reduce major adverse cardiac events vs medical therapy alone, but improved angina burden and quality of life if they had angina at baseline (ISCHEMIA, NEJM 2020).

- It is not clear if routine revascularization in combination with GDMT reduces rates of death or ischemic events.
- Based on observational data, many treat symptomatic patients with proximal left anterior descending artery disease or multivessel disease with an initial strategy of revascularization plus GDMT given the large area of ischemia [25, 26]. The guidelines generally support CABG over PCI for the intention of improving survival in these cases [1, 27, 28].

Key Learning Points

- The most useful preliminary predictors of clinically significant CAD are age, sex, type of chest pain, and comorbid conditions including tobacco use, hyperlipidemia, hypertension, family history of premature CAD, and diabetes mellitus.
- Nearly all patients should have a non-invasive functional (exercise or pharmacologic stress test with ECG, echo, or nuclear imaging) or anatomic (CCTA) assessment for CAD. The type of non-invasive test is determined using pre-test probability of CAD, resting ECG, and the ability to exercise.
- The clinician should consider moving directly to coronary angiography in a limited subset of patients.

- The goals of treatment are to minimize adverse cardiovascular outcomes and death and reduce symptoms. These goals can involve independent pharmacotherapy.
- All patients should have guideline-directed medical therapy to reduce the risk for mortality and relieve symptoms.
- Consider revascularization in conjunction with a specialist for patients at high risk for mortality, especially those with persistent symptoms despite GDMT.

References

1. Fihn SD, Gardin JM, Abrams J, Berra K, Blankenship JC, Dallas AP, et al. 2012 ACCF/AHA/ACP/AATS/PCNA/SCAI/STS guideline for the diagnosis and management of patients with stable ischemic heart disease. J Am Coll Cardiol. 2012;60(24):e44–e164.
2. Grundy SM, Stone NJ, Bailey AL, Beam C, Birtcher KK, Blumenthal RS, et al. 2018 AHA/ACC/AACVPR/AAPA/ABC/ACPM/ADA/AGS/APhA/ASPC/NLA/PCNA guideline on the management of blood cholesterol: a report of the American College of Cardiology/American Heart Association task force on clinical practice guidelines. J Am Coll Cardiol. 2018;10:25709.
3. Pryor DB, Shaw L, Harrell FE, Lee KL, Hlatky MA, Mark DB, et al. Estimating the likelihood of severe coronary artery disease. Am J Med. 1991;90(5):553–62.
4. Genders TSS, Steyerberg EW, Alkadhi H, Leschka S, Desbiolles L, Nieman K, et al. A clinical prediction rule for the diagnosis of coronary artery disease: validation, updating, and extension. Eur Heart J. 2011;32(11):1316–30.
5. Douglas PS, Hoffmann U, Patel MR, Mark DB, Al-Khalidi HR, Cavanaugh B, et al. Outcomes of anatomical versus functional testing for coronary artery disease. N Engl J Med. 2015;372(14):1291–300.
6. Investigators SCOT-HEART, Newby DE, Adamson PD, Berry C, Boon NA, Dweck MR, et al. Coronary CT angiography and 5-year risk of myocardial infarction. N Engl J Med. 2018;379(10):924–33.

7. Fihn SD, Blankenship JC, Alexander KP, Bittl JA, Byrne JG, Fletcher BJ, et al. 2014 ACC/AHA/AATS/PCNA/SCAI/STS focused update of the guideline for the diagnosis and management of patients with stable ischemic heart disease: a report of the American College of Cardiology/American Heart Association task force on practice guidelines, and the American Association for Thoracic Surgery, preventive cardiovascular nurses association, Society for Cardiovascular Angiography and Interventions, and Society of Thoracic Surgeons. J Am Coll Cardiol. 2014;64(18):1929–49.
8. Gulati M, Shaw LJ, Bairey Merz CN. Myocardial ischemia in women: lessons from the NHLBI WISE study. Clin Cardiol. 2012;35(3):141–8.
9. Marinescu MA, Löffler AI, Ouellette M, Smith L, Kramer CM, Bourque JM. Coronary microvascular dysfunction, microvascular angina, and treatment strategies. JACC Cardiovasc Imaging. 2015;8(2):210–20.
10. Marzilli M, Merz CNB, Boden WE, Bonow RO, Capozza PG, Chilian WM, et al. Obstructive coronary atherosclerosis and ischemic heart disease: an elusive link! J Am Coll Cardiol. 2012;60(11):951–6.
11. Bittencourt MS, Hulten E, Ghoshhajra B, O'Leary D, Christman MP, Montana P, et al. Prognostic value of nonobstructive and obstructive coronary artery disease detected by coronary computed tomography angiography to identify cardiovascular events. Circ Cardiovasc Imaging. 2014;7(2):282–91.
12. McClelland RL, Bild DE, Burke GL, Mukamal KJ, Lima JA, Kronmal RA. Alcohol and coronary artery calcium prevalence, incidence and progression: results from the multi-ethnic study of atherosclerosis (MESA). Am J Clin Nutr. 2008;88(6):1593–601.
13. Rossinen J, Partanen J, Koskinen P, Toivonen L, Kupari M, Nieminen MS. Acute heavy alcohol intake increases silent myocardial ischaemia in patients with stable angina pectoris. Heart Br Card Soc. 1996;75(6):563–7.
14. Dimsdale JE. Psychological stress and cardiovascular disease. J Am Coll Cardiol. 2008;51(13):1237–46.
15. Abdelhamid AS, Brown TJ, Brainard JS, Biswas P, Thorpe GC, Moore HJ, et al. Omega-3 fatty acids for the primary and secondary prevention of cardiovascular disease. Cochrane Database Syst Rev. 2018;18(7):CD003177.
16. Bhatt DL, Steg PG, Miller M, Brinton EA, Jacobson TA, Ketchum SB, et al. Cardiovascular risk reduction with Icosapent

ethyl for hypertriglyceridemia. N Engl J Med. 2019;380(1): 11–22.
17. Whelton PK, Carey RM, Aronow WS, Casey DE, Collins KJ, Himmelfarb CD, et al. 2017 ACC/AHA/AAPA/ABC/ACPM/AGS/APhA/ASH/ASPC/NMA/PCNA guideline for the prevention, detection, evaluation, and management of high blood pressure in adults: a report of the American College of Cardiology/American Heart Association task force on clinical practice guidelines. J Am Coll Cardiol. 2018;71(19):e127–248.
18. The SPRINT Research Group. A randomized trial of intensive versus standard blood-pressure control. N Engl J Med. 2015;373(22):2103–16.
19. Association, American Medical. Cardiovascular benefits of SGLT2 inhibitors and GLP-1 receptor agonists in type 2 diabetes. JAMA J Am Med Assoc. 2019;321(17):1720–1.
20. American Diabetes Association. 9. Pharmacologic approaches to glycemic treatment: standards of medical care in diabetes-2019. Diabetes Care. 2019;42(Suppl 1):S90–S102.
21. Fisher DP, Johnson E, Haneuse S, Arterburn D, Coleman KJ, O'Connor PJ, et al. Association between bariatric surgery and macrovascular disease outcomes in patients with type 2 diabetes and severe obesity. JAMA. 2018;320(15):1570–82.
22. Eikelboom JW, Connolly SJ, Bosch J, Dagenais GR, Hart RG, Shestakovska O, et al. Rivaroxaban with or without aspirin in stable cardiovascular disease. N Engl J Med. 2017;377(14):1319–30.
23. de Diego C, Vila-Córcoles A, Ochoa O, Rodriguez-Blanco T, Salsench E, Hospital I, et al. Effects of annual influenza vaccination on winter mortality in elderly people with chronic heart disease. Eur Heart J. 2009;30(2):209–16.
24. Yancy CW, Jessup M, Bozkurt B, Butler J, Casey DE, Colvin MM, et al. 2017 ACC/AHA/HFSA focused update of the 2013 ACCF/AHA guideline for the Management of Heart Failure: a report of the American College of Cardiology/American Heart Association task force on clinical practice guidelines and the Heart Failure Society of America. J Am Coll Cardiol. 2017;70(6):776–803.
25. Hachamovitch R, Hayes SW, Friedman JD, Cohen I, Berman DS. Comparison of the short-term survival benefit associated with revascularization compared with medical therapy in patients with no prior coronary artery disease undergoing stress myocardial perfusion single photon emission computed tomography. Circulation. 2003;107(23):2900–7.

26. Windecker S, Stortecky S, Stefanini GG, da Costa BR, da Costa BR, Rutjes AW, et al. Revascularisation versus medical treatment in patients with stable coronary artery disease: network meta-analysis. BMJ. 2014;348(jun23 8):g3859.
27. Patel MR, Calhoon JH, Dehmer GJ, Grantham JA, Maddox TM, Maron DJ, et al. ACC/AATS/AHA/ASE/ASNC/SCAI/SCCT/STS 2017 appropriate use criteria for coronary revascularization in patients with stable ischemic heart disease: a report of the American College of Cardiology Appropriate use Criteria Task Force, American Association for Thoracic Surgery, American Heart Association, American Society of Echocardiography, American Society of Nuclear Cardiology, Society for Cardiovascular Angiography and Interventions, Society of Cardiovascular Computed Tomography, and Society of Thoracic Surgeons. J Am Coll Cardiol. 2017;69(17):2212–41.
28. Farkouh ME, Domanski M, Sleeper LA, Siami FS, Dangas G, Mack M, et al. Strategies for multivessel revascularization in patients with diabetes. N Engl J Med. 2012;367(25):2375–84.
29. Katz D, Gavin MC. Stable ischemic heart disease. Ann Intern Med. 2019;171(3):ITC17.

Chapter 3
Atrial Fibrillation and Atrial Flutter

Vladimir Kaplinskiy and Eli V. Gelfand

Abbreviations

AF	Atrial Fibrillation
AV	Atrioventricular
CTI	Cavo-tricuspid isthmus
DAPT	Dual antiplatelet therapy
DCCV	direct current cardioversion
INR	International normalized ratio
LAA	Left Atrial Appendage
LV	Left ventricle
TEE	Transesophageal echocardiogram

Terminology

- Paroxysmal AF spontaneously terminates within 7 days of onset.

V. Kaplinskiy (✉)
Beth Israel Deaconess Medical Center,
Harvard Medical School, Boston, MA, USA
e-mail: vkaplins@bidmc.harvard.edu

E. V. Gelfand
Department of Cardiology, Beth Israel Deaconess Medical Center,
Harvard Medical School, Boston, MA, USA

B. J. Wells et al. (eds.), *Handbook of Inpatient Cardiology*,
https://doi.org/10.1007/978-3-030-47868-1_3

- Persistent AF lasts for >7 days and requires an intervention to restore sinus rhythm.
- Permanent or chronic AF is persistent AF which has been refractory to intervention or for which intervention to restore sinus has eventually been deemed futile/inappropriate.
- Conversion pause: transient bradycardia caused by delayed sinus node recovery following transition from atrial fibrillation to sinus rhythm.
- Tachy-brady Syndrome refers to co-existence of rapid rhythm (i.e., rapid ventricular heart rate during periods of atrial fibrillation) and bradycardia (i.e. conversion pauses and/or sinus bradycardia).

Epidemiology of Atrial Fibrillation

- Risk Factors for AF include: Age, hypertension, diabetes, obstructive sleep apnea, pulmonary disease, abnormal left ventricular systolic function, myo- and pericarditis, acute illness, alcohol intake, hyperthyroidism, surgery (especially cardiac surgery) [1].
- AF is rarely a manifestation of cardiac ischemia.

Consequences of Atrial Fibrillation

- Common symptoms of AF include palpitations, dyspnea, chest pain and fatigue.
- Stroke.
- Patients whose ventricular filling is largely dependent on the atrial kick, such as those with diastolic LV dysfunction or restrictive cardiomyopathy, may develop systemic hypoperfusion due to loss of atrial contraction.
- Sustained rapid ventricular rates in AF beyond 7–10 days may lead to a tachycardia-induced cardiomyopathy.
- Syncope is often a manifestation of a conversion pause.

- If a patient with atrial fibrillation is found to have a regular ventricular rhythm without clear atrial activity ("regularized" AF), this can be a manifestation of complete heart block and should prompt an urgent cardiology consultation.

Thromboembolic Risk

- Given difficulty in establishing AF burden, paroxysmal and chronic AF should generally be approached similarly in terms of risk of thromboembolism.
  - Controversy exists regarding this and very brief episodes of AF detected incidentally, for example upon interrogation of an implanted pacemaker, and may prompt a discussion with a cardiologist about the value of anticoagulation on a patient-specific basis.
- CHA_2DS_2-VASc score is a commonly used risk score to estimate the risk of thromboembolism (Table 3.1).
  - (C) Congestive heart failure (+1); (H) Hypertension (+1); (A) Age (65–74, +1; 75 or greater, +2); (D) Diabetes mellitus (+1); (S) History of stroke (+2); (VA) vascular disease, including history of coronary artery disease or peripheral vascular disease (+1); (Sc) Female gender (+1).

Evaluation of Patients with New Atrial Fibrillation

- Evaluate whether the patient is hemodynamically stable and needs rapid restoration of sinus rhythm.
- Assess for: acute illness, recent surgery, alcohol use, history of structural heart disease, hyperthyroidism.
- Assess the risk factors for thromboembolism.
- Perform transthoracic echocardiogram to assess ventricular and valvular function.

TABLE 3.1 Risk of stroke in patients with atrial fibrillation [2]

CHA2DS2VASc score	Risk of stroke per 100 years at risk
0	0.2
1	0.6
2	2.2
3	3.2
4	4.8
5	7.2
6	9.7
7	11.2
8	10.8
9	12.2

- Patients with cryptogenic stroke or other arterial thromboembolic event without explanation should be considered for long-term cardiac monitoring to assess for occult AF.

Anticoagulation for Atrial Fibrillation

- To reduce the risk of stroke, anticoagulation is recommended for any patient with CHA2DS2VASc score ≥ 2.
  - Anticoagulation should be strongly considered for any patient with a score = 1 if this is not based solely on gender.
- Prior pulmonary vein isolation or MAZE procedure does not eliminate the risk of stroke and anticoagulation should not be discontinued solely on the basis of having undergone the procedure.
- Aspirin has no evidence of prevention of stroke and should not be used as monotherapy for stroke prevention.

- Aspirin plus Clopidogrel has some benefit in stroke prevention but is inferior to the use of an anticoagulant [3].

- Non-vitamin K anticoagulants (Table 3.2) are considered first-line in the treatment of AF (except for patients with mechanical heart valves, moderate or severe rheumatic mitral stenosis and advanced renal disease) [4].
  - Rivaroxaban.
  - Dabigatran.
  - Apixaban.
  - Edoxaban.
- If warfarin is used for stroke prevention in atrial fibrillation, INR goal is 2.0–3.0.
- For patients on warfarin, time in therapeutic range of >60% has been shown to achieve stroke risk reduction [5].
- In cases of severe bleeding:
  - Patients on warfarin can be treated with vitamin K, fresh frozen plasma and prothrombin complex concentrates.
  - Novel reversal agents are available for direct oral anticoagulants.

    Andexanet alfa for rivaroxaban and apixaban.

    Idarucizumab for dabigatran.
- In cases when anticoagulation needs to be interrupted for a procedure.
  - Bridging anticoagulation should generally be pursued for patients on Warfarin if CHADS2 score ≥ 5, there is a history of prior stroke, and for those patients with AF who also have mechanical heart valves. Bridging should be considered for patients with AF who have additional stroke risks, such as low LV ejection fraction.
  - Patients on non-vitamin K-dependent anticoagulants generally do not require bridging anticoagulation [6].
- In patients with indication for dual antiplatelet therapy (DAPT) after percutaneous coronary interventions.
  - Rivaroxaban 15 mg/day + Clopidogrel showed equivalent level of cardiovascular mortality compared with warfarin + DAPT, with less bleeding. (PIONEER trial) [7].

Table 3.2 Common anticoagulants for atrial fibrillation

Anticoagulant	Mechanism	Common Dosing	Bleeding Risk (per year; vs. Warfarin)	Reversal Agent	Considerations
Dabigatran [13]	Direct thrombin inhibitor	150 mg PO BID[a]	Major: 3.1% vs. 3.4% Intracranial: 0.1% vs. 0.3%	Idarucizumab	
Apixaban [14]	Factor Xa inhibitor	5 mg PO BID[b]	Intracranial: 0.2% vs. 0.5% Major: 2.1% vs. 3.1%	Andexanet	Shown to be safe in end-stage renal disease
Rivaroxaban [15]	Factor Xa inhibitor	20 mg PO daily (with evening meal)[c,d]	Intracranial: 0.5% vs. 0.8% Fatal: 0.2% vs. 0.5%	Andexanet	Must be taken with a > 500 kCal meal

Edoxaban [16]	Factor Xa inhibitor	60 mg PO daily[e]	Major: 2.8% vs. 3.4% Intracranial: 0.4% vs. 0.9%	Contraindicated if creatinine clearance>95 mL/min

[a]A dose of 110 mg BID can be considered (off-label) in patients with high bleeding risk. Lower doses (i.e. 75 mg BID) may be necessary in patients with reduced renal function

[b]A dose of 2.5 mg BID is indicated in patients with any 2 of the following: Age ≥ 80 years, body weight ≤ 60 kg, or serum creatinine ≥1.5 mg/dL

[c]Post-percutaneous coronary intervention with stent placement and non-valvular AF, a dose of 15 mg daily in combination with an appropriate antithrombotic regimen (i.e. Clopidogrel ∓ Aspirin) is typically used

[d]A dose of 15 mg daily is typically used in patients with creatinine clearance of 15-50 mL/minute

[e]Dose should be reduced (i.e. 30 mg daily) for patients with creatinine clearance of 15–50 mL/minute

  - A regimen that included Apixaban and Clopidogrel resulted in less bleeding and fewer hospitalizations without significant difference in stroke compared to regimens that included Warfarin, Aspirin or both (AUGUSTUS trial) [8].
- Surgical or percutaneous left atrial appendage (LAA) exclusion should be considered in patients for whom long-term anticoagulation is either not feasible or associated with unacceptable bleeding risk.
  - Watchman percutaneous LAA occlusion system is currently FDA-approved, but notably still requires full anticoagulation for 45 days following implantation.
  - Surgical ligation can be done as a standalone procedure or as part of other cardiac surgery.

Heart Rate Control in Atrial Fibrillation

- Randomized trials generally show no significant difference in mortality or incidence of stroke between rate control and rhythm control strategies in AF (AFFIRM trial) [9].
  - Highly symptomatic patients may have been underrepresented.
  - Mortality may have been increased by discontinuation of anticoagulants in the rhythm control group.
- Ventricular heart rate in AF is determined by multiple factors, such as balance between sympathetic and parasympathetic stimulation, medications which affect atrioventricular (AV) nodal conduction, and metabolic derangements (i.e. thyroid dysfunction).
  - Slow ventricular rate (i.e. less than 60 beats/minute) suggests slow AV conduction.
  - Very rapid ventricular rate (i.e. greater than 200 beats/minute) suggests the presence of an accessory pathway.
- Uncontrolled elevation in ventricular rate has been associated with the development of cardiomyopathy.
- Goal heart rate is generally <110 beats/minute.

- RACE II Trial randomized patients to lenient (<110 bpm) vs. strict (<80 bpm) rate control. There was no difference in three-year incidence of cardiovascular death, HF hospitalization, stroke, systemic embolism, bleeding and life-threatening arrhythmia. However, results may not be generalizable since: the "lenient" group may have been treated more aggressively than expected (i.e. mean heart rate 86 bpm at 12 months), the trial included only patients with permanent AF and it took place in the outpatient setting [10].

- Therapies for control of heat rate include (Table 3.3):

TABLE 3.3 Common heart rate control medications for atrial fibrillation

Medication Class	Medication	Acute Dosing	Considerations
Beta blocker	Metoprolol	2.5-5 mg IV over 2 minutes; may be repeated every 5 minutes up to a total of 15 mg	May be particularly effective in AF in high catecholamine states. Typically followed by oral beta blocker such as Atenolol, Metoprolol, Timolol, Pindolol, Nadolol, Bisoprolol or Carvedilol. Monitor for bronchospasm, hypotension, worsening heart failure, bradycardia.
	Esmolol	Bolus of 0.5 mg/kg IV over 1 minute; followed by 50 μg/kg/min	
	Propranolol	Bolus 1 mg/minute IV	

(continued)

TABLE 3.3 (continued)

Medication Class	Medication	Acute Dosing	Considerations
Calcium channel blocker	Diltiazem	Bolus 0.25 mg/kg IV over 2 minutes, followed by 0.35 mg/kg over 2 minutes; followed by infusion of 5-15 mg/hour	Monitor for hypotension, worsening heart failure, bradycardia
	Verapamil	Bolus 5-10 mg IV over 2–3 minutes; may be repeated every 15–40 minutes; followed by maintenance infusion of 5-20 mg/hour	
Cardiac glycoside	Digoxin	0.25–0.5 mg IV over several minutes; repeat 0.25 mg IV every 6 hours to a maximum of 1.5 mg over 24 hours; followed by oral maintenance dose of 0.125–0.25 mg per day	Generally reserved for patients who do not respond to beta blocker to calcium channel blocker.

  - Calcium channel blockade with non-dihydropyridine calcium channel blockers (i.e. Verapamil or Diltiazem).
  - Beta blockade; particularly in patients with high adrenergic tone (i.e. post-operate AF).
  - Enhancement of vagal tone with Digoxin.
- Caution must be exercised with the use of calcium channel blockers or beta blockers in patients with significantly reduced ejection fraction and/or in whom there is concern for low cardiac output state, since they can exert negative inotropic effects and precipitate hypotension, bradycardia, and/or cardiogenic shock.
- Reversible causes of tachycardia (i.e. hypovolemia, sepsis) should be identified.

Rhythm Control in Atrial Fibrillation

- Spontaneous cardioversion will occur in 69% of patients within the first 48 h of AF and early electrical cardioversion may not improve maintenance of sinus rhythm at 4 weeks compared with expectant management [11].
  - AV nodal blocking agents do not promote restoration of sinus rhythm.
- Pharmacotherapy can restore sinus rhythm in up to 50% of cases.
- Electrical cardioversion (DCCV) is effective at restoring sinus rhythm in up to 90% of patients [12].
  - Risks of DCCV include: burn at location of pads, bradycardia and post-cardioversion pulmonary edema.
  - Ensure euvolemia in patients with volume overload prior to DCCV to reduce chance of AF recurrence.
  - Following restoration of sinus rhythm, there is gradual recovery in mechanical atrial function over a period of 3 weeks.
  - Prior to cardioversion (pharmacologic or electrical), the risk of stroke should be assessed.

    In patients who are definitely known to have developed new atrial fibrillation with in <48 hours, cardio-

version may typically be performed without assessment for intracardiac thrombus (anticoagulation should be initiated prior to cardioversion).
A transesophageal echocardiogram (TEE) should be pursued to exclude a thrombus in the left atrial appendage in any patient who has been in AF >48 hours or in whom timing of AF onset is less certain (unless the patient is in a severely hemodynamically unstable state due to AF).

Clinical Pearl
Consider reducing the dose of AV nodal-blocking medications prior to cardioversion

- Anticoagulation should be maintained for at least 4 weeks after cardioversion in all patients. Thereafter, the need for chronic anticoagulation should be determined based on risk factors, as described earlier.
- Monitor for post-DCCV pulmonary edema and myocardial dysfunction due to transient stunning (typically lasting <48 hours).
- Non-pharmacologic therapies (i.e. pulmonary vein isolation or AV node ablation with pacemaker placement) may need to be considered for patients with AF refractory to medical therapy.

Antiarrhythmic Therapy

- Procainamide, Ibutilide and Amiodarone are approved for pharmacologic cardioversion, but success rates are lower than with direct-current cardioversion.
- Choice of antiarrhythmic medication (Table 3.4) is determined by the presence of structural heart disease, coronary artery disease and renal disease.

Table 3.4 Common antiarrhythmic medications for atrial fibrillation

Class	Medications	Mechanism	Appropriate for	Contraindications	Monitoring parameters	Common Adverse Reactions
1a	Procainamide Disopyramide	Na + channel blockade K+ channel blockade Prolong action potential	Patients without structural heart disease Hypertrophic cardiomyopathy (Disopyramide)	Coronary artery disease Structural heart disease	QTc interval CBC LFTs	Disopyramide: anticholinergic effects and should be avoided in patients with prostate symptoms and glaucoma Agranulocytosis Quinidine Thrombo-cytopenia, granulomatous hepatitis, myasthenia gravis Procainamide: Agranulocytosis, lupus-like reaction

(continued)

Table 3.4 (continued)

Class	Medications	Mechanism	Appropriate for	Contraindications	Monitoring parameters	Common Adverse Reactions
1c	Flecainide Propafenone	Na + channel blockade	Patients without structural heart disease	Coronary artery disease Structural heart disease		Flecainide: Associated with interstitial lung disease Propafenone: Agranulocytosis and lupus-like syndrome
III	Amiodarone Sotalol Dronedarone Dofetilide	K+ channel blockade Sotalol and Amiodarone have beta blocker effect Amiodarone also blocks Na + and Ca2+ channels		-Sotalol and Dofetilide contraindicated with renal impairment -Dronedarone contraindicated in patients with CHF	Amiodarone: Liver, thyroid and pulmonary function should be checked every 6 months	Amiodarone: Interstitial lung disease Thyroid disease Transaminitis

- Type 1c agents (propafenone and flecainide) may be used in patients without structural heart disease.
  These should be used in combination with an AV nodal-blocking agent to avoid the organization of atrial flutter with 1:1 conduction.
- Sotalol, dofetilide and amiodarone may be used in patients with coronary artery disease.
- Amiodarone may be used in patients with structural heart disease.
- Dronedarone is contraindicated in patients with congestive heart failure.
- Due to risk of pharmacologic cardioversion, these agents should not be used in patients in whom duration in AF is not known and who had not been on therapeutic anticoagulation for at least 4 weeks (unless an LAA thrombus is excluded by transesophageal echocardiogram).

Clinical Pearl
Amiodarone and disopyramide may be particularly effective in patients with hypertrophic cardiomyopathy.

Atrial Flutter

- Results from rapid regular atrial depolarizations at approximately 300 beats/minute and often leads to a pattern of regular intermittent conduction via the AV node.
- Lower incidence than atrial fibrillation.
- Two general categories of atrial flutter:
  - Typical atrial flutter: Macro reentrant circuit around the cavo-tricuspid isthmus (CTI) in the right atrium. Involves either a counterclockwise pattern of rotation ("sawtooth" appearance, with inferior direction in the inferior ECG leads) or a "clockwise" circuit with positive flutter waves in the inferior ECG leads.

  - Atypical atrial flutter: A reentrant circuit that can involve any region of the right or left atria (often around an area of scar). Can be difficult to distinguish from a focal atrial tachycardia.
- Risk of thromboembolism extrapolated from atrial fibrillation and approach to anticoagulation should be guided by the same risk stratification scores (i.e. CHA_2DS_2-VASc).
- Heart rate control is often more difficult to achieve, and patients may benefit from earlier consideration of electrical cardioversion, ablation and/or initiation of anti-arrhythmic.
- Definitive treatment with ablation is preferred for most patients (particularly those with typical atrial flutter).

When Should a Cardiology Consultation Be Considered

- Symptomatic AF with difficulty controlling heart rate and/or hemodynamic compromise.
- Consideration of cardioversion or ablation.
- Initiation of new antiarrhythmic.
- Complex anticoagulation decisions in patients with high-risk AF and bleeding.

Key Learning Points

1. Patients with atrial fibrillation should have evaluation for reversible risk factors, including thyroid dysfunction, pericarditis and sleep apnea.
2. Assessment of stroke risk factors should be considered prior to initiation of an antiarrhythmic medication or non-emergent electrical cardioversion.
3. Patients who are taking antiarrhythmic medications, have undergone ablation procedures, MAZE surgery or left atrial appendage occlusion may still be at risk for thromboembolism. Anticoagulation should be guided by general stroke risk factors and bleeding risk.

References

1. Zimetbaum PJ, Josephson ME. Practical clinical electrophysiology: Lippincott Williams & Wilkins; Philadelphia, PA. 2017. 352 p.
2. Friberg L, Rosenqvist M, Lip GYH. Evaluation of risk stratification schemes for ischaemic stroke and bleeding in 182 678 patients with atrial fibrillation: the Swedish atrial fibrillation cohort study. Eur Heart J. 2012;33(12):1500–10.
3. ACTIVE Investigators, Connolly SJ, Pogue J, Hart RG, Hohnloser SH, Pfeffer M, et al. Effect of clopidogrel added to aspirin in patients with atrial fibrillation. N Engl J Med. 2009;360(20):2066–78.
4. January CT, Wann LS, Calkins H, Chen LY, Cigarroa JE, Cleveland JC Jr, et al. 2019 AHA/ACC/HRS focused update of the 2014 AHA/ACC/HRS guideline for the management of patients with atrial fibrillation: a report of the American College of Cardiology/American Heart Association task force on clinical practice guidelines and the Heart Rhythm Society in collaboration with the Society of Thoracic Surgeons. Circulation. 2019;140(2):e125–51.
5. Connolly SJ, Pogue J, Eikelboom J, Flaker G, Commerford P, Franzosi MG, et al. Benefit of oral anticoagulant over antiplatelet therapy in atrial fibrillation depends on the quality of international normalized ratio control achieved by centers and countries as measured by time in therapeutic range. Circulation. 2008;118(20):2029–37.
6. Douketis JD, Spyropoulos AC, Duncan J, Carrier M, Le Gal G, Tafur AJ, et al. Perioperative management of patients with atrial fibrillation receiving a direct oral anticoagulant. JAMA Intern Med. 2019. Available from: https://doi.org/10.1001/jamainternmed.2019.2431.
7. Gibson CM, Mehran R, Bode C, Halperin J, Verheugt F, Wildgoose P, et al. An open-label, randomized, controlled, multicenter study exploring two treatment strategies of rivaroxaban and a dose-adjusted oral vitamin K antagonist treatment strategy in subjects with atrial fibrillation who undergo percutaneous coronary intervention (PIONEER AF-PCI). Am Heart J. 2015;169(4):472–8.
8. Lopes RD, Heizer G, Aronson R, Vora AN, Massaro T, Mehran R, et al. Antithrombotic therapy after acute coronary syndrome or PCI in atrial fibrillation. N Engl J Med. 2019;380(16):1509–24.

9. Wyse DG, Waldo AL, DiMarco JP, Domanski MJ, Rosenberg Y, Schron EB, et al. A comparison of rate control and rhythm control in patients with atrial fibrillation. N Engl J Med. 2002;347(23):1825–33.
10. Van Gelder IC, Groenveld HF, Crijns HJGM, Tuininga YS, Tijssen JGP, Alings AM, et al. Lenient versus strict rate control in patients with atrial fibrillation. N Engl J Med. 2010;362(15):1363–73.
11. Pluymaekers NAHA, Dudink EAMP, Luermans JGLM, Meeder JG, Lenderink T, Widdershoven J, et al. Early or delayed cardioversion in recent-onset atrial fibrillation. N Engl J Med. 2019;380(16):1499–508.
12. Abu-El-Haija B, Giudici MC. Predictors of long-term maintenance of normal sinus rhythm after successful electrical cardioversion. Clin Cardiol. 2014;37(6):381–5.
13. Connolly SJ, Ezekowitz MD, Yusuf S, Eikelboom J, Oldgren J, Parekh A, et al. Dabigatran versus warfarin in patients with atrial fibrillation. N Engl J Med. 2009 Sep 17;361(12):1139–51.
14. Granger CB, Alexander JH, McMurray JJV, Lopes RD, Hylek EM, Hanna M, et al. Apixaban versus warfarin in patients with atrial fibrillation. N Engl J Med. 2011;365(11):981–92.
15. Patel MR, Mahaffey KW, Garg J, Pan G, Singer DE, Hacke W, et al. Rivaroxaban versus warfarin in nonvalvular atrial fibrillation. N Engl J Med. 2011;365(10):883–91.
16. Giugliano RP, Ruff CT, Braunwald E, Murphy SA, Wiviott SD, Halperin JL, et al. Edoxaban versus warfarin in patients with atrial fibrillation. N Engl J Med. 2013;369(22):2093–104.

Chapter 4
Supraventricular Tachycardia

George Black and Faisal Merchant

Abbreviations

AT	Atrial Tachycardia
AF	Atrial Fibrillation
AVN	Atrioventricular Node
AVNRT	Atrioventricular Nodal Reentrant Tachycardia
AVRT	Atrioventricular Reentrant Tachycardia
ECG	Electrocardiogram
JT	Junctional Tachycardia
MAT	Multifocal Atrial Tachycardia
PAC	Premature Atrial Contraction
PVC	Premature Ventricular Contraction
ST	Sinus Tachycardia
SVT	Supraventricular Tachycardia
TIA	Transient Ischemic Attack
VT	Ventricular Tachycardia
VF	Ventricular Fibrillation

G. Black (✉) · F. Merchant
Division of Cardiology, Emory University, Atlanta, GA, USA
e-mail: gbblack@emory.edu; faisal.merchant@emory.edu

B. J. Wells et al. (eds.), *Handbook of Inpatient Cardiology*,
https://doi.org/10.1007/978-3-030-47868-1_4

Supraventricular Tachycardia

Definition, Incidence and Prevalence

- Supraventricular tachycardia (SVT) is typically a regular, narrow complex tachycardia although underlying conduction disease (bundle branch blocks), aberrant conduction and, rarely, antegrade conduction (atrium to ventricle) through an accessory pathway will result in wide complex tachycardia.
- 90% of SVTs include a reentrant mechanism between the atria and the ventricle.
- Atrioventricular nodal reentrant tachycardia (AVNRT) comprises 60% of reentrant tachycardias, 30% are atrioventricular reentrant tachycardias (AVRT) and the remaining 10% are atrial tachycardias (AT).
- ATs increase in frequency in older patients (>50 years old) and AVRT becomes less common.
- SVT occurs in about 35 cases in 100,000 patient years with a prevalence of 2.25 per 1000 patients [2].
- For the purposes of this chapter we will exclude atrial fibrillation (AF) and atrial flutter as they are addressed in a separate chapter.

Interventions for SVT

Vagal Maneuvers

- During any intervention for SVT the patient should be connected to a continuous 12-lead ECG to aid in diagnosis of the arrhythmia.
- Vagal maneuvers, including carotid sinus massage (CSM) and the Valsalva maneuver (VM), increase the parasympathetic tone which slows conduction through the atrium and the atrioventricular node (AVN).

- Vagal maneuvers should be first line treatment for patients who are in SVT with stable hemodynamics.
- The VM involves inhaling followed by exhaling against a closed glottis for at least 10–15 seconds. The patient is generally in a supine or semi-recumbent position. The modified VM, which involves supine repositioning and passive leg raise at the end of strain, is significantly more effective at converting patients out of SVT [1].
- CSM, which is less efficacious than VM, may also be attempted. The patient should be in the supine position with the neck extended. The carotid sinus is located inferior to the angle of the mandible at the level of the thyroid cartilage. Constant pressure should be applied for 5–10 seconds. Contraindications to CSM include stroke or transient ischemic attack (TIA) within the last 3 months and presence of a carotid bruit [4].

Clinical Pearl
During any intervention for SVT the patient should be connected to a continuous 12-lead ECG to aid in diagnosis of the arrhythmia.

Adenosine

- Adenosine decreases the heart rate and slows conduction through the AVN, albeit briefly as the half-life is <10 seconds.
- IV Adenosine should be administered rapidly, over 1 to 2 seconds, followed by a rapid flush of normal saline. A 3-way stopcock may expedite the delivery of the flush. The patient should be in the supine position. The recommended initial dose through a peripheral IV is 6 mg followed by 12 mg.
- Adenosine should always cause transient atrioventricular (AV) block. If the bolus of adenosine fails to do so, then it

was not administered fast enough, or the patient requires a higher dose.
- Adenosine must be used with the utmost caution in cardiac transplant recipients as the denervated heart is incredibly sensitive to this medication and this may lead to profound bradycardia or asystole.

Electrical Cardioversion

- Patients with SVT who are hemodynamically unstable should undergo immediate synchronized electrical cardioversion.

> **Clinical Pearl**
> Patients with SVT who are hemodynamically unstable should undergo immediate synchronized electrical cardioversion.

Approach to the Patient with SVT

12-Lead Electrocardiogram (ECG)

- Obtaining a 12-lead ECG is paramount for the diagnosis of SVT as P waves may not be evident on telemetry.
- The RP relationship refers to the interval between the R wave and the ensuing P wave and can aid in the diagnosis of SVT. In a short RP tachycardia, the P wave will closely follow the R wave (RP < PR), whereas the P wave will be closer to the ensuing R wave in long RP tachycardia (RP > PR).

Response to Adenosine

- SVTs that are adenosine responsive include AVNRT, AVRT, junctional tachycardia (JT), and some focal ATs.
- Any AVN dependent SVT will terminate with an adequate bolus of IV adenosine.

- Adenosine may be diagnostic as the delay in conduction through the AVN may reveal discrete atrial activity.

AV Nodal Reentrant Tachycardia

- AVNRT is more common in women than men and the ventricular rate is generally between 180 beats per minute (BPM) and 200 BPM, although this may range from 110 BPM to >250 BPM.
- AVNRT requires dual AV nodal physiology, in which patients have a fast and slow pathway within the AVN. The fast pathway allows for rapid conduction but has a long recovery period. The slow pathway results in slower conduction but a shorter recovery time.

Typical AVNRT

- In typical AVNRT, or "slow-fast" conduction, a premature atrial contraction (PAC) will be conducted antegrade through the slow pathway as the fast pathway is refractory from the previous sinus beat. During this period of slow conduction, the fast pathway will repolarize and allow for retrograde conduction (ventricle to atrium) of the impulse. Thus, the retrograde P will be very close in proximity to the QRS complex (short RP interval). Conversely, a premature ventricular contraction (PVC) may conduct up the fast pathway and start the tachycardia.
- P waves may appear as a pseudo-r' pattern in the anterior precordial leads. Retrograde P waves may also appear as pseudo-S waves in the inferior leads (Fig. 4.1). An inferiorly directed retrograde P wave axis (upright in leads II, III and aVF) excludes AVNRT.
- Vagal maneuvers should be first line for the treatment of acute AVNRT, followed by adenosine. Adenosine should successfully terminate AVNRT with appropriate dosing

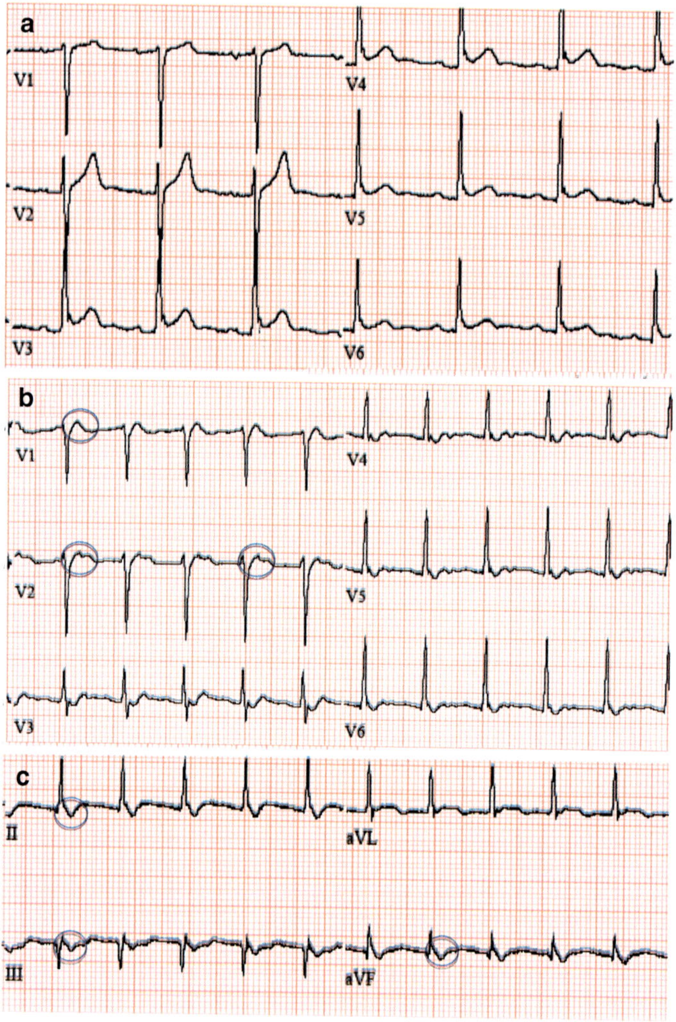

FIGURE 4.1 (**a**) This image demonstrates the precordial leads from the baseline ECG of a 32 year-old male who was later found to have typical AVNRT. (**b**) During tachycardia in the same patient a pseudo-r' pattern (retrograde P wave) develops conferring a short RP interval. (**c**) Note the superior axis of the retrograde P waves in the inferior leads during tachycardia, causing pseudo-S waves

and administration. Synchronized cardioversion is highly recommended for both stable and unstable patients who have failed to convert with vagal maneuvers and adenosine. However, IV nodal blockade is a reasonable option in hemodynamically stable patients.

Atypical AVNRT

- Atypical AVNRT, or "fast-slow" conduction, involves antegrade conduction down the fast pathway with retrograde conduction up the slow pathway. The retrograde P wave will be delayed due to the longer conduction time through the slow pathway resulting in a long RP tachycardia (Fig. 4.2).
- The treatment algorithm for atypical AVNRT is identical to that of typical AVNRT.

AV Reentrant Tachycardia

- AVRT requires an accessory pathway outside of the AVN to complete the reentrant circuit. Accessory pathways are termed manifest if they conduct antegrade, which will demonstrate ventricular pre-excitation in sinus rhythm with a delta wave on the ECG (Fig. 4.3). Manifest pathways may conduct impulses antegrade, retrograde or both. Those pathways that only conduct retrograde, termed concealed pathways, will not produce a delta wave.

Pre-Excited Atrial Fibrillation

- AF is particularly dangerous in patients with manifest pathways as this can lead to rapid conduction to the ventricle and degenerate to ventricular fibrillation (VF). For those with pre-excited AF (Fig. 4.4), procainamide or ibutilide are first line treatment for stable patients. *IV digoxin,*

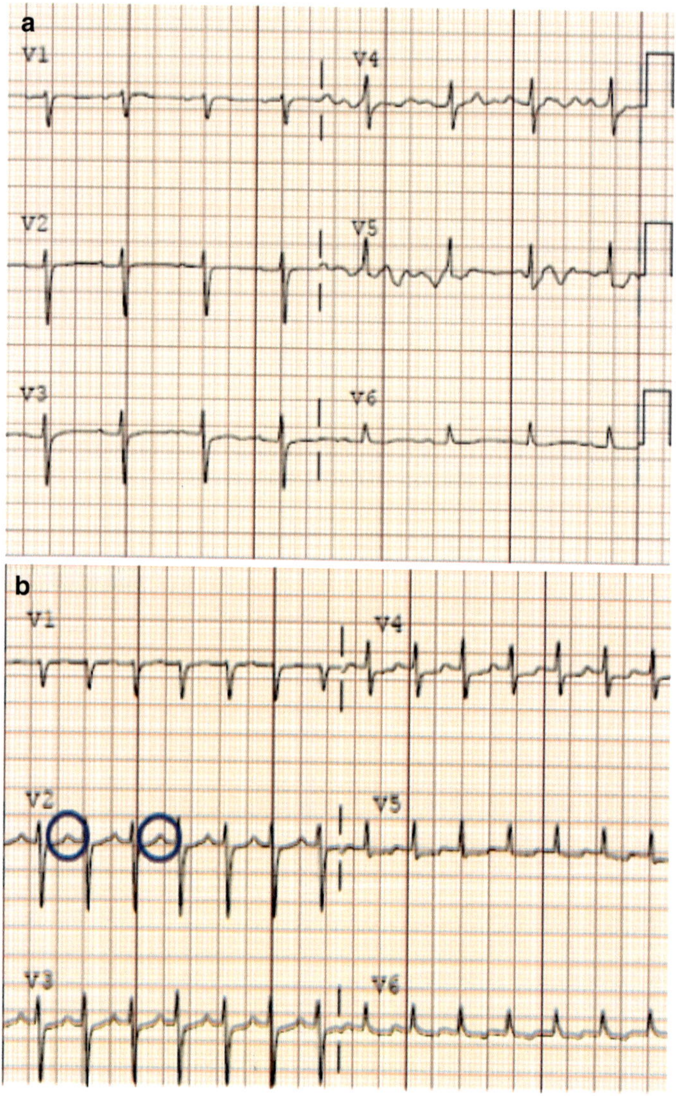

FIGURE 4.2 (**a**) The ECG on the left represents the precordial leads from a patient with atypical or "fast-slow" AVNRT which was captured in the precordial leads on the right. (**b**) The RP interval, which is evident with the retrograde p waves in the anterior leads, is longer than the PR interval

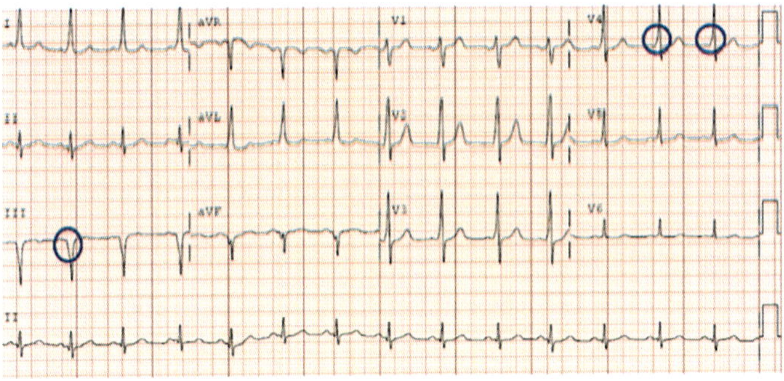

FIGURE 4.3 A 34 year-old male presented with syncope and was noted to have ventricular pre-excitation on the above 12-lead ECG. Note the short PR interval in sinus rhythm and the delta waves in the precordial and inferior limb leads

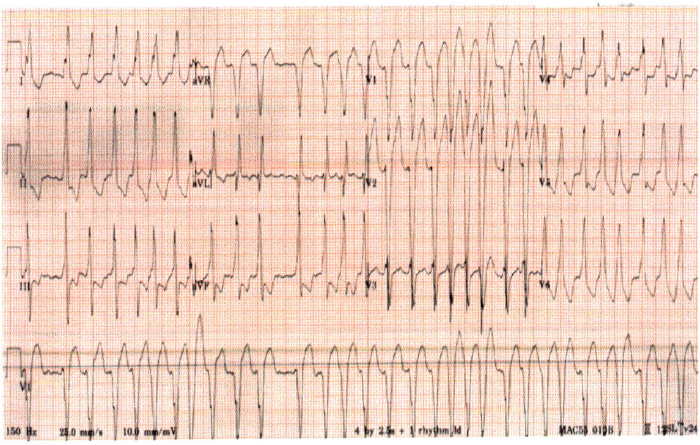

FIGURE 4.4 12-lead ECG from a 32 year-old male with pre-excited atrial fibrillation

IV amiodarone, beta blockers, diltiazem and verapamil are harmful in the acute treatment of pre-excited AF [3].

- For patients who have pre-excited AF and are hemodynamically unstable immediate synchronized cardioversion should be performed.

Orthodromic AVRT

- Orthodromic AVRT involves antegrade conduction through the AVN with retrograde conduction through the accessory pathway. The resultant ECG demonstrates a narrow complex tachycardia (the delta wave will resolve as the accessory pathway will be refractory following retrograde conduction), barring aberrant conduction, with a short RP interval. The RP interval will typically be longer than AVNRT as the accessory pathway is extranodal.
- Vagal maneuvers and adenosine, which should terminate the tachycardia, are first line therapies for AVRT. If the tachycardia persists cardioversion can be considered. If the patient is stable and does not have evidence of pre-excitation on the baseline ECG then IV beta blockers, diltiazem or verapamil may terminate the tachycardia. However, these drugs, including adenosine, should be avoided if there is evidence of pre-excitation given their potential to precipitate AF with rapid conduction to the ventricle. Therefore, cardioversion should be available.

Antidromic AVRT

- Antidromic, AVRT only occurs in 5-10% of patients with accessory pathways. Antidromic AVRT involves antegrade conduction down the accessory pathway resulting in a wide complex tachycardia as the antegrade depolarization does not propagate through the His-Purkinje system. It may be difficult to discern from ventricular tachycardia (VT).
- When suspected the treatment for atypical AVRT is identical to that of typical AVRT.

Atrial Tachycardia

Focal Atrial Tachycardia

- Atrial tachycardias are regular atrial rhythms with a single focus or small (<2 cm) microreentrant circuits that produce atrial rates generally between 100 and 250 BPM. AT can arise from specific sites in the atria and commonly occur in structurally normal hearts.
- Like other automatic mechanisms, ATs may display a gradual onset and offset or "warm up" and "warm down" over 3–4 beats if the patient is on telemetry [5]. On the other hand, ATs may start abruptly as in Fig. 4.5.
- ATs may conduct 1:1 to the ventricle, although this relationship varies, and generally appear as long RP tachycardias on the 12 lead ECG. However, the RP interval will be short in patients with first degree AV block. Further, due to the decremental property of the AVN (more frequent stimulation causes slower conduction through the node), the delay through the node may not be apparent in sinus rhythm.
- The P wave axis should at least demonstrate subtle differences when compared to sinus rhythm (Fig. 4.6). A consistent PP interval, the duration between consecutive P

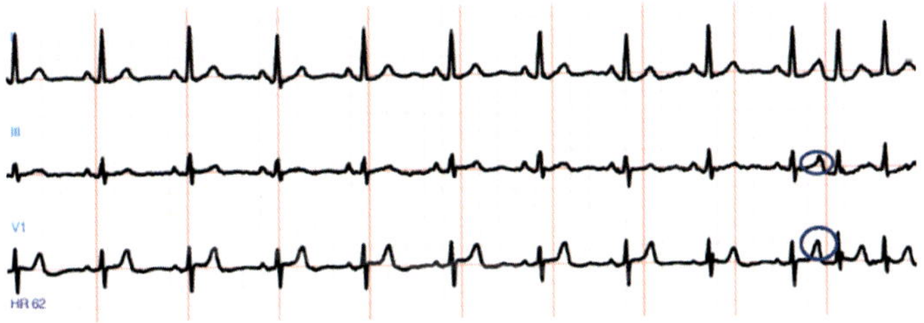

Figure 4.5 This 3-lead telemetry strip captured the onset of atrial tachycardia from a patient admitted for palpitations. Note the change in the T wave with the superimposed P wave, conferring a long RP interval, as well as the abrupt increase in the rate

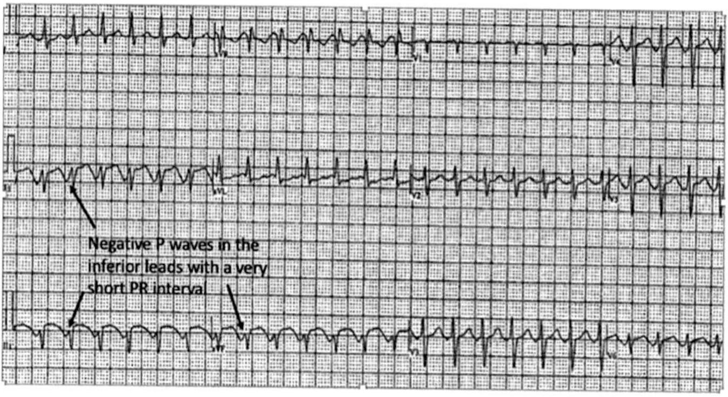

FIGURE 4.6 This 68 year-old male experienced recurrent tachycardia which was captured on this 12-lead ECG. The P wave axis is superior, opposite of that in sinus rhythm, in this long RP tachycardia. The patient was taken to the electrophysiology lab where he was found to have a focal AT emanating from the ostium of the coronary sinus

waves, despite variable PR and RP intervals on the ECG during tachycardia suggests AT.

- Transient AV block following the administration of adenosine may demonstrate persistent atrial activity without ventricular conduction, allowing differentiation of AT from AVNRT and AVRT. On the other hand, depending upon the mechanism of the AT, adenosine may terminate the tachycardia, although AV block usually occurs before termination of the arrhythmia.
- If AT is diagnosed, IV beta blockers, diltiazem or verapamil are first line therapies for the acute treatment of hemodynamically stable patients.

Multifocal Atrial Tachycardia

- Multifocal atrial tachycardia (MAT) involves multiple atrial foci and manifests as 3 distinct P wave morphologies with a ventricular rate of >100 BPM on the ECG. This arrhythmia usually occurs in older, critically ill patients with severe pulmonary or cardiac disease.

- IV metoprolol may be used in the acute setting to slow the ventricular rate, although it should be avoided in patients with severe pulmonary disease. IV verapamil is relatively successful at converting patients with MAT to sinus rhythm.

Junctional Tachycardia

- JT arises from the atrioventricular junction, specifically the perinodal tissue and His bundle. P waves may appear before, after or even within the QRS complex with a ventricular rate > 100 BPM. Thus, JT may appear on the ECG as a short or long RP tachycardia.
- JT is more common in infants and children and rarely occurs in adults. This arrhythmia may be seen in adults after valve surgery and tends to be transient [5].
- IV beta blockers, diltiazem, verapamil or procainamide are reasonable options for the treatment of acute JT.

Clinical Pearls

- During any intervention for SVT the patient should be connected to a continuous 12-lead ECG to aid in diagnosis of the arrhythmia.
- Patients with SVT who are hemodynamically unstable should undergo immediate synchronized electrical cardioversion.
- Adenosine should always cause transient atrioventricular (AV) block. If the bolus of adenosine fails to do so, then it was not administered fast enough or the patient requires a higher dose.
- IV digoxin, IV amiodarone, beta blockers, diltiazem and verapamil are potentially harmful in the acute treatment of pre-excited AF.
- Adenosine should be avoided in patients with pre-excited AF and heart transplant recipients.

Key Learning Points

1. Supraventricular tachycardia (SVT) is typically a regular, narrow complex tachycardia although underlying conduction disease, aberrant conduction and, rarely, antegrade conduction (atrium to ventricle) through an accessory pathway will result in wide complex tachycardia.
2. Any SVT that is dependent on the AV node, such as AVNRT and AVRT, should terminate with an adequate bolus of adenosine.
3. Adenosine can be a diagnostic and therapeutic intervention for SVT as it may terminate the arrhythmia or block AV conduction, allowing for visualization of discrete atrial activity. However, this medication should be used with extreme caution or avoided in patients who have received an orthotopic heart transplant those patients with evidence of ventricular pre-excitation.

References

1. Appelboam A, Reuben A, Mann C, Gagg J, Ewings P, Barton A, et al. Postural modification to the standard Valsalva manoeuvre for emergency treatment of supraventricular tachycardias (REVERT): a randomised controlled trial. Lancet. 2015;386(10005):1747–53. https://doi.org/10.1016/s0140-6736(15)61485-4.
2. Garcia MA, Macle L, Khairy P. Electrophysiology for clinicians. Minneapolis: Cardiotext Publishing; 2012.
3. Page RL, Joglar JA, Caldwell MA, Calkins H, Conti JB, Deal BJ, et al. 2015 ACC/AHA/HRS guideline for the management of adult patients with supraventricular tachycardia. J Am Coll Cardiol. 2016;67(13):e27–e115. https://doi.org/10.1016/j.jacc.2015.08.856.
4. Shen W, Sheldon RS, Benditt DG, Cohen MI, Forman DE, Goldberger ZD, et al. 2017 ACC/AHA/HRS guideline for the evaluation and management of patients with syncope: a

report of the American College of Cardiology/American Heart Association task force on clinical practice guidelines and the Heart Rhythm Society. Circulation. 2017;136(5):e60–e122. https://doi.org/10.1161/cir.0000000000000499.
5. Zipes DP, Jalife J, Stevenson WG. Cardiac electrophysiology: from cell to bedside. Philadelphia, PA: Elsevier; 2018.

Chapter 5
Ventricular Arrhythmias

Soroosh Kiani and Michael S. Lloyd

Terminology and Definitions

- *Ventricular Tachycardia (VT)*: three or more beats at a rate of >100 bpm that:
  - originate in the tissue below the level of the *atrio-ventricular (AV) node* and are independent of its activity [1].
  - These tissues can include the ventricular myocardium as well as portions of the His-Purkinje system [2].

There are several important qualifiers when describing ventricular arrhthmias [3]:

- Based on the length and frequency of the arrhythmia.
  - *Premature Ventricular Contraction* (PVC): one or two consecutive beats originating in the ventricular tissue independent of activity of the AV node.
  - *Non-sustained VT* (NSVT): > = 3 beats, but less than 30 seconds, with spontaneous termination.

S. Kiani (✉) · M. S. Lloyd
Department of Medicine, Division of Cardiology, Section of Electrophysiology and Pacing, Emory University School of Medicine, Atlanta, GA, USA
e-mail: skiani@emory.edu; soroosh.kiani@emory.edu

B. J. Wells et al. (eds.), *Handbook of Inpatient Cardiology*,
https://doi.org/10.1007/978-3-030-47868-1_5

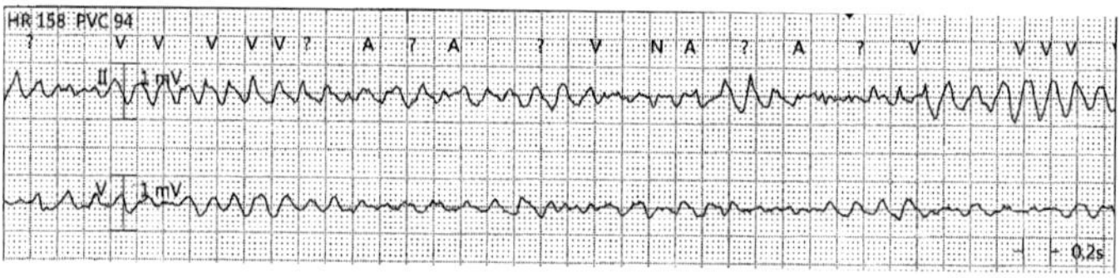

FIGURE 5.1 An example of VF on telemetry

- *Sustained VT*: >30 seconds of continuous VT or VT requiring termination in <30 seconds due to hemodynamic compromise.
- *VT/VF Storm*: > = 3 episodes of sustained VT or VF, or appropriate ICD shocks, within 24 hours.

- Based on the QRS morphology.
  - *Monomorphic*: VT with a single, stable QRS morphology with no, or minimal variation beat to beat.
  - *Polymorphic*: Changing or multiple QRS morphologies present from beat to beat.
  - *Torsade de Pointes (or "Torsades")*: A specific case of polymorphic VT occurring in the context of a long QT interval, often bradycardia dependent and occurring after a "long-short" initiating sequence (and long coupling interval to the first VT beat).
  - *Ventricular Fibrillation (VF)*: Very rapid and highly irregular electrical activity, usually with a ventricular rate of >300 bpm. The QRS complexes can often be of low amplitude (Fig. 5.1).

Epidemiology

- *Premature Ventricular Contractions (PVC) and NSVT.*
  - Prevalence typically increases with age and are very common those >age 50 [4].
  - *Frequent PVCs*: 1 PVC per standard 12-lead ECG or > 30 PVCs per hour [5].

    Frequent PVCs and NSVT: associated with a higher overall risk of poor cardiovascular outcomes and mortality and should prompt further investigation [5, 6].

- *Sustained VT and VF.*
  - There is a very strong association with VT and VF with acute coronary syndromes (ACS) including *myocardial infarction* (MI) [7, 8].

Clinical Pearl
- Typically, VTs associated with ACS are *polymorphic* [3].

  - 50% of all people with out-of-hospital cardiac arrests will have significant coronary artery disease.
  - 50% of all out of hospital arrests due to VF that also survive to hospital admission are found to have MI.
  - Among patients have acute MI, between 5–10% will have sustained VT or VF before or after hospital admission.
  - Patients without ACS but *with* structural heart disease (e.g. scar due to prior MI, non-ischemic cardiomyopathies, congenital heart disease, prior cardiac surgery, or significant valvular disease) are also at risk of scar-related VT which can degenerate into VF [9, 10]. In these cases, the VT is typically *monomorphic* [3].

    Monomorphic VT in the absence of structural disease is often referred to as *idiopathic* and is less common [1, 9].
  - Patients without structural disease are rarely at risk for polymorphic VT and VF. In this population polymorphic VT is usually related to an underlying channelopathy, long-QT syndrome, or may be idiopathic [3, 10].

Mechanisms of Ventricular Ectopy and Tachycardia

A detailed review of the underlying mechanisms of PVCs and VT is beyond the scope of this chapter. In brief, these include:

- *Increased Automaticity*, leading to spontaneous activity (i.e. PVCs or VT), often in ischemic tissue.

- *Reentry* [11], which is the most common mechanism of sustained VT in the context of structural heart disease and underlying scar [3].
- *Triggered Activity* resulting in "early afterdepolarizatoins" [1] which may lead to VT in the context of long QT syndromes and "delayed afterdepolarizations" [12] which are thought to be important triggers in numerous conditions including idiopathic VT, digoxin toxicity and heart failure [3].

Diagnosis of Ventricular Tachycardia

- Manifest as wide complex tachycardias (WCT) as a result of their sites of origin.
- Wide QRS complexes: duration of 120 ms or greater [13].
- The differential diagnosis of WCT is discussed in Chap. 4.
- Distinguishing VT from other WCT can be challenging at times, even among experienced clinicians.

Clinical Pearl

As a general rule, *all WCT should be treated at VT until definitively proven otherwise* [3]. There are several reasons for this approach.

- VT is the most common etiology of WCT) in general, representing up to 80% of cases [14].
- VT is usually more likely to be life threatening than other WCTs. Therefore, when there is doubt, consideration should be given to VT.
- Therapies for acute VT are often effective and, while not always first line, appropriate for other WCTs. However, the reverse is not always true and may indeed be dangerous as common therapies for SVTs (beta blockers, calcium channel blockers, or adenosine) can lead to hemodynamic deterioration or precipitate VF in the setting of VT [2].

The Surface ECG

Multiple systems and algorithms have been proposed to help distinguish monomorphic VT from other WCTs [14–17].

- The most common of these is the Brugada algorithm [17].
- A more recent alternative is the so-called Vereckei algorithm which may have a higher sensitivity and specificity than the former [15].

While different in their details, most of these systems utilize similar and important themes from the surface ECG (Fig. 5.3) [2, 14–17]:

1. *Rate and regularity,* per se, *are not helpful in distinguishing VT from other WCTs*. There is a great deal of overlap in rates in SVTs and VT. Likewise, both are frequently regular, and VT can be irregular at its onset. However, a great deal of irregularity would suggest atrial fibrillation with underlying bundle branch block or aberrancy [2].
2. *AV dissociation* (Fig. 5.2), *especially with more QRS complexes than p-waves* (i.e. *faster ventricular rate than atrial rate) is very specific for VT* [2, 14].
3. *The presence of fusion or capture beats are highly suggestive of VT.*
   - *Fusion beats* are a fused complex of both a native QRS and ventricular beat.
   - *Capture beat* is a sinus beat that conducts normally and "captures" the ventricle and temporarily usurps the ventricular arrhythmia.
4. *VT tends to produce "unusual" QRS morphologies.* If the QRS morphology is consistent with a typical right or left bundle branch block (or a right bundle branch block with a

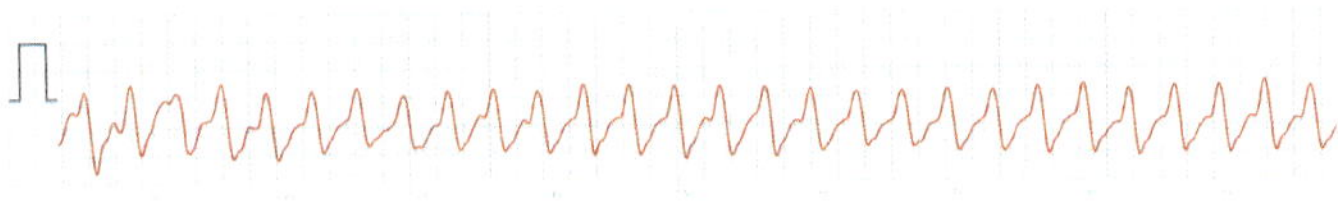

FIGURE 5.2 A smartphone device captured this WCT which was sustained monomorphic VT. Careful examination shows p-wave which march out independently of the QRS complexes

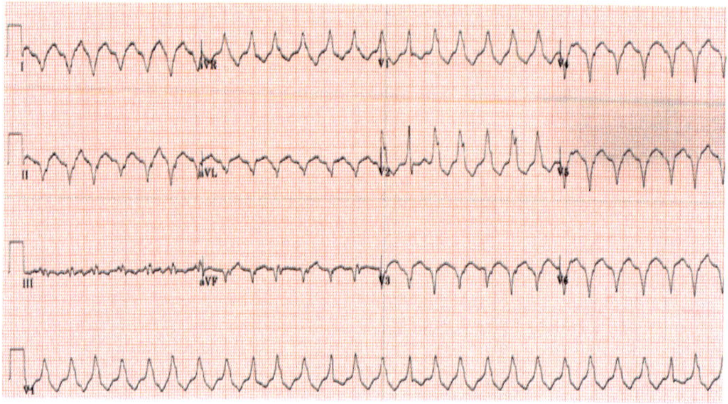

FIGURE 5.3 Surface ECG of a patient in sustained monomorphic VT. Many of the features that distinguish VT from other WCTs are present in this example. These include AV dissociation, slurred initial deflection of the QRS complexes (evident in the precordial leads), an atypical right bundle branch pattern in V1 (an RSr' pattern), a very wide QRS, a large positive R wave in aVR, and a "northwest axis" see in the limb leads, as well as a fusion beat (seen best as the first beat in leads V1 and V2)

left anterior or posterior fascicular block), then the rhythm is less likely to be VT [2].

- *Atypical bundle branch morphologies* (e.g. *qR, RSr' or monomorphic R-wave in V1) suggest VT.*
- *Very wide QRS complexes (>160 ms for LBBB or > 140 ms for RBBB) suggest VT.*
- *A change from one bundle branch morphology in native rhythm to another in tachycardia suggests VT.*
- *Paradoxically, a narrower QRS in tachycardia than in sinus suggests VT.*

5. *QRS complexes in VT tend to have a slow or slurred initial deflection.* The initial site of ventricular activation of VT is the *ventricular myocardium*, and not His-Purkinje system. As a result, the initial wave front is slower than usual, producing a slow initial deflection on the ECG.
6. *An initial R-wave, especially if wide, in aVR represents myocardial activation in an atypical pattern and suggests VT.*

Supraventricular-to-ventricular activation propagates down the intraventricular septum and then the rest of the ventricular myocardium and tends to produce a net vector *away* from lead aVR.

- This normal pattern of activation should also result in R waves in some precordial leads. Thus, *the absence of RS complexes in any precordial lead suggest VT.*

7. Similarly, *a QRS axis that is "northwest"* (i.e. *-90° to +/–180°*) *suggest VT.*

Inpatient Management of Ventricular Tachycardia

The focus of this chapter will be on acute inpatient management of sustained or hemodynamically significant VT. Primary and secondary prevention are discussed in Chap. 7 (ICD, CRT).

- *The initial management of all tachyarrhythmias, VT or otherwise, should adhere to American Heart Association Advanced Cardiac Life Support (ACLS) guidelines* [3, 18–21].
- An in-depth review of ACLS guidelines is beyond the scope of this chapter. However, some key points are included below in the setting of unstable VT or VF:
  - High quality CPR should be administered to all patients with cardiac arrest per ACLS guidelines.

    In patients with polymorphic VT or VF, defibrillation, vasopressor therapy and IV lidocaine, can be considered in addition to CPR.
  - Any unstable VT should be promptly cardioverted with a maximum energy direct-current shock. Should the rhythm persist, IV amiodarone should be administered.
  - Patients with polymorphic VT or VF, and with evidence of ST-elevation MI should be considered for urgent cardiac catheterization and revascularization.

  - An urgent consult to a Cardiovascular specialist should be pursued in this context.
- *Stable Sustained Monomorphic VT:*
  - *Initial evaluation*: should include.
    focused history and physical exam,
    12-lead ECG

Clinical Pearl
Taking a moment to obtain a 12-lead ECG is invaluable to cardiology consultants in order for proper localization, diagnosis, and targeted treatment of VT.

- Blood work to evaluate for electrolytes and metabolic panel, cardiac enzymes, etc. should be sent.

Clinical Pearl
Electrolytes should be corrected as soon as possible. However, pharmacologic or electrical therapy (see below) should not be delayed while waiting for blood work to come back - this workup can be done in parallel to therapy.

- *Therapeutic Considerations*: For patients in stable, sustained monomorphic VT, electrical [22] or pharmacologic cardioversion [3] is reasonable.
  - If electrical cardioversion is pursued as a first line therapy, it should be done with adequate sedation.
- *Typical pharmacologic agents* include [3, 22–27]:
  - *Amiodarone* (150 mg over 10 minutes followed by IV drip at 1 mg/min for 6 hours, then 0.5 mg/min).
    Bolus of amiodarone can precipitate hypotension and should be done with close monitoring.
  - *Procainamide* (20–50 mg/min with maximum dose of 15–75 mg/kg).

Close blood pressure monitoring (q5–10 min) is required as hypotension can ensue on procainamide.

Indications to terminate this therapy including:

- Hypotension.
- QRS widening by >50% of baseline width.

– *Lidocaine* (1–1.5 mg/kg at a rate of 25–50 mg/min) with repeated lower doses as needed (0.5–0.75 mg/kg) every 5–10 minutes.

May be less effective than sotalol in this context but has less risk of hypotension and pro-arrythmia.

– *Sotalol* (1–1.5 mg/kg at a rate of 10–20 mg/min) with blood pressure, heart rate, and telemetry monitoring (due to a risk of torsades due to QTc prolongation).

Should be avoided if baseline QTc is >500 ms.

Less commonly used in clinical practice in the US.

- *Preventative Therapy*
  - Treatment of any underlying factors, including treatment of heart failure, cardiac ischemia, offending medications (i.e. QT prolonging medications), and electrolyte disturbances should be undertaken whenever possible.
  - Beta Blockers are first line to prevent further ventricular arrythmias and should be used barring contraindication.
  - Antiarrhythmic Drug (AAD) Options:

    Antiarrhythmic therapy may be needed to manage arrythmia burden, decrease the risk of defibrillator therapies, and control symptoms [3].

    Amiodarone and sotalol are mainstays of therapy, though certainly not exclusive options for prevention of future ventricular arrhythmias.

Clinical Pearl

AAD therapy can often be nuanced, and is associated with risks of serious adverse events [1] and should be managed by a cardiovascular specialist whenever possible.

Key Learning Points

1. Understanding how to characterize various types of ventricular ectopy is critical in order to appropriately triage the electrical stability of the patient and deliver appropriate therapy.
2. Distinguishing VT from other WCTs can be challenging but understanding key features unique to VE are often helpful.
3. All WCT should be treated as VT until definitively proven otherwise.
4. The initial management of all tachyarrhythmias, VT or otherwise, should adhere to American Heart Association Advanced Cardiac Life Support (ACLS) guidelines whenever possible.

References

1. Buxton AE, Calkins H, Callans DJ, et al. ACC/AHA/HRS 2006 key data elements and definitions for electrophysiological studies and procedures: a report of the American College of Cardiology/American Heart Association task force on clinical data standards (ACC/AHA/HRS writing committee to develop data standards on electrophysiology). J Am Coll Cardiol. 2006;48(11):2360–96.
2. Issa ZF. *Clinical arrhythmology and electrophysiology : a companion to Baunwald's heart disease*. 3rd ed. Philadelphia: Elsevier; 2018.
3. Al-Khatib SM, Stevenson WG, Ackerman MJ, et al. 2017 AHA/ACC/HRS guideline for management of patients with ventricular arrhythmias and the prevention of sudden cardiac death: executive summary: a report of the American College of Cardiology/American Heart Association task force on clinical practice guidelines and the Heart Rhythm Society. Heart Rhythm. 2018;15(10):e190–252.
4. Brodsky M, Wu D, Denes P, Kanakis C, Rosen KM. Arrhythmias documented by 24 hour continuous electrocardiographic moni-

toring in 50 male medical students without apparent heart disease. Am J Cardiol. 1977;39(3):390–5.

5. Ataklte F, Erqou S, Laukkanen J, Kaptoge S. Meta-analysis of ventricular premature complexes and their relation to cardiac mortality in general populations. Am J Cardiol. 2013;112(8):1263–70.
6. Lin CY, Chang SL, Chung FP, et al. Long-term outcome of non-sustained ventricular tachycardia in structurally normal hearts. PLoS One. 2016;11(8):e0160181.
7. Dumas F, Cariou A, Manzo-Silberman S, et al. Immediate percutaneous coronary intervention is associated with better survival after out-of-hospital cardiac arrest: insights from the PROCAT (Parisian Region Out of hospital Cardiac ArresT) registry. Circ Cardiovasc Interv. 2010;3(3):200–7.
8. Gupta S, Pressman GS, Figueredo VM. Incidence of, predictors for, and mortality associated with malignant ventricular arrhythmias in non-ST elevation myocardial infarction patients. Coron Artery Dis. 2010;21(8):460–5.
9. El-Sherif N, Smith RA, Evans K. Canine ventricular arrhythmias in the late myocardial infarction period. 8. Epicardial mapping of reentrant circuits. Circ Res. 1981;49(1):255–65.
10. Koplan BA, Stevenson WG. Ventricular tachycardia and sudden cardiac death. Mayo Clin Proc. 2009;84(3):289–97.
11. Cherry EM, Fenton FH, Gilmour RF Jr. Mechanisms of ventricular arrhythmias: a dynamical systems-based perspective. Am J Physiol Heart Circ Physiol. 2012;302(12):H2451–63.
12. Priori SG, Chen SR. Inherited dysfunction of sarcoplasmic reticulum Ca2+ handling and arrhythmogenesis. Circ Res. 2011;108(7):871–83.
13. Surawicz B, Childers R, Deal BJ, Gettes LS. AHA/ACCF/HRS recommendations for the standardization and interpretation of the electrocardiogram. Circulation. 2009;119(10):e235–40.
14. Vereckei A. Current algorithms for the diagnosis of wide QRS complex tachycardias. Curr Cardiol Rev. 2014;10(3):262–76.
15. Vereckei A, Duray G, Szénási G, Altemose GT, Miller JM. Application of a new algorithm in the differential diagnosis of wide QRS complex tachycardia. Eur Heart J. 2007;28(5):589–600.
16. Vereckei A, Duray G, Szénási G, Altemose GT, Miller JM. New algorithm using only lead aVR for differential diagnosis of wide QRS complex tachycardia. Heart Rhythm. 2008;5(1):89–98.
17. Brugada P, Brugada J, Mont L, Smeets J, Andries EW. A new approach to the differential diagnosis of a regular tachycardia with a wide QRS complex. Circulation. 1991;83(5):1649–59.

18. Hazinski MF, Nolan JP, Billi JE, et al. Part 1: executive summary: 2010 international consensus on cardiopulmonary resuscitation and emergency cardiovascular care science with treatment recommendations. Circulation. 2010;122(16 Suppl 2):S250–75.
19. Link MS, Berkow LC, Kudenchuk PJ, et al. Part 7: adult advanced cardiovascular life support: 2015 American Heart Association guidelines update for cardiopulmonary resuscitation and emergency cardiovascular care. Circulation. 2015;132(18 Suppl 2):S444–64.
20. Neumar RW, Shuster M, Callaway CW, et al. Part 1: executive summary: 2015 American Heart Association guidelines update for cardiopulmonary resuscitation and emergency cardiovascular care. Circulation. 2015;132(18 Suppl 2):S315–67.
21. Soar J, Donnino MW, Maconochie I, et al. 2018 international consensus on cardiopulmonary resuscitation and emergency cardiovascular care science with treatment recommendations summary. Resuscitation. 2018;133:194–206.
22. Link MS, Atkins DL, Passman RS, et al. Part 6: electrical therapies: automated external defibrillators, defibrillation, cardioversion, and pacing: 2010 American Heart Association guidelines for cardiopulmonary resuscitation and emergency cardiovascular care. Circulation. 2010;122(18 Suppl 3):S706–19.
23. Kowey PR, Levine JH, Herre JM, et al. Randomized, double-blind comparison of intravenous amiodarone and bretylium in the treatment of patients with recurrent, hemodynamically destabilizing ventricular tachycardia or fibrillation. The Intravenous Amiodarone Multicenter Investigators Group. Circulation. 1995;92(11):3255–63.
24. Waxman HL, Buxton AE, Sadowski LM, Josephson ME. The response to procainamide during electrophysiologic study for sustained ventricular tachyarrhythmias predicts the response to other medications. Circulation. 1983;67(1):30–7.
25. Naccarelli GV, Jalal S. Intravenous amiodarone. Another option in the acute management of sustained ventricular tachyarrhythmias. Circulation. 1995;92(11):3154–5.
26. deSouza IS, Martindale JL, Sinert R. Antidysrhythmic drug therapy for the termination of stable, monomorphic ventricular tachycardia: a systematic review. Emerg Med J. 2015;32(2):161–7.
27. Ho DS, Zecchin RP, Richards DA, Uther JB, Ross DL. Double-blind trial of lignocaine versus sotalol for acute termination of spontaneous sustained ventricular tachycardia. Lancet. 1994;344(8914):18–23.

Chapter 6 Bradyarrhythmias and AV Block

Amole O. Ojo and Alfred E. Buxton

Abbreviations

AV	Atrioventricular
bpm	Beat per minute
CHB	Complete heart block
ECG	Electrocardiogram
HR	Heart rate
SA	Sinoatrial
SND	Sinus node dysfunction

Sinus Bradycardia

Definition

- By convention, sinus bradycardia is defined as a heart rate (HR) less than 60 beats per minute (bpm) with a normal P wave vector on the electrocardiogram (ECG).

A. O. Ojo (✉) · A. E. Buxton
Department of Medicine, Cardiovascular Division, Beth Israel Deaconess Medical Center, Harvard Medical School, Boston, MA, USA
e-mail: aoojo@bidmc.harvard.edu; abuxton@bidmc.harvard.edu

B. J. Wells et al. (eds.), *Handbook of Inpatient Cardiology*,
https://doi.org/10.1007/978-3-030-47868-1_6

- Others have advocated for definition of a HR less than 50 bpm, given sinus rates between 50 and 60 bpm may reflect physical conditioning and not sinus node pathology.

Causes

- Medication use: beta blockers, calcium channel blockers, antiarrhythmic medications, digoxin, ivabradine, lithium, clonidine, methyldopa, opioids and sedatives, etc.
- Myocardial ischemia (especially involving right coronary distribution as the SA artery originates from RCA in about 60% of people, typically due to increased vagal tone and often transient).
- Hypothyroidism.
- Obstructive sleep apnea (HR may be less than 30 beats per minute during apneic episodes).
- Hypothermia.
- Increased intracranial pressure.
- Enhanced vagal tone (triggered by stimuli such as vomiting, coughing, bowel movement, urination, and Valsalva maneuver).
- Infections such as Lyme carditis.
- Highly conditioned athletes (due to increase in vagal tone induced by exercise conditioning, typically asymptomatic).
- Sinus node dysfunction (SND, described in detail later in this chapter).

Clinical Pearl
In normal healthy adults, sinus bradycardia is a frequent finding, especially during sleep when HR may drop as low as 30 beats per minutes, with pauses up to 2 seconds [1].

Clinical Presentation

- Sinus bradycardia is usually asymptomatic.
- Typical symptoms include lightheadedness, fatigue, exertional dyspnea, or chest discomfort and presyncope.

> **Clinical Pearl**
> There is no specific HR below which everybody develops symptoms, as cardiac output varies depending on ability to augment stroke volume depending on underlying conditions or comorbidities.

Diagnosis/ECG Features

- ECG shows positive/upright P wave in leads I, II, aVL, and a negative/inverted P wave in lead aVR as a result of right atrial depolarization prior to left atrial depolarization as well as HR less than 60 bpm.
- Differentiate sinus bradycardia from other bradyarrhythmias such as atrioventricular (AV) block by establishing a 1:1 relationship between P waves and QRS complexes on the ECG.

Treatment

- Treatment is not indicated in patients who are asymptomatic.
- For hemodynamically unstable patients, consider atropine. The initial dose of atropine is 0.5 mg IV and it can be repeated every 3–5 minutes for a total of 3 mg. If symptoms do not improve with atropine, consider temporary transcutaneous or transvenous pacing or medications such as dopamine and epinephrine. However, also consider that

the symptoms may not be due to sinus bradycardia (depending on how slow the sinus rate is).

- For hemodynamically stable patients, look for etiology of the sinus bradycardia and treat accordingly.
- Withhold medications that may be causing the sinus bradycardia, if symptoms are documented to be a result of sinus bradycardia. However, a pacemaker may be indicated if the medication is mandatory for the treatment of comorbid conditions.

Clinical Pearl
In patients with symptomatic bradycardia because of calcium channel blocker overdose, consider intravenous calcium; in those with beta-blocker overdose, consider glucagon, and in those with digoxin toxicity, consider digoxin Fab antibody fragment.

Sinus Pauses or Arrest

- This is due to intermittent failure of the SA node to generate impulse.
- It may be due to intrinsic SND or related to medications.
- The ECG shows absence of a P wave at the expected time and can last from 2 seconds to several minutes (Fig. 6.1).
- The duration of the pause should have no arithmetical relationship to the prior PP interval. This can manifest as a delay of the next P wave (sinus pause) or complete absence of a P wave with escape rhythm/beats (sinus arrest).

Sinoatrial Exit Block

- This occurs when there is interference with impulse conduction from the SA node to the atria.

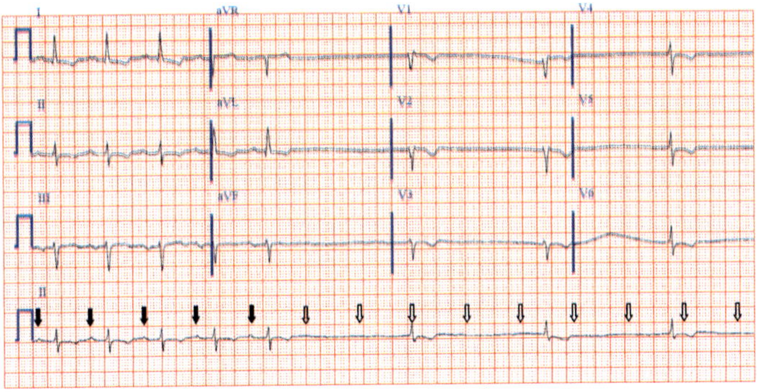

FIGURE 6.1 ECG showing sinus arrest on the right hand of the tracing with junctional escape rhythm. No P wave is seen at the expected time (hollow arrows)

- It can be due to medications, increased vagal activity, infiltrative, ischemic, or inflammatory diseases.
- SA exit block can be first degree, second degree, or third degree, following the convention for AV block.
  - First-degree SA exit block

    There is slowing of impulse exit to the atrium but still with 1:1 conduction. However, the ECG looks normal. It can only be diagnosed using special intracardiac recordings.
  - Second-degree SA exit block.

    Type I (Wenckebach type) – ECG shows progressively decreasing PP intervals prior to a dropped P wave; the pause is less than two PP intervals.

    Type II – ECG shows that the PP surrounding the pause is a multiple of the basic sinus rate [3] (Fig. 6.2).
  - Third-degree SA exit block

    No impulse reaches the atrium from the SA node and this gives appearance of no P waves. The ECG is indistinguishable from the ECG of sinus arrest. There may be either an atrial, junctional, or ventricular rhythm. P waves may be absent or be of a different morphology, depending on the location of a possible subsidiary atrial pacemaker.

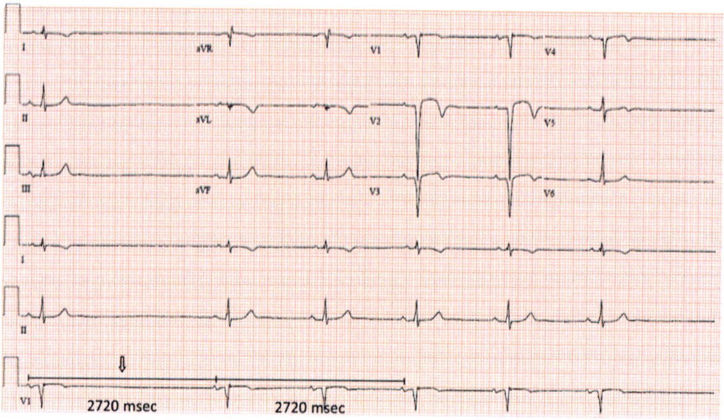

FIGURE 6.2 ECG showing SA exit block Mobitz type II. The pause is twice the PP intervals. The hollow arrow showed where the expected P wave was meant to be

Sinus Node Dysfunction (SND)

Definition

- SND, historically known as sick sinus syndrome, is due to dysfunction of the sinoatrial node. It is often related to age-dependent fibrosis of the SA node and the surrounding atrial myocardium.
- It can lead to abnormalities of SA node and atrial impulse formation and propagation and can manifest as various bradycardia or pause-related syndromes.
- It can also manifest as chronotropic incompetence – inability to proportionally increase HR in response to increase in physiological demands during physical activities.
- Period of bradycardia can alternate with period of tachycardia (atrial tachyarrhythmias) as part of tachycardia-bradycardia syndrome.

Clinical Presentation

- Patients frequently present with symptoms of lightheadedness, fatigue, presyncope, syncope, exertional chest discomfort, or dyspnea and palpitations in those with tachycardia-bradycardia syndrome.
- Symptoms are often intermittent and progressive in frequency and severity.

Diagnosis/ECG Features

- Diagnosis is made based on surface ECG in those suspected of SND. Electrophysiology study is of low yield and very rarely indicated.
- ECG can show
  - Inappropriate sinus bradycardia (with HR often less than 50 bpm).
  - Sinus pauses.
  - Sinus arrest and SA exit block, with or without appropriate escape rhythms.
  - Ectopic atrial bradycardia.
  - Isorhythmic dissociation when the atrial rate is slower than the ventricular rate from a junctional or ventricular rhythm.
- Patients may also develop atrial tachyarrhythmias – most commonly atrial fibrillation but atrial flutter and atrial tachycardia can also occur.
- More than 50% of the patients with SND have alternating periods of bradycardia and tachycardia [2], possibly because the pathologic process that affects the SA node also affects the atria.
- It is very important to establish a correlation between symptoms and the rhythm at the time of the symptoms. Ambulatory ECG/event monitoring can be very helpful in doing this. The type of monitor to be used is dictated by the frequency of patient's symptoms.

- Reversible causes such as medications and myocardial ischemia need to be identified and treated as indicated. Other differential diagnoses to be considered include neurocardiogenic syncope with a predominant cardioinhibitory component and carotid sinus hypersensitivity.
- Exercise stress tests can be helpful in identifying SND and to exclude myocardial ischemia and can help to identify patients with chronotropic incompetence.

Treatment

- Patients with SND are rarely hemodynamically unstable for prolonged periods. If hemodynamically unstable, use the ACLS protocol including pharmacologic intervention with medications such as atropine, dopamine, epinephrine, or isoproterenol. Transcutaneous and transvenous pacing are other options. Long-term treatment is the same as patients who were hemodynamically stable.
- Long-term treatment of SND typically entails consult/referral for pacemaker implantation.

Atrioventricular Block

Definition

- AV conduction disturbances may manifest as conduction delay in the AV node and/or infranodal structures, intermittent failure of impulse conduction from the atria to the ventricles, or complete AV block.

Causes

- Infiltrative cardiomyopathies (consider evaluation for cardiac sarcoidosis in patients with AV block who are younger than 60 years).
- Certain muscular dystrophies.

- Myocardial infarction; Myocarditis.
- Increase in vagal tone (can be seen in athletes).
- Medications (such as calcium channel blockers, digoxin).
- Post-cardiac surgery.
- Infection such as Lyme carditis (obtain history of potential exposure to ticks), acute rheumatic fever.
- Endocarditis with abscess formation.
- Lev's or Lenegre's disease (fibrosis and/or calcification of the conduction system).

Clinical Presentation

- Patients with first-degree AV delay and second-degree AV block Mobitz type I are usually asymptomatic.
- Patients with higher degree AV block (Mobitz II second-degree block or complete heart block) may also be asymptomatic or present with symptoms such as fatigue, exercise intolerance, dyspnea, chest pain, presyncope, syncope, or much less often cardiac arrest.

Treatment

- Patients with first- or second-degree AV block rarely require acute intervention.
- Patients with very slow heart rates in the setting of complete heart block may be given atropine only if there is ECG evidence that the block is in the AV node.
- Hemodynamically unstable patients should receive temporary cardiac pacing.
- Dopamine or isoproterenol may be administered if the ability to implant a temporary pacemaker is delayed.
- For hemodynamically stable patients, reversible causes of AV block should be excluded prior to implantation of a permanent pacemaker. Please see the Chap. 7 on pacemakers for indications. Cardiology should be consulted for patients with symptomatic second-degree or higher degree AV block.

Prolonged PR Interval (First-Degree AV Block)

- It is more appropriate to use the term "AV delay" as there is no true AV block. This is due to slowed AV conduction, which most commonly occurs in the AV node but can also occur in the His-Purkinje system.
- It is defined as PR > 0.20 seconds on the ECG. Given that the PR interval includes intra-atrial conduction (P wave) and the PR segment, AV delay can also be due to a delay in right atrial conduction.

Second-Degree AV Block

- Mobitz type I (Wenckebach): There is progressive delay of each subsequent impulse in the AV node (rarely in the His-Purkinje system) until the AV node fails to conduct the impulse to the ventricle.
  - ECG shows progressive lengthening of the PR interval until a P wave is not followed by a QRS complex. All PP intervals are equal (unless the Wenckebach is due to heightened vagal tone – then the PP intervals may increase prior to block). The PR interval after the blocked P wave is less than the PR interval immediately preceding the blocked P wave (Fig. 6.3). Sometimes the PR interval does not show progressive increase prior to block, but the post-block PR interval is always shorter. It is one of the causes of grouped beating on the ECG.
- Mobitz type II: this usually reflects disease of the His-Purkinje system. The block almost always occurs below the AV node, within the His bundle or both bundle branches. There is no change in the PR interval prior to or after the blocked P wave (Fig. 6.4).
  - It has a higher risk of progression to complete heart block and permanent pacemaker implantation is usually indicated [4] even in asymptomatic patients, as, if CHB develops, the escape rhythm is almost always ventricular, which is likely to be slow.
- *High-grade AV block:* This is an advanced form of second-degree AV block Mobitz type II. ECG shows

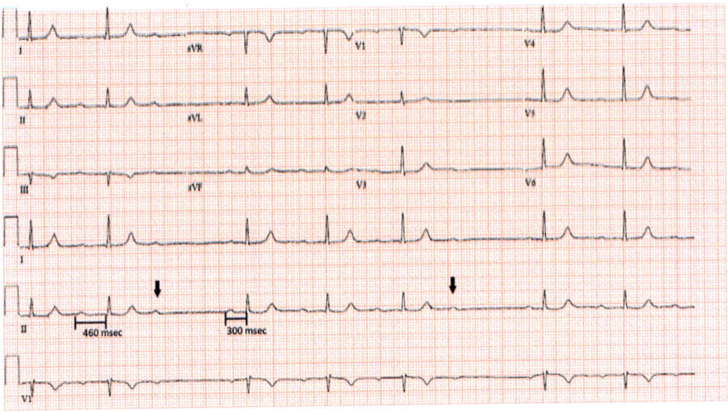

FIGURE 6.3 ECG showing second-degree AV block Mobitz type I (Wenckebach). Solid arrows show P waves that did not conduct to the ventricles

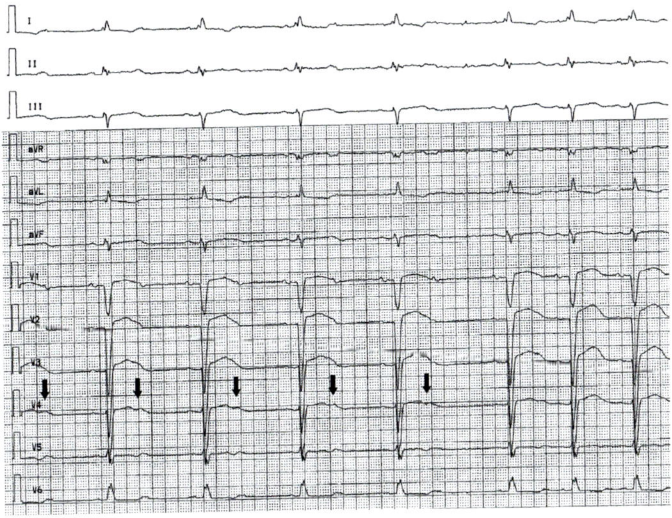

FIGURE 6.4 Initial part of the ECG shows 2:1 AV block which improved to 1:1 AV conduction by the end of the ECG with carotid sinus massage which proved this to be a second-degree AV block Mobitz II. Solid arrows showed the P waves that did not conduct to the ventricles

more than one successive non-conducted P wave, leading to several consecutive P waves without subsequent QRS complexes (Fig. 6.5).

- *2:1 AV block:* Based on ECG alone, it is not possible to determine if this is Mobitz type I or Mobitz type II as every other P wave is non-conducted (Fig. 6.6). Maneuvers that can be helpful in differentiating the two are listed in Table 6.1.

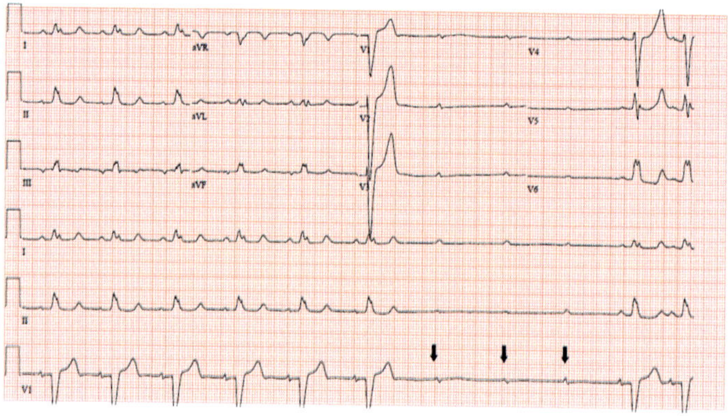

Figure 6.5 ECG showing high-grade AV block with three consecutive non-conducted P waves at the end of the tracing (solid arrows)

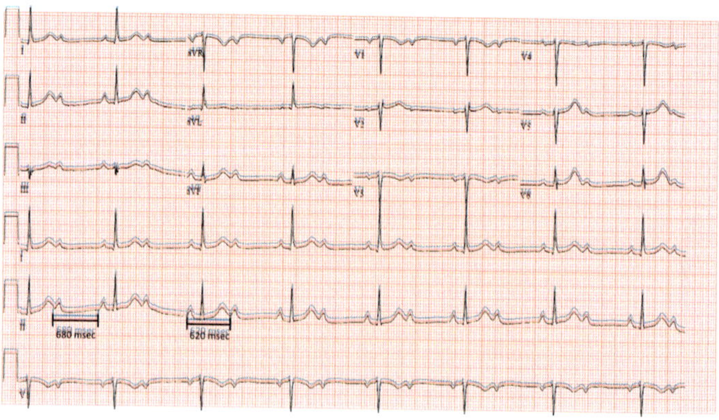

Figure 6.6 ECG showing 2:1 AV block. Ventriculophasic sinus arrhythmia is also noted on this tracing with the two PP waves surrounding a QRS complex occurring at a faster rate compared to two PP waves without an intervening QRS complex

Table 6.1 Shows maneuvers that may help to differentiate Mobitz type I from Mobitz type II in 2:1 AV block

	Response to exercise	Response to carotid sinus massage	Response to Atropine	QRS width	PR interval of the conducted P wave
Mobitz type 1	Improves*	Worsens*	Improves	Often normal	Usually prolonged
Mobitz type II	Worsens	Improves	Worsens	Often wide, with bundle branch block suggestive of underlying His-Purkinje disease	Usually normal

Table 6.1 shows how to differentiate Mobitz type I from Mobitz type II in 2:1 AV block. *The Mobitz type I block will only improve with exercise or worsen with carotid sinus massage if it occurs in the AV node. If it is occuring in the bundle branches or His bundle, the typical response will not be obsereved.

Third-Degree AV Block

- This is also known as complete heart block (CHB).
- There is complete failure of impulse conduction from the atria to the ventricles.
- The PR intervals are irregularly variable as there is complete dissociation of the P waves from the QRS complexes, and the atrial rate may be faster than the rate of the escape rhythm (Fig. 6.7).
- Depending on the location of the block, the escape rhythm may be junctional (QRS complexes resemble the baseline sinus rhythm) or ventricular (wide QRS complexes that often do not resemble typical right or left bundle branch block).

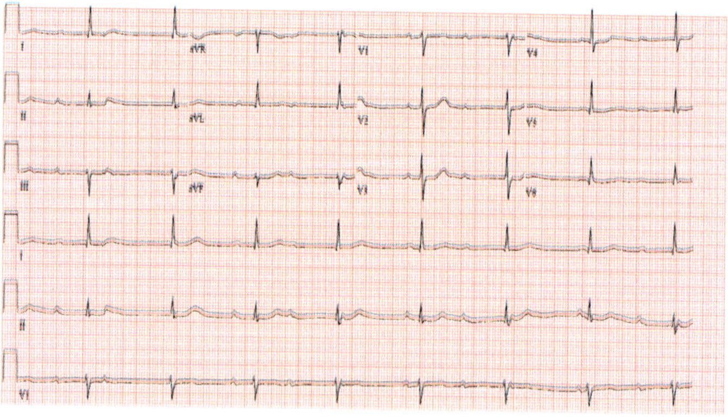

FIGURE 6.7 ECG showing complete heart block with junctional escape rhythm. Note the regular ventricular rate and lack of stable relation between P waves and QRS complexes

Paroxysmal AV Block

- Defined as abrupt and unexpected development of AV block leading to a period of ventricular asystole until a properly timed escape or premature beat can reset the membrane potential to normal and allow for AV conduction.
- This may be due to an increased rate of spontaneous Phase 4 depolarization in diseased His-Purkinje tissue, as well as abrupt spontaneous conduction failure [5].
- Patients frequently have evidence of right or left bundle branch block or intraventricular conduction delay at baseline [6].

Ventriculophasic Sinus Arrhythmia

- It manifests as intermittent differences in the PP intervals based on their relationship to the QRS complex.
- The two P waves surrounding a QRS complex occur at a slightly faster rate compared to two P waves without an intervening QRS complex (Fig. 6.6).
- It may be seen in second- or third-degree AV block with intermittent or constant failure of antegrade conduction through the AV node.
- Proposed mechanisms include phasic changes in baroreceptor-mediated vagal input to the SA node, mechanical effect of ventricular systole on the SA node (which enhances nodal automaticity), and effect of pressure changes caused by ventricular systole.

Key Learning Points

- Careful review of the electrocardiogram is paramount to determine diagnosis and possible therapies for bradyarrhythmias.
- Asymptomatic patients with bradycardia or sinus pauses should not be implanted with a pacemaker. They should be followed closely.

References

1. Bjerregaard P. Mean 24 hour heart rate, minimal heart rate and pauses in healthy subjects 40–79 years of age. Eur Heart J. 1983;4(1):44.
2. Rubenstein JJ, Schulman CL, Yurchak PM, DeSanctis RW. Clinical spectrum of the sick sinus syndrome. Circulation. 1972;46(1):5.
3. O'keefe Jr. JH, Hammill SC, Freed MS, Pogwizd SM. The complete guide to ECGs: a comprehensive study guide to improve ECG interpretation skills. 3rd ed. Burlington, Jones and Bartlett; 2008.
4. Kusumoto FM, Schoenfeld MH, Barrett C, et al. 2018 ACC/AHA/HRS guideline on the evaluation and management of patients with bradycardia and cardiac conduction delay: a report of the American College of Cardiology/American Heart Association task force on clinical practice guidelines and the Heart Rhythm Society. Heart rhythm. 2018;S1547–5271(18):31127–5.
5. Josephson ME. Josephson's clinical cardiac electrophysiology: techniques and interpretations. 5th ed. Philadelphia, Wolters Kluwer; 2016.
6. Lee S, Wellens HJ, Josephson ME. Paroxysmal atrioventricular block. Heart Rhythm. 2009;6(8):1229–34.

Chapter 7
Pacemakers, Defibrillators, and Cardiac Resynchronization Therapy

Hakeem Ayinde, Muhie Dean Sabayon, and Michael S. Lloyd

Abbreviations

ACLS	Advanced cardiac life support
ATP	Anti-tachycardia pacing
CIED	Cardiac implantable electronic device
CRT	Cardiac resynchronization therapy
ECG	Electrocardiogram
ICD	Implantable cardioverter-defibrillator
MRI	Magnetic resonance imaging
PMT	Pacemaker-mediated tachycardia
VF	Ventricular fibrillation
VT	Ventricular tachycardia

H. Ayinde (✉) · M. S. Lloyd
Department of Cardiac Electrophysiology, Emory University, Atlanta, GA, USA
e-mail: hayinde@emory.edu; hakeem.o.ayinde@emory.edu; mlloyd2@emory.edu

M. D. Sabayon
Clinical Cardiac Electrophysiology, Emory University Hospital, Atlanta, GA, USA
e-mail: muhie.dean.sabayon@emory.edu

B. J. Wells et al. (eds.), *Handbook of Inpatient Cardiology*,
https://doi.org/10.1007/978-3-030-47868-1_7

Introduction

- About 1.2–1.4 million cardiac implantable electronic devices (CIEDs) are implanted annually worldwide for indications ranging from bradycardia, tachycardia, and heart failure to the prevention of sudden cardiac death.
- Many patients with CIEDs will be hospitalized for cardiac and non-cardiac conditions.
- It is important that the internist understands normal function of pacemakers and defibrillators, and is further able to identify abnormal CIED function that would necessitate consultation with a cardiologist.

Components/Hardware

- A transvenous pacemaker or defibrillator consists of:
  - A pulse generator that is implanted subcutaneously or submuscularly in the pectoral area of the chest. The generator contains the battery, circuitry, and capacitors (Fig. 7.1a).
  - Around 1–3 leads connecting the pulse generator to chambers of the heart via the subclavian vein. A lead consists of insulated conductor cables (Fig. 7.1b, c).
- A deviation from above convention is the leadless pacemaker (Micra, Medtronic), which is fully implanted in the right ventricle (Fig. 7.1d).

Identification

- Pacemakers and Implantable Cardioverter-Defibrillators (ICDs) can be differentiated by the size of the pulse generator and the appearance of the leads on chest X-ray.
- ICD pulse generators are at least twice the size of pacemaker generators (Fig. 7.1a).
- ICD leads have one or two shock coils that can be seen on chest X-ray (Fig. 7.2a).

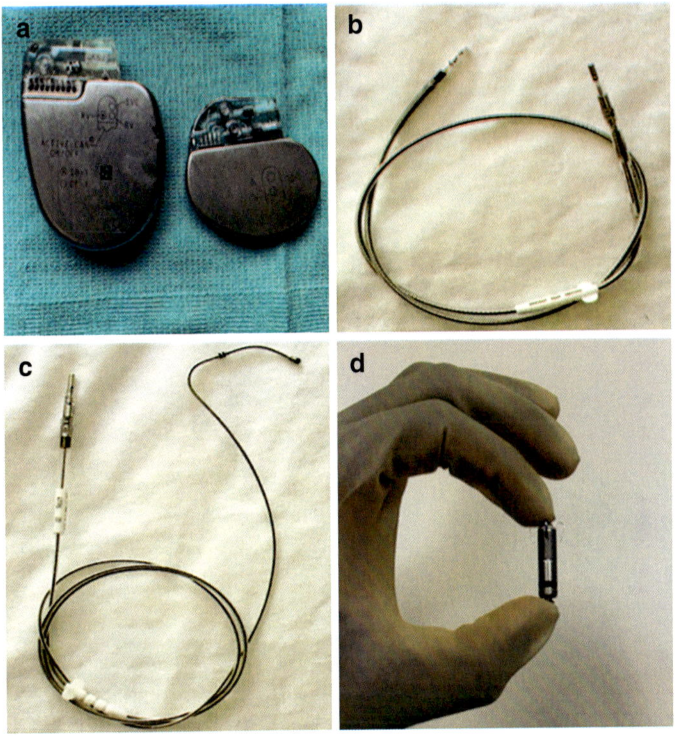

FIGURE 7.1 (**a**) Side by side comparison of a single chamber ICD and a dual chamber pacemaker. (**b**) An active fixation pacemaker lead with proximal pin and distal electrodes shown. (**c**) A left ventricular pacemaker lead. (**d**) A leadless pacemaker showing the tines used for attachment to the right ventricle

- A cardiac resynchronization therapy (CRT) device or biventricular pacemaker/defibrillator system can be identified by the presence of an additional left ventricular lead that runs through the coronary sinus and its branches (Fig. 7.2a, see also Fig. 7.1c).
- The subcutaneous ICD (Boston Scientific) is a defibrillator that is implanted on the left lateral chest wall and has a defibrillator lead located in the subcutaneous tissue of the anterior chest wall (Fig. 7.2c, d).

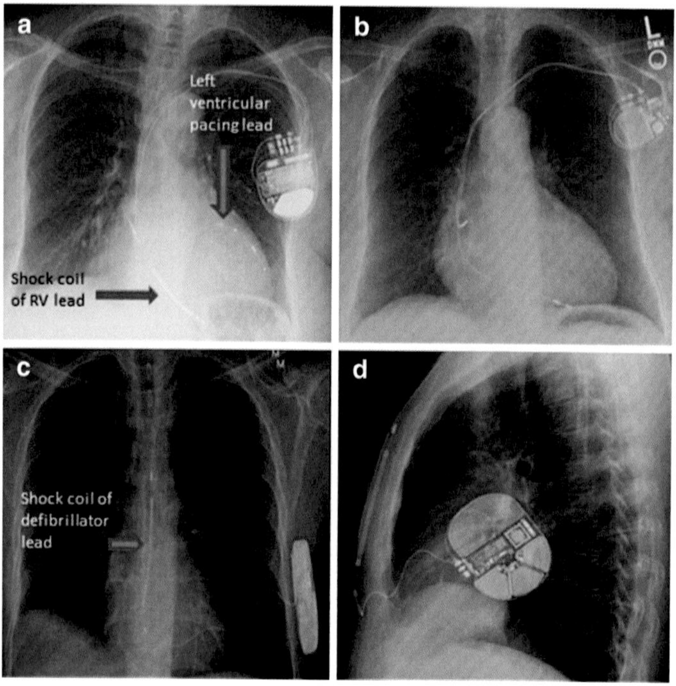

FIGURE 7.2 Postero-anterior chest X-ray appearance of a CRT-D (**a**) a dual chamber pacemaker (**b**) and postero-anterior and lateral image of a S-ICD (**c**, **d**) showing the subcutaneous location of the pulse generator and the defibrillator lead

Basic Concepts

- The primary function of a pacemaker is to treat bradycardia by pacing.
- The primary function of a defibrillator is to treat tachycardia by delivering anti-tachycardia pacing (ATP) or shock. All transvenous ICDs are capable of pacing.

Sensing and Pacing

- Sensing implies that the pacemaker can detect intrinsic electrical activity in the heart.
- *Sensitivity* is the minimum intrinsic activity (in voltage) that the pacemaker is programmed to detect. The pacemaker is programmed sensitive enough to appropriately detect all intrinsic activity while filtering out artifact.
- Pacemakers respond to a sensed signal by either inhibiting or triggering pacing.
- Pacing implies that the pacemaker delivers an electrical stimulus.
- *Capture* occurs when a pacing stimulus leads to depolarization of myocardial tissue and myocardial contraction.
- *Capture threshold* is the minimum pacing stimulus strength needed to consistently depolarize myocardium. The pacing output is usually programmed at a safety margin above the capture threshold.

Pacemaker Codes

- Pacemaker nomenclature is often presented in a four-letter code (Table 7.1).
- DDDR programming implies the pacemaker will pace in both chambers, sense in both chambers, respond to sensing by either inhibiting or triggering pacing, and change pacing rate in response to physical activity (rate modulation). Figure 7.3 presents the four modes of DDD pacing.
- VVI programming implies the pacemaker will pace in the ventricle, sense ventricular signals, and respond to sensing by inhibiting pacing output.
- Indication for pacemaker will determine its programming.
  - Patients in sinus rhythm with dual chamber pacemaker for AV block may be programmed DDD.

Table 7.1 Modified NASPE/BPEG[a] generic code for anti-bradycardia and multi-chamber pacing

I (Chamber Paced)	II (Chamber Sensed)	III (Response to Sensing)	IV Rate Modulation
A – Atrial Paced	A – Atrial Sensed	I – Inhibited	R – Rate Responsive
V – Ventricular Paced	V – Ventricular Sensed	T – Triggered	
D – Dual (A + V)	D – Dual (A + V)	D – Dual (I + T)	
O – None	O – None	O – None	

[a]North American Society of Pacing and Electrophysiology/British Pacing and Electrophysiology Group

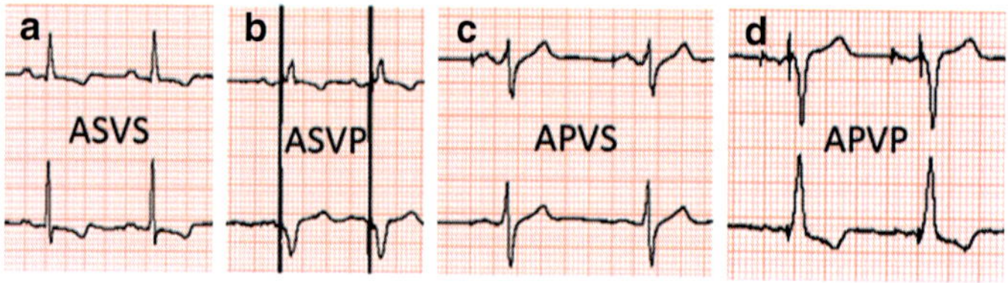

Figure 7.3 The four modes of DDD pacing: (**a**) Atrial sensed-Ventricular sensed. (**b**) Atrial paced-Ventricular sensed. (**c**) Atrial paced-Ventricular sensed. (**d**) Atrial paced-Ventricular paced

- Patients with single chamber ventricular pacemaker/ICD who do not need regular pacing may be programmed backup VVI.
- Rate response is usually enabled for patients with sinus node dysfunction.

Clinical Pearl

Pacemakers are usually programmed to pace in the ventricle only when necessary. This is because chronic right ventricular pacing has been shown to cause cardiomyopathy. However, CRT devices are programmed to maximize ventricular pacing in order to deliver resynchronization benefit.

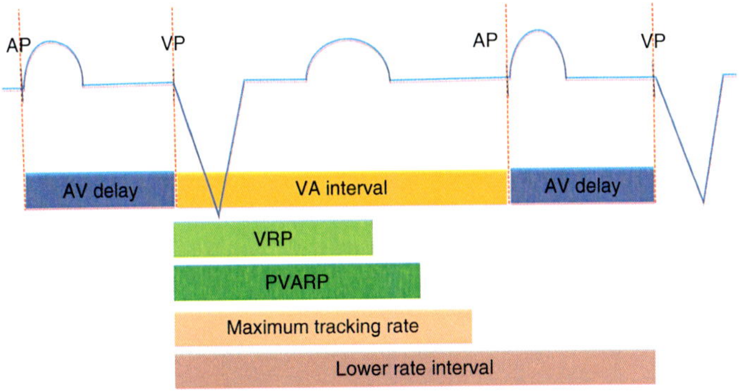

FIGURE 7.4 Timing cycle of a dual chamber pacemaker programmed DDD. AV atrio-ventricular, VA ventriculo-atrial, VRP ventricular refractory period, PVARP post-ventricular atrial refractory period

Timing Cycles

- Timing cycles ensure regular pacemaker function. It is important to understand basic definitions:
  - Lower Rate Limit (LRL): Pacemaker begins pacing when heart rate falls below this rate. In dual chamber pacemakers, LRL is equivalent to the V-V interval (Fig. 7.4). V-V interval = AV delay + VA interval
  - AV delay: Analogous to the PR interval. It is usually programmed long enough to allow for intrinsic AV conduction in single or dual chamber pacemakers.
  - Upper rate limit (URL): Also known as the maximum tracking rate, is the fastest rate that a pacemaker will pace.

Basic Troubleshooting

- Pacemaker malfunction can be seen occasionally. However, when pacemaker malfunction is suspected on ECG, it is more commonly due to pseudo-malfunction.
- True sensing and pacing abnormalities that are commonly discerned on ECG or telemetry frequently manifest as unexpected pacing or loss of pacing.

- Causes of unexpected pacing: Undersensing, atrial arrhythmia, pacemaker-mediated tachycardia (PMT), anti-tachycardia pacing (ATP). See Fig. 7.5a–d.
- Unexpected loss of pacing: Oversensing, loss of capture, failure to output. See Fig. 7.6a, b.

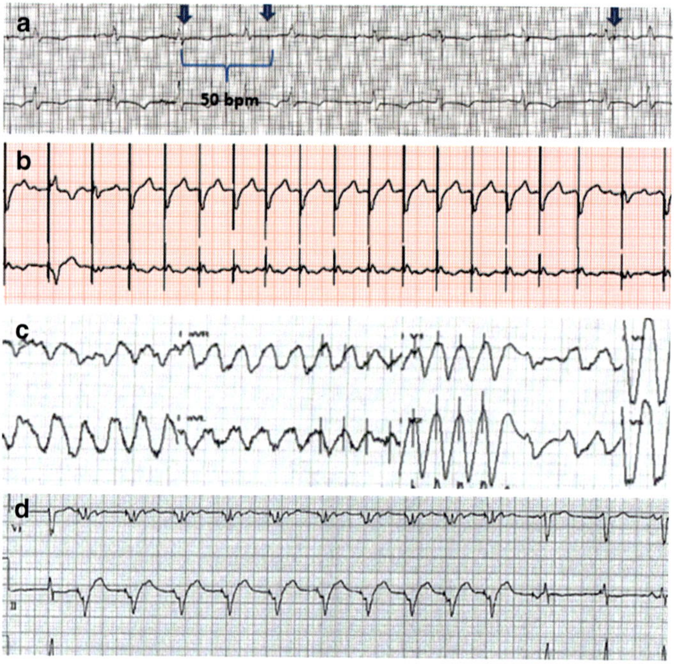

FIGURE 7.5 Examples of episodes of unexpected pacing. (**a**). Atrial undersensing. Intrinsic p waves are not sensed as atrial pacing (blue arrows) continues at the programmed rate of 50 bpm. (**b**). Atrial fibrillation with tracking at the upper rate limit of 130 bpm. Dual chamber pacemakers are programmed to automatically switch to a non-tracking mode (DDI) when atrial fibrillation develops. (**c**). ATP during VT. ATP did not terminate VT in this case. (**d**). PMT often starts with a PVC with retrograde conduction to the atrium. A dual chamber pacemaker senses the atrial signal and paces in the ventricle, again with retrograde conduction to the atrium. This initiates an endless loop tachycardia The pacemaker identified the PMT and terminated it appropriately. *ATP anti-tachycardia pacing, VT ventricular tachycardia, PMT pacemaker-mediated tachycardia, PVC premature ventricular complex

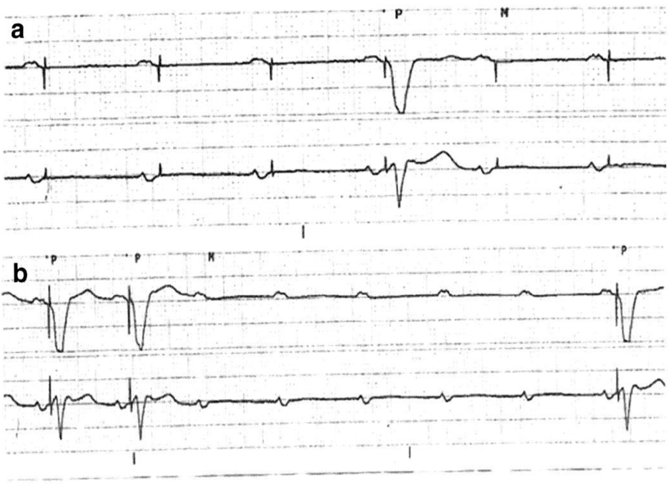

FIGURE 7.6 Examples of episodes of failure of pacing. (**a**) Loss of ventricular capture in a dual chamber pacemaker. Spikes after the p waves denote ventricular pacing which fail to capture the ventricle. (**b**) Ventricular asystole due to failure of ventricular output. Interrogation showed that ventricular output was inhibited because of oversensing of noise on the ventricular lead (not shown)

Magnet Response

- CIEDs are programmed to respond to magnets in specific ways.
- When a magnet is applied over a pacemaker pulse generator that has good battery life, the pacemaker will usually be reprogrammed to asynchronous pacing, i.e., DOO or VOO, at a pacing rate of 85–100 bpm (depending on the manufacturer). This means all sensing is disabled.
- Once the magnet is removed from the chest wall, the pacemaker resumes prior programmed function.
- A magnet will reprogram a CRT-D or ICD by only temporarily disabling tachycardia therapies (ATP and shock). The programmed pacing function will not be affected. For example, if the ICD was programmed DDD, that function will remain active. Tachycardia therapies will resume once

the magnet is removed. A patient who receives a flurry of inappropriate shocks (for example, due to inappropriate sensing of noise on a fractured lead) may receive immediate relief with a magnet as this will prevent further shocks.

Clinical Pearl
A magnet will temporarily reprogram a pacemaker to asynchronous mode. The magnet will reprogram a CRT-D or ICD by temporarily turning off the tachycardia therapies while unaffecting the pacing function. Previous programming is restored once magnet is removed

Clinical Indications

- Pacemakers are generally implanted for bradycardia. Common manifestations of sinus and AV node dysfunction that require pacemaker implantation are listed in Table 7.2.
- ICDs are implanted for the primary prevention of sudden cardiac death in high-risk patients, or for secondary prevention in patients who have experienced sustained VT or VF.
- Certain familial conditions (e.g., hypertrophic cardiomyopathy, long QT syndrome) can present with increased risk of sudden cardiac death, requiring ICD implantation.
- CRT can improve symptoms and reduce mortality in symptomatic patients with cardiomyopathy and left ventricular conduction delay.
- Majority of well-selected patients experience symptom improvement with CRT. Class I indication for CRT is sinus rhythm, left bundle branch block (LBBB), QRS duration at least 150 ms, LVEF ≤35% and NYHA II, III, or ambulatory IV symptoms despite optimal medical therapy for at least 3 months.

TABLE 7.2 Common indications for permanent pacemaker

Sinus node dysfunction
Symptomatic sinus bradycardia
Symptomatic sinus pauses
Symptomatic chronotropic incompetence (failure to mount age-appropriate heart rate increase with activity)
Required medication use causing symptomatic sinus bradycardia
Atrioventricular node/His-Purkinje disease
High-grade or complete AV block
Mobitz type II 2nd-degree AV block, with or without symptoms
Symptomatic Mobitz type I 2nd-degree AV block
Alternating bundle branch block
AV node ablation for rate control of atrial arrhythmia
Other indications
Neurocardiogenic syncope associated with bradycardia or carotid sinus hypersensitivity
Sustained pause-dependent VT, with or without QT prolongation

MRI Safety of CIED

- MRI generates magnetic and radiofrequency fields that can interact with or damage CIED.
- Potential consequences of CIED exposure to MRI include arrhythmias due to inductive current in leads, tissue heating, changes in sensing or capture thresholds, electromagnetic interference, power-on reset, battery depletion, and irregular reed switch behavior.
- More recently, MR conditional systems have been designed to mitigate the potential hazards of MRI exposure.
- A MR conditional system is a specific combination of a CIED generator and attached leads that have been

approved by the FDA for use under specific MRI conditions.

- When the system is not specified to be MRI conditional; or there are different manufacturer generator and leads present; or fractured, epicardial, or abandoned leads present, then the system is MRI non-conditional.
- Hospitals have a standardized workflow in place for imaging MRI conditional and non-conditional systems.
- The CIED would need to be reprogrammed prior to MRI. MRI conditional systems have a 'MRI-mode' that can be programmed for safety. Features that would need to be deactivated prior to MRI for non-conditional systems include rate response, anti-tachycardia therapies, noise response, magnet response, and other specialized features. Pacemaker-dependent patients would need to be programmed to asynchronous pacing mode.
- Patients should be monitored with ECG and pulse-oximetry during MRI.
- Personnel skilled in performing ACLS and in reprogramming CIED should be readily available.
- An external defibrillator and CIED programmer should be close by the MRI suite.

Implantation and Perioperative Considerations

- CIEDs are usually implanted by experienced physicians under sterile conditions in the electrophysiology laboratory.
- The procedure is frequently done under conscious or deep sedation and may take 1–3 hours, depending on complexity.
- Transvenous systems are most commonly implanted in the left prepectoral area. After the area is sterilized and draped, local anesthesia is applied to the skin. A small incision is made and venous access is obtained via cephalic vein cut-down or needle puncture of the axillary or subcla-

vian vein. The leads are advanced into the appropriate cardiac chambers and secured in place. The leads are then connected to the generator, which is implanted in a subcutaneous or submuscular pocket that was created in the upper anterior chest area. The incision is closed using multiple layers of absorbable suture and covered in sterile dressing.

- Peri-procedural complications are rare, including bleeding and pocket hematoma, pneumothorax, cardiac perforation, and tamponade. Post-operative complications (days to weeks from implant) include infection, wound dehiscence, lead dislodgement, and pocket hematoma.
- Perioperative anticoagulation management is at the discretion of the implanting physician. However, physicians usually suspend heparin and enoxaparin the day prior to procedure because of increased risk of bleeding. In patients with mechanical valves or other indication for warfarin, it is often safe to perform the procedure with therapeutic INR. Anti-platelets are usually continued for the procedure.

Clinical Pearl
Heparin and enoxaparin should be discontinued the day prior to pacemaker implantation and usually restarted after 48 hours from implant to prevent pocket hematoma. It is often safe to continue warfarin peri-procedurally, keeping INR within therapeutic range.

Indications for Device Interrogation and Consultation

- CIEDs are usually interrogated on a routine basis in clinic and/or remotely via a home monitoring system that uses telephone or cellular network.

TABLE 7.3 Common indications for inpatient CIED interrogation

Syncope
Palpitations
ICD shock
Suspect device malfunction such as abnormal sensing or pacing
Arrhythmias when ECG diagnosis is unclear
Auditory or vibratory alarms
Decompensated heart failure (assess for arrhythmia, percentage of CRT pacing)

- CIEDs do not need to interrogated in the hospital except if there is concern for an arrhythmia or device malfunction.
- Common indications for inpatient device interrogation are listed in Table 7.3.
  - Syncope can indicate a tachyarrhythmia or device malfunction such as oversensing or failure of pacing, leading to asystole.
  - Palpitations may be a manifestation of an arrhythmia or device-related tachycardia such as PMT.
  - In patients presenting with heart failure, precipitants of decompensation such as atrial or ventricular arrhythmias may be gleaned by interrogation.
  - A single ICD shock is usually due to appropriate therapy for VT/VF. However, when patients have multiple ICD shocks, they can be appropriate for recurrent VT/VF, or inappropriate shocks for an atrial arrhythmia/SVT, or device malfunction such as lead fracture.
  - Patients may complain of auditory or vibratory alarms from their CIED. Alerts are commonly due to low battery voltage, arrhythmia episodes, and abnormalities in lead function.

Conclusion

Pacemakers, defibrillators, and cardiac resynchronization therapy offer different forms of therapy for bradycardia, tachycardia, prevention of sudden cardiac death, and heart failure management. The internist should be familiar with common indications and basic function of these devices, and understand when to request expert consultation.

Key Learning Points

1. Basic pacemaker function includes both sensing intrinsic cardiac signals and pacing.
2. Commonly, pacemaker/ICD malfunction presents as unexpected episodes of pacing or no pacing when expected.
3. Certain symptoms such as syncope, ICD shock, or ECG abnormalities that suggest pacemaker malfunction warrant inpatient device interrogation and possibly cardiology consultation.

Chapter 8
Acute Decompensated Heart Failure

Donya Mohebali and Edward W. Grandin

Abbreviations

ADHF	Acute decompensated heart failure
PND	Paroxysmal nocturnal dyspnea
JVP	Jugular venous pressure
HJR	Hepatojugular reflex
PCWP	Pulmonary capillary wedge pressure
CXR	Chest X-ray
ECG	Electrocardiogram
LFTs	Liver function tests
BNP	B-type natriuretic peptide
NT-proBNP	N-terminal pro-B-type natriuretic
CI	Cardiac index
ACEi	Angiotensin converting enzyme inhibitors
ARB	Angiotensin II receptor blocker

D. Mohebali (✉)
Department of Medicine, Division of Cardiology, Beth Israel Deaconess Medical Center, Boston, MA, USA
e-mail: dmohebal@bidmc.harvard.edu

E. W. Grandin
Department of Medicine, Beth Israel Deaconess Medical Center, Boston, MA, USA
e-mail: wgrandin@bidmc.harvard.edu

B. J. Wells et al. (eds.), *Handbook of Inpatient Cardiology*,
https://doi.org/10.1007/978-3-030-47868-1_8

ARNI	Angiotensin neprolysin inhibitor
CO	Cardiac output
RAAS	Renal angiotensin aldosterone system

Background/Epidemiology

- Acute decompensated heart failure (HF) is associated with major morbidity and mortality [1] and is the leading cause of hospital readmission [2, 3].
- Sixty-day mortality following a heart failure exacerbation is estimated as high as 20% [4].

Definition of Acute Decompensated Heart Failure

- Acute decompensated heart failure (ADHF) is a clinical syndrome of new or worsening HF resulting in pulmonary and/or systemic venous congestion with or without an associated decrease in cardiac output and requiring urgent therapy with IV diuretics and initiation/dose titration of HF medications.

Causes of Acute Decompensated Heart Failure

- The potential causes of acute decompensated heart failure (ADHF) are summarized in Table 8.1.

Diagnosis of Acute Decompensated Heart Failure

- The rapid diagnosis of ADHF is key to initiate appropriate treatment.
- Failure to recognize this condition results in inflation of treatment costs and need for mechanical support [5, 6].

Table 8.1 Triggers of acute decompensated heart failure

Myocardial insults/ ischemia	Ischemia Myocardial infarction Myocarditis Stress-induced cardiomyopathy Peripartum cardiomyopathy
Arrhythmia and electrical disturbances	Tachyarrhythmias: Atrial fibrillation, atrial tachycardia Other arrhythmias: Premature ventricular contractions Related: Right ventricular, decreased proportion of cardiac resynchronization therapy Bradyarrhythmia: Complete heart block, sinus node dysfunction, medication excess
Valvular	Obstructive left-sided valvular disease: Aortic stenosis, mitral stenosis Regurgitant disease: Aortic regurgitation, mitral regurgitation Tricuspid regurgitation with isolated right ventricular failure Complications of mechanical or prosthetic valves: Valve thrombosis or perforation of prosthetic valve leaflet Infectious: Endocarditis
Pericardial disease	Pericardial syndrome: Tamponade or constriction
Nonadherence	Non-compliance with diuretic and other heart failure regimen Dietary non-compliance, i.e., increased sodium and fluid intake
Toxins/new medications	Alcohol use Drug use such as cocaine Supplements and/or stimulants Non-steroidal anti-inflammatory medications
Worsening renal function	Acute kidney injury Progressive chronic renal disease Dialysis dependence with inadequate volume removal or inaccurate dry weight

Key Historical Clinical Features in the Diagnosis of Acute Decompensated Heart Failure

- There are many symptoms/signs of ADHF (Tables 8.2, 8.3, and 8.4).
- Dyspnea on exertion is the most sensitive (negative likelihood ratio 0.45, 95% confidence interval [CI] 0.35–0.67) [7].
- Paroxysmal nocturnal dyspnea is most specific (positive likelihood ratio 2.6, 95% CI 1.5–4.5) [7].
- Orthopnea is associated with elevated pulmonary capillary wedge pressure (PCWP) ≥ 28 mmHg [8].

Table 8.2 Clinical pearls for the assessment of jugular venous pressure

Start by assessing the JVP with patient sitting upright at 90 degrees in order to evaluate for a very high JVP
The JVP should be assessed at various angles supine, 30 degrees, 45 degrees, etc.
If not elevated when supine, check to see if it becomes elevated with the abdominojugular response
If it is difficult to find, you can inspect both sides of the neck with the patient looking straight ahead as sometimes the JVP may be better visualized on the left side of the neck rather than on the right
To differentiate from the carotid artery, pulsations should not be palpable and vary with respiration

Table 8.3 Findings of intravascular versus extravascular congestion

Intravascular congestion	Extravascular congestion
JVP elevation S3 Pulmonary rales Hepatojugular reflex Pulmonary edema	Lower extremity edema Ascites Weight gain Pleural effusions

Table 8.4 Historical, physical exam, and laboratory findings in acute decompensated heart failure

Elevated filling pressures	Low output
Orthopnea	Mental confusion
Paroxysmal nocturnal dyspnea	Cool extremities
Bendopnea	Narrow pulse pressure/fractional pulse pressure
JVP +/– peripheral edema	Elevated lactate
Hepatojugular reflex	Acute kidney injury
Pulmonary Rales/ pleural effusion	Metabolic acidosis
S3 gallop	Transaminitis

- Symptoms of left-sided HF: shortness of breath, orthopnea, paroxysmal nocturnal dyspnea (PND).
- Symptoms of right-sided HF: nausea, abdominal fullness, decreased appetite, lower extremity edema.
- Bendopnea is dyspnea when bending forward at the waist and is associated with increased filling pressures and adverse HF outcomes, including increased mortality and HF admissions [9, 10].
- In patients with HF, identify prior "dry weight" and triggers of their exacerbation including medication noncompliance, new medications (such as beta blockade), or increased sodium/fluid intake.
- A new "dry weight" may need to be established as guided by the physical examination.

Key Physical Exam Findings in the Diagnosis of Acute Decompensated Heart Failure

- Assessing congestion, including intravascular and extravascular congestion, is critical to the evaluation and management of patients with ADHF (Table 8.3).

- Elevated jugular venous pressure (JVP) ≥ 10 cm H_2O is the MOST useful assessment and can estimate right atrial pressure to guide therapy. See Table 8.2 for tips on assessing JVP.

Clinical Pearl
In most patients, ↑ JVP is a surrogate for ↑ left-sided filling pressures. In approximately one-third of patients, JVP may appear normal, despite ↑ left-sided filling pressures. Similarly, in some cases, ↑ JVP may be a result of isolated ↑ right-sided filling pressures with normal left-sided filling pressures.

- ↑ JVP, an S3 gallop, or both are associated with ↑ risk of HF hospitalization and death [11].
- The presence of hepatojugular reflex (HJR) as defined by a sustained ↑ in JVP > 3 cm (in the absence of RV failure) during 10 seconds of continuous pressure on the abdomen with abrupt fall after pressure released predicts PCWP >15 mmHg and indicates worse prognosis [12].
- Signs of low cardiac output on examination: narrow systemic pulse pressure (systolic blood pressure (SBP) – diastolic blood pressure (DBP)) typically <30 mmHg, low fractional pulse pressure (SBP–DBP/SBP) < 0.25, decreased carotid pulse volume, and cool extremities.
- Pulmonary rales, pleural effusion, and peripheral edema can be seen in ADHF.

Clinical Pearl
In chronic HF, patients may not have rales secondary to a compensatory increase in pulmonary lymphatic drainage and may have clear lung fields on radiographic imaging despite elevated filling pressures.

- Peripheral edema alone should not be used as a sign of increased filling pressures. The specificity of peripheral edema is increased in the presence of JVP elevation [13].

Key Tests in the Diagnosis of Acute Decompensated Heart Failure

- Laboratory testing, CXR, ECG, and echocardiogram are key in the evaluation of patients presenting with ADHF.
- Laboratory testing: CBC, renal function/chemistry, liver function tests (LFTs), B-type natriuretic peptide (BNP), or N-terminal pro-B-type natriuretic (NT-proBNP), troponin level, lactate level, and thyroid function tests.
- > 40% of patients hospitalized with ADHF have abnormal LFTs secondary to hepatic congestion [14].
- A low level of BNP or NT-proBNP rules out HF in most cases (similar assays—NT-proBNP sixfold ↑ than BNP).
- In patients presenting to ED with shortness of breath, a BNP > 100 pg/mL had a sensitivity 90% (95% CI 88%–92%), specificity 76% (95% CI 73%–79%), PPV 79% (95% CI 76%–81%), and NPV 89% (95% CI 87%–91%) for predicting a diagnosis of HF [15].

Clinical Pearl

BNP may be normal in some patients (particularly obese women, HFpEF) despite ↑ filling pressures [16]. If physical exam indicates ↑ filling pressures, a normal BNP should not exclude the diagnosis of HF.

- BNP at discharge predicts 1-year mortality and/or rehospitalization among HF patients. Risk of adverse clinical outcomes increases with increasing levels of BNP [17].
- Pulmonary edema on CXR increases the likelihood of ADHF 12-fold [7].
- ECG can detect ischemia, prior myocardial infarction, or arrhythmia contributing to patient's presentation.
- Transthoracic echocardiography to assess LV systolic function, right ventricular function, and valvular function and to estimate filling pressures and pulmonary artery pressure.

Classification and Treatment of Acute Decompensated Heart Failure

Classification of Acute Decompensated Heart Failure

- It is important to appropriately estimate cardiac filling pressures and perfusion to provide treatment. The "Stevenson classification" is used to categorize volume status as wet versus dry and perfusion status as warm versus cold (Fig. 8.1) [18].
- "Wet" is defined as PCWP ≥22 mm Hg and "cold" as a cardiac index (CI) ≤2.2 L/min/m^2.

	Congestion	
Inadequate Perfusion	No	Yes
No	Warm and Dry	Warm and Wet Treatment: Diuretics
Yes	Cold and Dry	Cold and Wet Treatment: Diuretics+Inotropes or Vasodilators

FIGURE 8.1 Classification of acute decompensated heart failure

- For patients who are "warm and wet," treat with diuresis + optimization of guideline-directed medical therapy (GDMT) for heart failure with reduced ejection fraction (HFrEF, EF ≤40%).
- In patients who are "cold and wet," improve cardiac output and systemic perfusion with inotropes and/or systemic vasodilators and decongest with diuretics or occasional ultrafiltration for patients with inadequate response to diuretics. Therapy can be tailored to hemodynamic goals by measurements from a pulmonary artery catheter.
- Clinical criteria for cardiogenic shock (CS):
  - Signs of end-organ hypoperfusion: ↓ urine output (< 30 ml/hr), ↑ creatinine, cold extremities, mental confusion, ↑ LFTS and lactate.

    OR
  - SBP < 90 mmHg for ≥30 minutes OR need for vasoactive medications to maintain SBP ≥ 90 mmHg. Note: patients can be in CS without hypotension.

    AND
  - Obvious cardiac etiology (e.g., acute myocardial infarction) or invasive hemodynamics demonstrating low cardiac output (CI ≤ 2.2 L/min/m^2) AND ↑ PCWP ≥15 mmHg.
  - *If symptoms of cardiogenic shock are suspected, cardiology consultation should be promptly obtained for management and determination of the need for more advanced therapies including vasodilators, inotropes, and/or mechanical circulatory support.*

Treatment of Acute Heart Failure with Reduced Ejection Fraction

- *Congestion/diuretics*
  - Use intravenous loop diuretics for diuresis goal in daily increments with monitoring of electrolytes/renal function.
  - High-dose loop diuretics (2.5× above their home dose) has been shown to achieve more effective diuresis and relief of symptoms compared to low doses but is often associated with modest, transients increases in creatinine [19].

- Loop diuretics are administered as bolus dosing (typically 6–8 hours apart) or as a bolus followed by continuous infusion. Randomized trial of bolus versus continuous loop diuretics failed to show clear difference in outcomes [19].
- If response to loop diuretics is inadequate, loop diuretic can be supplemented by thiazide diuretics (metolazone or chlorthalidone).
- For significant hypochloremic metabolic alkalosis (due to the retention of bicarbonate to maintain anionic balance in the setting of large-volume chloride loss through the urine), aggressive chloride repletion, typically via potassium chloride or occasionally magnesium chloride, can be helpful. Occasionally, a carbonic anhydrase inhibitor (e.g., acetazolamide) can be used to promote bicarbonate loss and augment diuresis.
- For severe hyponatremia (Na <120) and clinical congestion, vasopressin receptor antagonists (e.g., tolvaptan) can be used.

Clinical Pearl
For patients with ongoing intravascular congestion, diuretic dosing should not be withheld due to hypotension, as many patients with HFrEF have low blood pressure at baseline.

- Place patients on daily 2-L fluid and 2-g sodium restriction.

Clinical Pearl
Once euvolemia is achieved, transition to an oral diuretic regimen and monitor for at least 24 h to ensure adequacy. For example, if a patient required 80 mg IV Lasix twice daily for diuresis in a 24-h period, an oral dose decrement of 50% of the intravenous dose would be torsemide 40 mg twice daily (Table 8.5).

- *Neurohormonal Antagonists/Guideline-Directed Medical Therapy*

TABLE 8.5 Conversion of oral to intravenous (IV) loop diuretics

Loop diuretic	PO (mg)	IV (mg)
Furosemide	40	20
Torsemide	20	20
Bumetanide	1	1

Beta Blocker Therapy

Clinical Pearl
For patients who don't have evidence of decreased cardiac output (e.g., warm and wet), continue prior beta blocker (BB). If marginal blood pressure or profound volume overload is observed, reduce the BB dose by 50% until adequate diuresis is achieved. In cases of suspected cardiogenic shock, beta blockers should be stopped entirely.

- If BB is continued, long-acting form (i.e., metoprolol succinate) should be given unless there is a need for rapid dose titration, such as for a concomitant tachyarrhythmia like atrial fibrillation.

ACE Inhibitors (ACEi)/Angiotensin Receptor Blockers (ARBs)

- ACEis (e.g., captopril, lisinopril, enalapril) and ARBs (e.g., valsartan, losartan) inhibit the renin-angiotensin-aldosterone system (RAAS) and also cause vasodilation leading to left ventricular afterload reduction.
- In cases of acute kidney injury that typically improves with HF optimization, hydralazine and isordil dinitrate can be used for afterload reduction until renal function improves allowing transition back to ACEi/ARB.
- For patients who are warm and wet with only modest worsening of their renal function, ACEi/ARB can be continued.
- For patients where more rapid titration of afterload reduction is desired, such as patients with severe hypertension or reduced cardiac output with a high systemic vascular resistance, short-acting captopril can be used "and dosed

every 8 hours with dose increases after every 2–3 doses. Captopril can ultimately be converted into lisinopril in a 5:1 ratio.

Angiotensin Receptor Blocker/Neprilysin Inhibitors (ARNIs)

- When compared to traditional ACEi therapy in HFrEF patients with NYHA class II–III symptoms, sacubitril-valsartan has a superior survival benefit, reduction in HF hospitalization, and improved quality of life [20].
- When initiated among HFrEF patients admitted with ADHF, ARNI therapy compared to ACEi was safe and resulted in reduced rehospitalization for HF and greater reductions in NT-proBNP [21].
- Contraindications to starting ARNIs: history of angioedema, symptomatic hypotension, prior history of intolerance to other afterload-reducing agents like ACEi or ARBs, or hyperkalemia.
- ACEis must be STOPPED for 36 hours prior to starting an ARNI to avoid the risk of life-threatening angioedema and hypotension and can occur with concomitant ACE and neprilysin inhibition.
- No wash-out period is required when transitioning from an ARB to ARNI.
- Due to augmented natriuretic peptide signaling, ARNI can result in increased natriuresis/diuresis, so the dose of concomitant loop diuretic may need to be reduced.
- The most common side effects are symptomatic hypotension, cough, hyperkalemia, and worsening renal function.
- Prior authorization typically required and co-pay may be cost prohibitive for some patients.
- Sacubitril-valsartan did not result in lower rates of HF hospitalization or death from cardiovascular causes among patients with HFpEF, although there were strong trends toward reduced HF hospitalization and better NYHA class particularly among women and patients with mid-range LVEF (45–55%) [22].

Hydralazine/Isosorbide Dinitrate (H/ISDN)

- Vasodilator combination that has been shown to reduce mortality in HFrEF, particularly among African-American patients [23].
- Helpful alternative to ACEi/ARB/ARNI in patients with severe renal dysfunction.
- H/ISDN should be added alongside ACEi/ARB in HFrEF patients with adequate BP after maximizing ACEi/ARB. There are no robust studies using ARNI plus H/ISDN.

Mineralocorticoid Receptor Antagonists (MRAs)

- MRAs (e.g., spironolactone, eplerenone) block the effects of aldosterone and are associated with improved survival in HFrEF (see Table 9.2 chronic HF chapter).
- Ameliorate potassium loss that is provoked by loop diuretics, particularly during aggressive inpatient diuresis.

Vasodilators

- In patients with a low-output state (e.g., cold and wet), intravenous arterial vasodilators such as nitroprusside and high-dose intravenous nitroglycerin can be used, in addition to the oral options listed previously (Table 8.6).
- Nitroprusside is a potent arterial vasodilator and works rapidly. Adverse effects include cyanide toxicity, which is more likely at higher doses (>3 mcg/kg/min) and with concomitant renal dysfunction.

Table 8.6 Hemodynamic effects of inodilators and vasodilators

	PCWP	**SVR**	**CO**
Nitroglycerin	↓↓	↔↓	↑ ↔ ↓
Nitroprusside	↓↓	↓↓	↑↑
Milrinone	↓↓	↓↓	↑↑
Dobutamine	↓	↓	↑↑

Inodilators

- Dobutamine and milrinone are inodilators which increase contractility and reduce vascular resistance (Table 8.6).
- Dobutamine is a beta-agonist with rapid onset and is not renally cleared (better for patients with acute kidney injury). Can provoke arrhythmias.
- Milrinone acts as a phosphodiesterase-3 (PDE-3) inhibitor with slower onset of action (~12 hours to reach steady state) and is generally a more potent vasodilator. It is renally cleared, so should be avoided in patients with severe renal impairment.

Guideline-Directed Medical Therapy (GDMT)

- GDMT in HFrEF should be optimized once euvolemia is achieved and typically consists of the following classes of medications: beta-blockers, ACEi/ARB/ARNI, MRAs, and H/ISDN. The uptitration of these medications to target doses is typically achieved gradually in the outpatient setting. Refer to the chronic heart failure chapter (Table 9.2) for target doses of these medications.

Treatment of Acute Heart Failure with Preserved Ejection Fraction (HFpEF)

- The most important therapy is decongestion with the use of IV diuretics.
- Spironolactone is helpful and may reduce HF hospitalizations [24].
- Anti-hypertensive therapy should be administered to achieve normotension. ACEi/ARB can be used but neurohormonal antagonists (e.g., BB and RAAS inhibitors) do not have the same benefit as seen in HFrEF.
- Severe pulmonary congestion can sometimes develop abruptly in HFpEF patients from rapid increases in blood pressure. Patients with severe pulmonary edema can benefit from continuous positive pressure ventilation (CPAP).

Criterion for Consideration of Right Heart Catheterization and/or Cardiology Consultation

- Diagnostic uncertainty regarding the diagnosis of HF or intracardiac filling pressures based upon the clinical examination.
- Signs/symptoms of HF with normal BNP.
- Worsening clinical status, such as worsening renal function or hypotension, despite what is felt to be appropriate medical therapy.
- Signs/symptoms of cardiogenic shock.
- Suspected or known severe pulmonary hypertension.

Discharge Considerations

- The discharge period is a critical time for patients with recent acute HF exacerbation.
- Prior to discharge the following factors are key:
  - Euvolemia, based upon clinical examination, with successful transition to oral diuretic dosing. A 24-hour trial period with an oral diuretic regimen is recommended.
  - In general, the diuretic dose at the time of discharge after an ADHF exacerbation should be higher than the prior dose, unless another clear precipitating factor was identified, such as diuretic non-adherence, arrhythmia, or new ischemia.
  - Identify and eliminate precipitating factors such as medication or dietary non-adherence. Consider consultation with a nutritionist.
  - Implementation of GDMT with plan for further optimization in the outpatient setting.
  - Education of patients and family members regarding home weight monitoring, symptoms of heart failure, medication doses and schedules, dietary restrictions,
  - Short interval post-discharge follow-up (within 1 week), interval lab testing to reassess renal function and elec-

trolytes, and clear communication with outpatient providers are key [25].
– Strongly consider referral to advanced HF provider in patients with recurrent admissions, intolerance to attempted GDMT (worsening symptoms or hypotension), young patients, and recent cardiogenic shock.

Key Learning Points

- ADHF is a condition with high morbidity/mortality.
- Prompt recognition of HF signs and symptoms is key for timely management.
- Initial recognition of congestion and low cardiac output via the physical examination allow for the appropriate classification and treatment of HF.
- Elevated BNP can help make the diagnosis of HF in patients with dyspnea, but BNP can be normal in a subset of HF patients and should not trump the physical exam and invasive hemodynamics.

References

1. Redfield MM. Heart failure – an epidemic of uncertain proportions. N Engl J Med. 2002;347:1442–4.
2. McCullough PA, Philbin EF, Spertus JA, et al. Confirmation of a heart failure epidemic: findings from the Resource Utilization Among Congestive Heart Failure (REACH) study. J Am Coll Cardiol. 2002;39:60–9.
3. Cuffe MS, Califf RM, Adams KF Jr, et al., Outcomes of a Prospective Trial of Intra-venous Milrinone for Exacerbations of Chronic Heart Failure (OPTIME-CHF) Investigators. Short-term intravenous milrinone for acute exacerbation of chronic heart failure: a randomized controlled trial. JAMA 2002;287: 1541–1547.
4. Binanay C, Califf RM, Hasselblad V, et al., ESCAPE Investigators and ESCAPE Study Coordinators. Evaluation study of congestive heart failure and pulmonary artery catheterization effectiveness: the ESCAPE trial. JAMA 2005;294:1625–1633.

5. Bales AC, Sorrentino MJ. Causes of congestive heart failure: prompt diagnosis may affect prognosis. Postgrad Med. 1997;101:44–6.
6. Wuerz RC, Meador SA. Effects of prehospital medications on mortality and length of stay in congestive heart failure. Ann Emerg Med. 1992;21:669–74.
7. Wang CS, Fitzgerald JM, Schulzer M, et al. Does this dyspneic patient in the emergency department have congestive heart failure. JAMA. 2005;294:1944–56.
8. Drazner MH, Hellkamp AS, Leier CV, et al. Value of clinician assessment of hemodynamics in advanced heart failure: the ESCAPE trial. Circ Heart Fail. 2008;1:170–7.
9. Baeza-Trinidad R, Mosquera-Lozano JD, El Bikri L. Assessment of bendopnea impact on decompensated heart failure. Eur J Heart Fail. 2017;19:111–5.
10. Thibodeau JT, Jenny BE, Maduka JO, et al. Bendopnea and risk of adverse clinical outcomes in ambulatory patients with systolic heart failure. Am Heart J. 2017;183:102–7.
11. Drazner MH, Rame JE, Stevenson LW, Dries DL. Prognostic importance of elevated jugular venous pressure and a third heart sound in patients with heart failure. N Engl J Med. 2001;345:574–81.
12. Ewy GA. The abdominojugular test: technique and hemodynamic correlates. Ann Intern Med. 1988;109:456–60.
13. Stevenson LW, Perloff J. The limited reliability of physical signs for estimating hemodynamics in chronic heart failure. JAMA. 1989;261:884–8.
14. Samksy MD, Dunning A, DeVore AD, Schulte PJ, Starling RC, Tang WH, Armstrong PW, Ezekowitz JA, Butler J, McMurray JJ, Teerlink JR, Voors AA, Metra M, Mentz RJ, O'Connor CM, Patel CB, Hernandez AF. Liver function tests in patient with acute heart failure and associated outcomes: insights from ASCEND-HF. Eur J Heart Fail. 2016;4:424–32.
15. Maisel AS, Krishnaswamy P, Nowak RM, Breathing Not Properly Multinational Study Investigators, et al. Rapid measurement of B-type natriuretic peptide in the emergency diagnosis of heart failure. N Engl J Med. 2002;347:161–7.
16. Venkatesh AJ, Loftus TM, Burke MA, Akhter N, Fonarrow GC, Gheorghiade M, Sha SJ. Prevalence, clinical phenotype, and outcomes associated with normal B-type natriuretic peptide levels in heart failure with preserved ejection fraction. Am J Cardiol. 2012;111:870–6.

17. Kociol RD, Horton JR, Fonarow GC, Reyes EM, Shaw LK, O'Connor CM, Felker M, Hernandez AF. Admission, discharge, or change in B-Type natriuretic peptide and long-term outcomes. Data from organized program to initiate lifesaving treatment in hospitalized patients with heart failure (OPTIMIZE-HF) linked to medicare claims. Circ Heart Fail. 2011;4:628–36.
18. Stevenson LW. Tailored therapy to hemodynamic goals for advanced heart failure. Eur J Heart Fail. 1999;1:251–7.
19. Felker GM, Lee KL, Redfield MM, et al. Diuretic strategies in patients with acute decompensated heart failure. N Engl J Med. 2011;364:797–805.
20. McMurray JJV, Packer M, Desai AS, et al. Angiotensin-neprilysin inhibition versus enalapril in heart failure. N Engl J Med. 2014;371:993–1004.
21. Velazquez EJ, Morrow DA, DeVore AD, Duffy CI, Ambrosy AP, McCague K, Rocha R, Braunwald E. Angiotensin-neprilysin inhibition in acute decompensated heart failure. N Engl J Med. 2019;380:539–48.
22. Solomon S, McMurray J, Anand I. Angiotensin-neprilysin inhibition in heart failure with preserved ejection fraction. N Engl J Med. 2019; https://doi.org/10.1056/NEJMoa1908655.
23. Taylor AL, et al. Combination of isosorbide dinitrate and hydralazine in blacks with heart failure. N Engl J Med. 2004;351:2049–57.
24. Pfeffer MA, Claggett B, Assmann SF, et al. Regional variation in patients and outcomes in the treatment of preserved cardiac function heart failure with an aldosterone antagonist (TOPCAT) trial. Circulation. 2015;131:34–42.
25. Fleming LM, Kociol RD. Interventions for heart failure readmissions: successes and failures. Curr Heart Fail Rep. 2014;11:178. https://doi.org/10.1007/s11897-014-0192-x.

Chapter 9
Chronic Heart Failure

Donya Mohebali and Marwa Sabe

Abbreviations

ARNIs	Angiotensin receptor-neprilysin inhibitors
BNP	Brain natriuretic peptide
BTT	Bridge to transplant therapy
CRT	Cardiac resynchronization therapy
GDMT	Guideline-directed medical therapy
HFmrEF	Heart failure with moderately-reduced ejection fraction
HFpEF	Heart failure with preserved ejection fraction
HFrecEF	Heart failure with recovered ejection fraction
HFrEF	Heart failure with reduced ejection fraction
ICD	Internal cardiac defibrillator
LBBB	Left bundle branch block
LV	Left ventricle
NYHA	New York Heart Association Classification
RAAS	Renin-angiotensin-aldosterone system
SGLT2	Sodium glucose co-transporter 2
TID	Three times daily
VAD	Ventricular-assist device

D. Mohebali (✉) · M. Sabe
Department of Medicine, Division of Cardiology, Beth Israel Deaconess Medical Center, Boston, MA, USA
e-mail: dmohebal@bidmc.harvard.edu; msabe@bidmc.harvard.edu

B. J. Wells et al. (eds.), *Handbook of Inpatient Cardiology*,
https://doi.org/10.1007/978-3-030-47868-1_9

Background/Epidemiology

- 6.5 Million Americans have heart failure (HF), and 10 million people will have HF by 2037 [1].
- >1 Million admissions per year [1].
- HF hospitalizations –50% from HF with reduced ejection fraction (HFrEF) and 50% from HF with preserved ejection fraction (HFpEF) [1].

Definition and Pathophysiology of Chronic Heart Failure (CHF)

- CHF is a clinical syndrome caused by structural defects in the myocardium resulting in the impairment of ventricular filling or ejection of blood.
- Causes include valvular disorders, rhythm abnormalities, persistently ↑ heart rate, coronary disease, or non-ischemic causes leading to supply-demand mismatch of blood for metabolic needs with elevation of pulmonary or systemic venous pressures.
- HFrEF results from poor contraction of the left ventricle (LV) with inadequate emptying leading to decreased ejection fraction. A higher preload required to maintain cardiac output ➔ the ventricle remodels over time becoming spherical and dilated.
- HFpEF ➔ LV filling is impaired ➔ ↑ LV end-diastolic pressure with normal global contractility and normal EF.
- In HF ➔ ↑ sympathetic tone (↑ norepinephrine release), ↑ HR, and ↑ myocardial contractility ➔ arterio-veno-constriction occurs.
- ↓ Renal blood flow ➔ activation of the renin-angiotensin-aldosterone system (RAAS). RAAS ➔ ↑ angiotensin II levels ➔ remodeling of the heart and peripheral vasculature ➔ ↑ vasopressin release➔ ↑ sodium and water retention ➔ ↑ peripheral vascular tone and hyponatremia seen in HF.
- Beta-1 receptors downregulated as the result of ↑ sympathetic activation ➔ impaired myocyte contractility and ↑ heart rate.

- Brain natriuretic peptide (BNP) released from ventricle due to ventricular stretching. BNP ➔ renal excretion of sodium, counter-regulatory effects on RAAS system, and catecholamine activation (blunted in HF as a result of receptor downregulation).

Classification of Heart Failure

- HFrEF: EF ≤40%.
- HFpEF: HF with EF >50%.
- HF with borderline EF: EF 41–49%. The ESC categorizes patients with EF of 40–49% as heart failure with moderately reduced ejection fraction (HFmrEF) [3].
- HF with improved or recovered EF (HFrecEF): HFrEF improved to >40%.

Treatment of Heart Failure Based Upon Stage of Heart Failure

Various stages of heart failure that help classify patients and guide treatment strategies (Table 9.1). Patient can move up and down class categorizations of heart failure, but once a person reaches a stage classification they cannot move back down a stage.

Treatment of Heart Failure with Reduced Ejection Fraction

- Therapy for HFrEF is aimed at targeting neurohormonal responses to prevent adverse remodeling with neurohormonal blockade and decongestion with loop diuretics. Beta blockade counteracts the upregulation of sympathetic tone that occurs.

Table 9.1 ACC/AHA stages of heart failure and NYHA Class [2]

ACC/AHA stages of heart failure	NYHA Class
A: No structural heart disease but at risk for heart failure with comorbidities such as HTN, DM, atherosclerotic disease, use of cardiotoxins, or family history of cardiomyopathy *Therapy goals:* Healthy lifestyle, prevention of vascular/coronary disease, and prevention of LV structural abnormalities *Treatment:* Angiotensin-converting enzyme inhibitors (ACEi)/aldosterone receptor blockers (ARB), diabetes treatment, and statins as appropriate	None
B: Structural heart disease but no heart failure such as previous MI, LV remodeling including LV hypertrophy, low EF without evidence of volume overload, or valvular disease *Therapy goals:* Prevention of HF symptoms and further cardiac remodeling *Treatment:* ACEi/ARB or beta blockers as appropriate. ICD, revascularization, or valvular surgery as appropriate	I: Asymptomatic
C: Structural heart disease with current or history of heart failure symptoms *Therapy goals:* HFpEF/HFrEF – control symptoms, prevent hospitalization/mortality *Treatment* for HFpEF: Diuresis. Follow guidelines for comorbidities such as hypertension, atrial fibrillation, coronary artery disease, and diabetes. MRAs may be useful in some patients *Treatment* for HFrEF: Diuresis, ACEi/ARBs/ARNIs, beta blockers, MRAs. For use in selected patients: hydralazine/isosorbide, digoxin, CRT, ICD	II: Mild heart failure; symptomatic with mild exertion III: Moderate heart failure; symptomatic with minimal exertion
D: Refractory heart failure needing advanced therapies (left ventricular assist device, OHT) *Treatment:* Advanced heart failure therapy like heart transplantation and/or ventricular assist device therapy, chronic inotropes, palliative care and hospice	IV: Severe heart failure; symptomatic at rest

Neurohormonal Antagonists/Guideline-Directed Medical Therapy (GDMT)

Beta Blocker (BB) Therapy

- Metoprolol succinate ➔ 34% reduction in all-cause mortality in patients with HFrEF (MERIT-HF, Lancet 1999) [4]. Mortality benefit with carvedilol and bisoprolol as well [5, 6]. See Table 9.2 for staring/target doses.
- When starting BB, monitor for signs of fatigue, shortness of breath, or HF exacerbation. If identified➔ reduce BB dose (typically by half) or discontinue all together.
- Attempt uptitration to maximally tolerated dose for mortality benefit.

ACE Inhibitors (ACEi)/Angiotensin Receptor Blockers (ARBs)

- ACEi ➔ reduce morbidity/mortality in HFrEF (RCT data).
- Enalapril ➔ 16% reduction in 4-year mortality in HFrEF and NYHA Class II-IV symptoms (SOLVD, NEJM 1991) [7].
- Other ACEi with mortality benefit: lisinopril and captopril [8, 9].
- When starting, caution in patients with ↓ systemic blood pressure, renal insufficiency, or ↑ potassium levels. Monitor for angioedema. Monitor renal function/potassium within 1–2 weeks of initiation and/or dose adjustment.
- ACEi side effects: cough secondary to inhibition of kininase ➔ ↑ levels of bradykinin.
- ARBs reduce morbidity/mortality in HFrEF, particularly when ACEi intolerant [9–11].
- ARBs do not inhibit kininase ➔ ↓ incidence of angioedema and cough.
- Monitor renal function/potassium within 1–2 weeks of initiation and/or dose adjustment. See Table 9.2 for starting/target doses.

TABLE 9.2 Guideline-directed medical therapy for heart failure with reduced ejection fraction

Drug	Initial daily doses	Max doses	Mean doses achieved in clinical trials	References
ACE inhibitors				
Captopril	6.25 mg BID	50 mg TID	122.7 mg QD	[9]
Enalapril	2.5 mg BID	10-20 mg BID	16.6 mg QD	[7]
Lisinopril	2.5–5 mg QD	20–40 mg QD	32.5–35 mg QD	[8]
ARBs				
Losartan	25–50 mg QD	50–150 mg QD	129 mg QD	[11]
Valsartan	20–40 mg BID	160 mg BID	254 mg QD	[10]
ARNI				
Sacubitril/valsartan	24/26 mg BID or 49/51 mg BID	97/103 mg BID	Target dose: 24/26 mg, 49/51 mg, or 97/103 mg BID	[12]
I_f channel inhibitor				
Ivabradine	5 mg BID	7.5 mg BID	6.5 mg BID at 1 year	[17]

Aldosterone antagonists				
Spironolactone	12.5–25 mg QD	25 mg QD or BID	26 mg QD	[15]
Eplerenone	25 mg QD	50 mg QD	42.6 mg QD	[16]
Beta blockers				
Bisoprolol	1.25 mg QD	10 mg QD	8.6 mg QD	[5]
Carvedilol	3.125 mg BID	50 mg BID	37 mg QD	[6]
Metoprolol succinate	12.5–25 mg QD	200 mg QD	159 mg QD	[4]
Isosorbide dinitrate and hydralazine				
Isosorbide dinitrate and hydralazine	20–30 mg isosorbide dinitrate/25–50 mg hydralazine TID or QD	40 mg isosorbide dinitrate TID with 100 mg hydralazine TID	N/A	[13]

Modified from the 2017 ACC Expert Consensus Decision Pathway for Optimization of Heart Failure Treatment [2]

Angiotensin Neprilysin Inhibitors (ARNIs)

- ARNI is an ARB combined with an inhibitor of neprilysin, an enzyme that degrades natriuretic peptide, bradykinin and other vasoactive peptides.
- Valsartan/sacubitril (Entresto) ➔ reduced composite endpoint of CV death or HF hospitalization by 20% in HFrEF and NYHA Class II-III (PARADIGM-HF, NEJM 2014) [12].
- Contraindications to starting ARNIs: angioedema, symptomatic hypotension, prior intolerance to ACEi or ARBs, or hyperkalemia.
- Starting dose is 24/26 mg twice daily (low dose). Goal uptitration to moderate 49/51 mg twice daily (intermediate dose), or 97/103 mg twice daily (high dose).

Clinical Pearl

- ACE is STOPPED for 36 hours prior to starting an ARNI; otherwise, there is an ↑ risk of life-threatening angioedema and hypotension.
- No wash-out period is required when transitioning from an ARB to an ARNI.
- Increased natriuresis/diuresis effect can be expected, so in some cases the loop diuretic dose can be reduced.
- Once an ARNI is started, monitor for symptomatic hypotension (0.9% of patients in PARADIGM-HF experienced symptomatic hypotension resulting in discontinuation of sacubitril-valsartan) [12].
- Monitor renal function/potassium within 1–2 weeks of initiation and/or dose adjustment. See Table 9.2 for starting/target doses.

Isosorbide Dinitrate (Isordil)/Hydralazine (Hydral)

- Combination of Isordil-Hydral ↓ all-cause mortality among blacks with HFrEF by ~40% and ↓ hospitalizations by ~33% when used as add-on agent in patients already on GDMT (A-HEFT, NEJM 2004) [13, 14].

- Mortality benefits of this class of agents extrapolated to other groups, particularly when renal insufficiency prohibits use of ACEi/ARBs. See Table 9.2 for starting/target doses.

Mineralocorticoid Receptor Antagonists (MRAs)

- MRAs such as spironolactone ➔ 30% reduction in all-cause mortality in HFrEF (EF <35%) and NYHA Class III-IV symptoms (RALES, NEJM 1999) [15].
- Avoid if creatinine >2.5 mg/dL, GFR <30 ml/min/1.73 m^2 and/or K >5 mEq/L.
- Baseline creatinine and potassium levels obtained prior to starting this medication and within 1 week of its initiation and/or dose titration.
- Eplerenone reduces risk of death and hospitalization in patients with HFrEF [16]. Consider in patients who develop gynecomastia with use of spironolactone. See Table 9.2 for staring/target doses.

Ivabradine

- Ivabradine blocks I_f current in the sinoatrial node➔ ↓ HR.
- Considered for reduction of HF hospitalization in symptomatic NYHA Class II-III stable chronic HFrEF (LVEF ≤35%) receiving GDMT including BB at maximally tolerated dose and sinus rhythm with resting HR of ≥70 beats per minute (SHIFT, Lancet 2015) [17].
- Starting dose: 5 mg BID with uptitration to 7.5 mg BID [17–19].

Digoxin

- Inhibits Na-K ATPase ➔ ↑ contractile state of the heart➔ ↑ inotropy and ↓ norepinephrine/plasma renin levels.
- In chronic compensated HF and LVEF ≤45% digoxin reduces hospitalization rates though *does not* impact mortality (DIG trial, NEJM 1997) [20].

Goals of Guideline-Directed Medical Therapy (GDMT)

- Once GDMT is maximized to highest tolerated doses, obtain repeat echocardiogram to evaluate for improvement in LV function. Pending results, consider other therapies like implantable cardioverter-defribillator (ICD) and cardiac resynchronization therapy (CRT) (see below).

Anemia and Heart Failure Guidelines

- Pursue standard work up for anemia to identify causal factor.
- In NYHA Class II and III, HF and iron deficiency (defined as ferritin <100 ng/mL or 100–300 ng/mL if transferrin saturation is <20%) with or without anemia (Hgb 9–13.5 g/dL) IV iron replacement (ferric carboxymaltose) is reasonable to improve functional status and quality of life [21, 22] with improvements in 6-min walk test distance, peak oxygen consumption, quality of life, and NYHA functional class. *Oral iron therapy has no effect on exercise capacity* [23]. May reduce hospitalization rates for heart failure and cardiovascular mortality [24].
- A prospective trial to investigate effects on morbidity and mortality is ongoing (HEART-FID).

Indications for Cardiac Resynchronization Therapy (CRT)

- CRT involves pacing the LV and RV to restore ventricular synchrony and improve LV systolic function and clinical outcomes for select patients.
- Class I indications for CRT: LVEF ≤35%, normal sinus rhythm, NYHA Class II-IV symptoms, left bundle branch block (LBBB), and QRS duration ≥150 ms [25].
- Re-assess LV function several months after CRT. Patients with improvement of LV function are considered to be responders.

Clinical Pearl
Patients continued on GDMT, even if LV function improves to >40%. Decreasing doses of loop diuretics may be needed with improved LV function.

- For patients with non-ischemic dilated cardiomyopathy, (LVEF) ≤35%, and associated heart failure (HF) with NYHA Class II or III status, ICD therapy for primary prevention of sudden cardiac death is recommended [25].

Patient Selection for Advanced Therapies

- If patients remain symptomatic despite maximal doses of GDMT, then advanced therapies should strongly be considered (Table 9.3) and include durable ventricular assist devices (VADs).
- Selection for destination therapy VAD therapy includes: Stage D HF with LVEF ≤25%, Peak V02 <14 ml/kg/min (or <50% age/sex predicted) on cardiopulmonary exercise testing *and* NYHA Class IV symptoms, despite optimal GDMT for at least 45/last 60 days, *or* Inotrope dependence for at least 14 days *or* dependence on mechanical support for at least 7 days.
- VAD devices can also be used as a bridge to transplantation.

Table 9.3 Reason to consider referral for advanced therapies

NYHA Class III symptoms despite optimal medical therapy and/or cardiac resynchronization therapy (CRT) or lack of response to CRT
Recurrent heart failure readmissions
Persistent hyponatremia
Worsening renal function
Inability to tolerate neurohormonal blockade (ACEi/ARB/Beta blocker)
Increasing diuretic requirement

Heart Failure with Moderate-Range Ejection Fraction (HFmREF)

- HFmREF: HF and ejection fraction from 40% to 49%.
- ~13–24% of all HF patients in the United States estimated at 1.6 million [26].
- Combination of mild HFrEF and HFpEF. Clinical characteristics similar to HFpEF. Comorbidities: COPD, diabetes, and hypertension [26]. Uncontrolled hypertension is a common precipitant for hospitalization.

Clinical Pearl
No therapies in HFmREF have been shown to improve outcomes in patients with randomized data. *Treat patients with optimization of comorbidities, particularly hypertension and screen for/treat coronary artery disease to prevent progression of HFmREF to HFrEF.*

- Diuretics used to relieve symptoms of congestion.

Heart Failure with Recovered Ejection Fraction (HFrecEF)

- HFrecEF: HFrEF that has improved to EF >40% [27].
- Patients not well understood.
- In clinical practice, treat similarly to HFrEF. Withdrawal of HF medications in this group with recovered EF results in relapse of HF [28].

Clinical Pearl
Even after LV recovery, patients are continued on GDMT unless not tolerated or side effects develop. Continue loop diuretics for decongestion, though may reduce dose.

Heart Failure with Preserved Ejection Fraction (HFpEF)

- GDMT in patients with HFpEF not robust.
- TOPCAT trial (treatment of preserved cardiac function heart failure with an aldosterone antagonist) ➔ *no difference* in primary composite outcome of CV mortality, aborted cardiac arrest, or HF hospitalization (3.3 years follow up) in patients on spironolactone with HFpEF (LVEF ≥45%, findings of HF, and either a HF hospitalization or elevated BNP).
- Spironolactone associated with "nominal" reduction in HF hospitalizations (12.0% vs. 14.2%, NNT 45) [29].
- Subgroup analysis ➔ significant reduction in the primary outcome for those in Americas but not Eastern Europe (attributed to suggested non-consumption of spironolactone given larger portion of undetectable metabolites in this population) [30].
- Secondary analysis limited to subjects from the Americas showed spironolactone therapy in women ➔ ↓ all-cause mortality in women (hazard ratio 0.66; $p = 0.01$) but not in men (p interaction = 0.02) [31].
- MRAs: ↓ HF hospitalizations in patients with an LVEF ≥45%, elevated BNP or HF admission in the last year (if eGFR >30, Cr <2.5 mg/dl and K <5.0 mEq/L) [31] according to 2017 ACC/AHA guidelines (class IIa recommendation).
- NEAT-HFpEF. isosorbide mononitrate led to less activity, no improvement in quality of life, and submaximal exercise in HFpEF [32]; therefore, try to stop in these patients unless used for another indication like angina or hypertension.

Diabetes and Heart Failure

- Empagliflozin, a sodium-glucose co-transporter-2 (SGLT2) inhibitor➔ 38% reduction in CV death and 35% reduction in HF hospitalization in patients with type II diabetes at

high risk for CV disease (EMPA-REG OUTCOME, NEJM 2015) [33].
- Consider addition of empagliflozin for management of type II diabetes and HF.
- In HFrEF, risk of worsening heart failure/death from cardiovascular causes is lower in patients on dapagliflozin than placebo, regardless of presence or absence of diabetes (DAPA-HF, NEJM 2019) [34].

Clinical Pearl
Patients may require lower doses of diuretics after SGLT2 initiation given the reduction in glucose reabsorption and ↑ urinary glucose excretion expected.

Mitral Regurgitation (MR) and Heart Failure

- Secondary MR develops as the result of dilated cardiomyopathy, ventricular dilation, mitral annular dilation, and impairment of leaflet coaptation.
- First-line treatment: GDMT.
- In moderate-to-severe or severe secondary MR with symptomatic despite maximal dose GDMT, transcatheter mitral valve repair shown ➔ ↓ hospitalization for HF and all-cause mortality within a 24-month follow-up period compared to medical therapy alone (COAPT, NEJM 2018) [35].
- Patients considered for transcatheter mitral valve repair evaluated by a multidisciplinary team (interventional cardiology, advanced heart failure, and cardiac surgery).

CardioMEMs Device

- Some patients with HFrEF at high risk for hospitalization and mortality despite GDMT.
- In HFrEF (LVEF ≤40%) and NYHA Class III symptoms, remote monitoring of pulmonary artery pressures using CardioMEMs heart sensor results in 28% ↓ HF hospital-

izations and a 47% trend towards lower mortality (CHAMPION, JACC 2017) [36].
- Refer to advanced heart failure clinicians for this device.

Key Learning Points
- Chronic HF is a condition with high morbidity/mortality.
- Treatment of HFrEF directed by the most evidence-based guidelines. HFpEF and HFmREF treatment guided by management of comorbidities like hypertension. HFrecEF treated like HFrEF. More studies are needed to better understand the pathophysiologic factors leading to HFpEF, HFmREF, and HFrecEF.
- Other management considerations for HFrEF patients include CRT, mitra-clip, or CardioMEMs devices.
- Consider advanced therapy options such as durable VADs or heart transplantation if NYHA Class IV symptoms despite optimal GDMT and/or CRT with recurrent HF readmissions, inability to tolerate GDMT, worsening renal function, or increasing diuretic requirements and worsening functional capacity.

References

1. Benjamin EJ, Virani CSS, Callaway CW, et al. ACC/AHA heart disease and stroke statistics 2018 update. Circulation. 2018;137:e67–e492.
2. Yancy CW, Jessup M, Bozkurt B, et al. 2017 ACC/AHA/HFSA focused update of the 2013 ACCF/AHA Guideline for the Management of Heart Failure. JACC. 2017;70:776–803.
3. Ponikowski P, Voors AA, Anker SD, et al. 2016 ESC guidelines for the diagnosis and treatment of acute and chronic heart failure: the Task Force for the diagnosis and treatment of acute and chronic heart failure of the European Society of

Cardiology (ESC) developed with the special contribution of the Heart Failure Association (HFA) of the ESC. Eur Heart J. 2016;37:2129–200.

4. Effect of metoprolol CR/XL in chronic heart failure: Metoprolol CR/XL Randomised Intervention Trial in Congestive Heart Failure (MERIT-HF). Lancet. 1999; 353:2001–7.
5. Authors CI. The Cardiac Insufficiency Bisoprolol Study II (CIBIS-II): a randomized trial. Lancet. 1999;353:9–13.
6. Packer M, Coats AJ, Fowler MB, et al. Effect of carvedilol on survival in severe chronic heart failure. NEJM. 2001;344:1651–8.
7. The SOLVD Investigators. Effect of enalapril on survival in patients with reduced left ventricular ejection fractions and congestive heart failure. NEJM. 1991;325:293–302.
8. Packer M, Poole-Wilson PA, Armstrong PW, et al. Comparative effects of low and high doses of the angiotensin-converting enzyme inhibitor, lisinopril, on morbidity and mortality in chronic heart failure. ATLAS Study Group. Circulation. 1999;100:2312–8.
9. Pitt B, Segal R, Martinez FA, et al. Randomized trial of losartan versus captopril in patients over 65 with heart failure (Evaluation of Losartan in the Elderly Study, ELITE). Lancet. 1997;349:747–52.
10. Cohn JN, Tognoni G, Investigators VHFT. A randomized trial of the angiotensin-receptor blocker valsartan in chronic heart failure. NEJM. 2001;345:1667–75.
11. Konstam MA, Neaton JD, Dickstein K, et al. Effects of high-dose versus low-dose losartan on clinical outcomes in patients with heart failure (HEAAL study): a randomised, double-blind trial. Lancet. 2009;374:1840–8.
12. McMurray JJV, Packer M, Desai AS, et al. Angiotensin-neprilysin inhibition versus enalapril in heart failure. NEJM. 2014;371:993–1004.
13. Taylor AL, Ziesche S, Yancy C, et al. Combination of isosorbide dinitrate and hydralazine in blacks with heart failure. NEJM. 2004;351:2049–57.
14. Cohn JN, Archibald DG, Ziesche S, et al. Effect of vasodilator therapy on mortality in chronic congestive heart failure. Results of a Veterans Administration Cooperative Study. NEJM. 1986;314:1547–52.
15. Pitt B, Zannad F, Remme WJ, et al. The effect of spironolactone on morbidity and mortality in patients with severe heart failure. Randomized Aldactone Evaluation Study Investigators. NEJM. 1999;341:709–17.

16. Zannad F, McMurry JJ, Krum H, van Veldhuisen DJ, et al. Eplerenone in patients with systolic heart failure and mild symptoms. N Engl J Med. 2011;364:11–21.
17. Swedberg K, Komajda M, Böhm M, et al. Ivabradine and outcomes in chronic heart failure (SHIFT): a randomised placebo-controlled study. Lancet. 2010;376:875–85.
18. Fox K, Ford I, Steg PG, et al. Ivabradine in stable coronary artery disease without clinical heart failure. NEJM. 2014;371:1091–9.
19. Fox K, Ford I, Steg PG, et al. Ivabradine for patients with stable coronary artery disease and left-ventricular systolic dysfunction (BEAUTIFUL): a randomized, double-blind, placebo-controlled trial. Lancet. 2008;372:807–16.
20. Gorlin R, et al. The effect of digoxin on mortality and morbidity in patients with heart failure. NEJM. 1997;336:525–53.
21. Anker SD, Colet CJ, Filippatos G, et al. Ferric carboxymaltose in patients with heart failure and iron deficiency. NEMJ. 2009;361:2436–48.
22. Ponikowski P, van Veldhuisen DJ, Comin-Colet J, et al. Beneficial effects of long-term intravenous iron therapy with ferric carboxymaltose in patients with symptomatic heart failure and iron deficiency. Eur Heart J. 2015;36:657–68.
23. Lewis GD, Malhorta R, Hernandez AF, et al. Effect of oral iron repletion on exercise capacity in patients with heart failure with reduced ejection fraction and iron deficiency. JAMA. 2017;317(19):1958–66.
24. Haehling S, Ebner N, Evertz R, et al. Iron deficiency in heart failure. JACC Heart Failure. 2019;7:36–46.
25. Epstein AE, DiMarco JP, Ellenbogen KA, et al. 2012 ACCF/AHA/HRS focused update incorporated into the ACCF/AHA/HRS 2008 guidelines for device based therapy of cardiac rhythm abnormalities: a report of the American College of Cardiology Foundation/American Heart Association Task Force on Practice Guidelines and the Heart Rhythm Society. JACC. 2013;61:e6–75.
26. Hsu JJ, Ziaeian B, Fonarow GC. Heart failure with mid-range (borderline) ejection fraction, clinical implications and future directions. JACC HF. 2017;11:763–71.
27. Florea VG, Rector TS, Anand IS, Oxon DP, Cohn JN. Heart failure with improved ejection fraction: clinical characteristics, correlates of recovery, and survival. Results from the Valsartan Heart Failure Trial. Circ Heart Fail. 2016;9:e003123.

28. Halliday BP, Wassall R, Lota AS, et al. Withdrawal of pharmacological treatment for heart failure in patients with recovered dilated cardiomyopathy (TRED-HF): an open-label, pilot, randomised trial. Lancet. 2018. ePub 2018-11-09:1–13.
29. Pitt B, Pfeffer MA, Assman SF, et al. Spironolactone for heart failure with preserved ejection fraction. NEJM. 2014;370:1383–92.
30. Pfeffer MA, Claggett B, Assmann SF, et al. Regional variation in patients and outcomes in the Treatment of Preserved Cardiac Function Heart Failure With an Aldosterone Antagonist (TOPCAT) trial. Circulation. 2015;131:34–42.
31. Merrill M, Sweitzer NK, Lindenfeld J, et al. Sex difference in outcomes and response to spironolactone in heart failure with preserved ejection fraction. J Am Coll Cardiol HF. 2019;7:228–38.
32. Redfield MM, Anstrom KJ, Levine JA, et al. Isosorbide mononitrate in heart failure with preserved ejection fraction. NEJM. 2015;373:2314–24.
33. Zinman B, Wanner C, Lachin JM, Fitchett D, Bluhmiki E, Hantel S, et al. Empagliflozin, cardiovascular outcomes, and mortality in Type 2 diabetes. NEJM. 2015;373:2117–28.
34. DAPA-HF, McMurray J, Solomon S, Inzucchi S, et al. Dapagliflozin in patients with heart failure and reduced ejection fraction. NEMJ. 2019; https://doi.org/10.1056/NEJMoa1911303.
35. Stone GW et al., for the COAPT Investigators. Transcatheter mitral- valve repair in patients with heart failure. N Engl J Med. 2018;379:2307–18.
36. Givertz MM, Stevenson LW, Costanzo MR, Bourge RC, Bauman JG, Ginn G, Abraham WT. Pulmonary artery pressure-guided management of patients with heart failure and reduced ejection fraction. JACC. 2017;70:1875–86.

Chapter 10
Management of Pulmonary Hypertension in the Hospital Setting

Vladimir Kaplinskiy, Cyrus Kholdani, and Debby Ngo

Abbreviations

ANA	Anti-nuclear antibody
BMPR2	Bone morphogenetic protein receptor 2
BNP	Brain natriuretic peptide
CCB	Calcium channel blocker
COPD	Chronic obstructive pulmonary disease
CT	Computed tomography
CTA	Computed tomography angiography
CTEPH	Chronic thromboembolic pulmonary hypertension
DNA	Deoxyribonucleic acid
ECG	Electrocardiogram
HIV	Human immunodeficiency virus

V. Kaplinskiy (✉)
Beth Israel Deaconess Medical Center, Harvard Medical School, Boston, MA, USA
e-mail: vkaplins@bidmc.harvard.edu

C. Kholdani · D. Ngo
Department of Pulmonary, Critical Care and Sleep Medicine, Beth Israel Deaconess Medical Center, Harvard Medical School, Boston, MA, USA

B. J. Wells et al. (eds.), *Handbook of Inpatient Cardiology*, https://doi.org/10.1007/978-3-030-47868-1_10

ILD	Interstitial lung disease
NO	Nitric oxide
OSA	Obstructive sleep apnea
PA	Pulmonary artery
PE	Pulmonary embolism
PFTs	Pulmonary function tests
PHTN	Pulmonary hypertension
PVOD	Pulmonary veno-occlusive disease
PVR	Pulmonary vascular resistance
RF	Rheumatoid factor
RH	Right heart
RHC	Right heart catheterization
RNA	Ribonucleic acid
RV	Right ventricle
SLE	Systemic lupus erythematosus
V/Q Scan	Ventilation/perfusion scan
WHO	World Health Organization

Terminology

- Pulmonary hypertension has recently been defined by a mean pulmonary artery (PA) pressure ≥ 20 mmHg [1].
- Pulmonary arterial hypertension (PAH) is defined as a mean PA pressure of ≥20 mmHg with a pulmonary vascular resistance (PVR) of ≥3 Woods Units or 240 dynes-sec/cm^5 units and a pulmonary artery wedge pressure of ≤15 mmHg.
- Pre-capillary PH refers to elevation of pressure within the pulmonary arterial system.
- Post-capillary PH refers to elevation of pressure within the pulmonary venous and/or capillary system.

Etiology of Pulmonary Hypertension

- PH is classified into five groups according to the World Health Organization (WHO), based on etiology and disease mechanisms [2]:

- *Group I*: Pulmonary arterial hypertension (PAH) involves the obstruction of pulmonary arterioles. The mechanism is not fully understood but involves proliferation of cells within all three layers of the vascular wall, leading to a decrease in the diameter of the pulmonary arteries. Fibrosis and microthrombosis is also seen on microscopic examination.
- The diagnosis of PAH requires a right heart catheterization (RHC) to exclude alternative etiologies.
- WHO Group 1 PAH is further subclassified as below:

  Idiopathic PAH: PAH with no underlying/associated etiology.

  Heritable PAH: PAH in the setting of one of the known causative genetic mutations such as that in the bone morphogenetic protein receptor 2 (BMPR2) gene.

  Connective Tissue Disease-Associated PAH: PAH in the setting of collagen-vascular diseases such as systemic lupus erythematosus (SLE), systemic sclerosis, or rheumatoid arthritis that can manifest with pulmonary vasculopathy.

  Congenital heart disease-Associated PAH: PAH in the setting of a known volume- or pressure-loading congenital heart defect such as an atrial or ventricular septal defect.

  Portopulmonary hypertension: PAH in the setting of portal hypertension, often with advanced liver disease and is thought to be related, in part, to an imbalance between vasoconstrictive and vasodilatory humoral factors.

  Infectious etiologies including *schistosomiasis* and human immunodeficiency virus (HIV) are associated with PAH.

  Drug/toxin-associated PAH: PAH secondary to prior exposure to certain implicated compounds, including chemotherapy agents (such as tyrosine kinase inhibitors), illicit substances (such as amphetamines and possibly cocaine), dietary supplements (such as fenfluramine, aminorex, benfluorex), and possibly herbal supplements such as "Quing-Dai" and rapeseed oil. *Pulmonary veno-occlusive disease (PVOD)* involves occlusion of the pulmonary venous system and can be seen in association with chemotherapeutic regimens (i.e., bleomycin, cisplatin, vincristine), organic solvents (i.e., trichloroethylene), and cigarette smoking.

- *Group II*: Refers to PH which results from left heart disease and is typically defined by a pulmonary capillary wedge pressure ≥ 15 mmHg. This can be due to either left ventricular systolic dysfunction, diastolic dysfunction, or valvular disease.
- *Group III*: PH is the result of primary airway diseases such as chronic obstructive pulmonary disease (COPD), interstitial lung disease (ILD), or sleep-disordered breathing. PH can result from hypoxia-mediated vasoconstriction and collagen deposition within the intimal layer.
- *Group IV*: Chronic thromboembolic pulmonary hypertension (CTEPH) refers to PH that results from chronic pulmonary embolization/thrombosis within the pulmonary arterial vasculature.
- *Group V*: Refers to PH occurring as a result of any number of miscellaneous conditions, such as glycogen storage diseases, congenital cardiomyopathies (excluding atrial septal defects), chronic kidney disease, Langerhans histiocytosis X, sarcoidosis, schistosomiasis, compression of pulmonary vessels (i.e., by malignant tumors), hematologic disorders (i.e., sickle cell anemia).

Clinical Consequences of Pulmonary Hypertension

- Clinical manifestations of pulmonary hypertension are non-specific and may include:

- Dyspnea/fatigue (most commonly)
- Hypoxia
- Lightheadedness
- Chest pain (due to right ventricular wall stress or coronary artery compression via enlarged PA)
- Peripheral edema
- Abdominal distension
- Right ventricular lift
- Ortner's syndrome (hoarseness due to palsy of the recurrent laryngeal nerve)
- Augmented P2 heart sound
- Jugular venous distension
- Right-sided S3 gallop
- Systolic murmur which increases with inspiration (due to tricuspid regurgitation)
- Widely split S2 sound
- Hepatomegaly or pulsatile liver [3].

- Severity of symptoms is defined by the World Health Organization on a scale of 1–4, with I indicating no significant limitation in physical activity and IV indicating severe symptoms with any activity or at rest (Table 10.1) [4].

Clinical Pearl
History of splenectomy and thyroid disorders appears to be associated with PH.

- Right Heart Failure Associated with Pulmonary Hypertension
  - PH is the most common cause of RHF, with a global prevalence estimate of 1%, increasing up to 10% in individuals aged >65 years [5].
  - The process of RH failure can be chronic, as with pulmonary hypertension from chronic heart and lung disease, most commonly as a result of gradual increase in RV afterload. The initial response is hypertrophy of the RV myocytes and maintenance of adequate cardiac output despite high right-sided filling pressures. Over

time, this can progress to RV myocyte fibrosis and RV hypokinesis, resulting in low pulmonary artery (PA) pressures despite a high pulmonary vascular resistance.

The possibility of acute PE should be considered in worsening right heart failure in PH.

Notably management of acute RV failure in a low RV afterload state (e.g., acute PE or acute RV infarct) is managed differently from decompensated RV failure from chronic PH.

- Reduced RV function can result in new or worsening tricuspid regurgitation (due to distension of the valve apparatus) and ventricular interdependence, whereby the interventricular septum may shift leftward. In some cases, this can impede left ventricular filling and result in hypotension/shock. In addition, this can lead to coronary sinus congestion and myocardial ischemia.
- Over time, hepatic and renal dysfunction can develop due to congestion.
- Due to their tenuous hemodynamic state, patients with advanced RV dysfunction and with signs of impending hemodynamic compromise may benefit from earlier invasive monitoring to assess their central venous pressure and pulmonary hypertension consult.
- Goals for decompensated right heart failure from pulmonary hypertension include the following [6]:

  Optimization of preload (see citation):

  - If low intravascular volume is suspected, volume resuscitation should be initiated.
  - However, when RV failure occurs in the setting of increased RV afterload, over resuscitation may result in displacement of the interventricular septum toward the LV and impaired LV diastolic filling. RV dilation increases free wall tension, resulting in increased oxygen demand and

decreased RV perfusion. In this setting, intravascular volume may need to be decreased via diuresis of dialysis.

Reduction of afterload

- Avoidance of hypoxia, hypercapnia, and acidemia may reduce pulmonary vasoconstriction.
- Initiation and/or addition of pulmonary vasodilators should be considered. Pulmonary vasodilators that may be available include inhaled nitric oxide (NO), Epoprostonal/Treprostinal, and Sildenafil.
- Pulmonary hypertension specialist consult is highly recommended for initiation of therapy.

Inotropic/vasopressor support

- Indicated to improve RV contractility and/or to maintain adequate mean arterial pressure.
- Dobutamine and milrinone are the preferred inotropes.
- Preferred vasopressors include vasopressin, levophed for mild hypotension, and epinephrine for moderate to severe systemic hypotension.
- Pulmonary hypertension or heart failure physician should be consulted before initiation of inotropic or vasopressor support.

Table 10.1 World Health Organization (WHO) functional classification for pulmonary hypertension [4]

Class	Functional classification
I	No limitation in physical activity
II	Slight limitation in physical activity. Symptoms with ordinary physical activity but not at rest
III	Marked limitation in physical activity. Symptoms with less than ordinary physical activity but not at rest
IV	Symptoms with any physical activity (or at rest)

Workup of Pulmonary Hypertension

- *Patients with new PH should undergo a thorough history, to assess for: drug use, smoking history, occupational exposures, family history, evaluation for symptoms of connective tissue disease or vasculitis, risk factors for immunodeficiency, travel history, and assessment for heart, liver and lung diseases.*
- Further workup should include
  - Chest X-ray
  - High-resolution chest CT (PA:Aorta ratio > 1 specific and sensitive for PH) [7]
  - Electrocardiogram (ECG) assessing for RV hypertrophy, right axis deviation, right bundle branch block, or other signs of right heart strain
  - Pulmonary function tests (PFTs)
  - Polysomnography
  - Ambulatory oximetry
- Transthoracic echocardiogram should be obtained to assess for signs of PH
  - Tricuspid regurgitant jet velocity > 2.8 m/s
  - Estimated PA systolic pressure > 35 mmHg
  - RV dilation
  - Flattening of the interventricular septum
  - Pulmonic insufficiency
  - Mid-systolic closure of the pulmonic valve
  - Pulmonary artery diameter > 2.5 cm.
- Phlebotomy for evaluation of new PH should include: BNP, LFTs, HIV, and, in the appropriate clinical context, labs to evaluate collagen-vascular diseases (ANA, RF, anti-centromere, anti-topoisomerase, anti-RNA polymerase III, anti-double stranded DNA, anti-Ro, anti-La).
- RHC should be considered

Clinical Pearl
Ventilation-perfusion (V/Q) scanning is the modality of choice to evaluate patients suspected of having CTEPH.

  - In order to confirm pulmonary hypertension in patients with low probability of PH but with high clinical suspicion
  - Clarify contribution of left heart disease to PH
  - Unexplained PH
  - Assess for intracardiac shunting
  - Test for vasoreactivity
- Pulmonary vasoreactivity testing (i.e., nitric oxide) should be performed on initial RHC, and it can be used to identify patients likely to respond to calcium channel blockers.
- RHC must be performed before initiating any pulmonary vasodilator therapy.
  - Vasoreactivity testing involves administration of a vasodilator, such as adenosine or nitric oxide and monitoring for a change in mean pulmonary artery pressure. A test is considered positive if there is a decrease in mean pulmonary artery pressure of ≥10 mmHg to a value below 40 mmHg with no decrease in cardiac output and minimal effect on systemic blood pressure.
  - Vasoreactivity testing is contraindicated if a patient has hypotension or severe functional limitation.
  - Only patients with a positive test should be treated for PAH with CCBs.
  - Vasoreactivity testing also provides an opportunity to evaluate left ventricular response to increased preload from increased pulmonary blood flow (i.e., PCWP response).

Therapy for Pulmonary Hypertension

- Oxygen supplementation, particularly in group III, can be beneficial in patients with PH (21% decrease in mortality in patients with COPD) [8].
- Diuresis is often helpful to improve symptoms in patients with PH, particularly in group II PH.
- Anticoagulation is the standard therapy for CTEPH, with consideration for surgical pulmonary thromboendarterectomy:
  - Warfarin is typically utilized, given the limited experience with other anticoagulants.
  - Conflicting evidence in patients with Group I PH, with some studies showing improvement in mortality (COMPERA) [9] and other evidence showing no survival advantage (REVEAL) [10].
- Calcium channel blockers (non-dihydropyridine preferred). Approximately 10% of Group 1 PAH are vasoreactivity responders [11] who demonstrate improved survival, functional class, and hemodynamics on CCB therapy.
- If there is a strong component of group II or III PH, pulmonary vasodilators (Table 10.2) should generally be avoided as they are not proven to be effective and may induce pulmonary edema and/or worsening ventilation-perfusion mismatch. Pulmonary vasodilators are also contraindicated in PVOD. Referral to a pulmonary hypertension specialist should be considered.
- Riociguat and macitentan have been studied and approved as PH-specific therapies in patients with CTEPH.
- Patients who are chronically on IV pulmonary vasodilators should be maintained on a stable dose of the infusion unless there is definitive contraindication. Interruptions and boluses of the infusion can be life-threatening in certain cases. A pulmonary hypertension specialist should be consulted for management of parenteral therapy.

Table 10.2 Pulmonary vasodilator therapy

Medication (generic)	Alternative name(s)	Mechanism of action	Indicated for	Adverse effects
Sildenafil (PO)	Revatio	Cyclic GMP phosphodiesterase type 5 inhibitor	PAH Improvement in symptoms [12]	Headache, flushing, indigestion
Tadalafil (PO)	Adcirca, Alyq	Cyclic GMP phosphodiesterase type 5 inhibitor	PAH Improvement in symptoms [13]	Headache, flushing, indigestion
Riociguat (PO)	Adempas	Guanylate cyclase stimulator	Group IV/CTEPH Improvement in symptoms [14] PAH Improvement in symptoms [15]	Hypotension, headache, dizziness, dyspepsia Contraindicated in pregnancy
Bosentan (PO)	Tracleer	Non-selective endothelin receptor antagonist	PAH Improvement in symptoms [16]	Hepatotoxicity, edema Contraindicated in pregnancy

(continued)

TABLE 10.2 (continued)

Medication (generic)	Alternative name(s)	Mechanism of action	Indicated for	Adverse effects
Macitentan (PO)	Opsumit	Non-selective endothelin receptor antagonist	PAH Mortality reduction [17] Group IV/CTEPH Improvement in PVR [18]	Hepatotoxicity, edema
Ambrisentan (PO)	Letairis	Selective endothelin receptor A antagonist	PAH Delayed disease progression [19]	Hepatotoxicity, edema
Epoprostenol (IV, IH)	Flolan; Veletri	Prostacyclin; Adenylate cyclase activation	PAH -Mortality benefit in PAH [20] Hemodynamic benefit in other types of WHO Group I PH [21]	Hypotension (mainly IV form), tachycardia, flushing, headache, ulceration, diarrhea, myalgia, arthralgia, limb pain, jaw pain

Treprostinil (PO, IV, SC, IH)	Remodulin	Prostacyclin analogue; Adenylate cyclase activation	PAH Hemodynamic and symptomatic improvement [22]	Hypotension, headache, diarrhea, nausea, myalgia, arthralgia, flushing, limb pain, jaw pain
Iloprost (IH)	Ventavis	Prostacyclin analog; Adenylate cyclase activation	PAH Improvement in symptoms [23]	Requires frequent administration Headache, diarrhea, nausea, myalgia, flushing, jaw pain
Selexipag (PO)	Uptravi	Non-prostanoid prostacyclin receptor agonist	PAH Reduction in hospitalizations and disease progression [24]	Headache, diarrhea, nausea, myalgia, flushing, jaw pain

Clinical Pearl
Patients with pulmonary hypertension are at high risk from surgical complications. Patients with moderate to severe pulmonary hypertension and/or moderate to severe RV dysfunction should be evaluated by pulmonary hypertension specialist for preoperative optimization recommendations.

Key Learning Points
- New PH warrants a broad evaluation for systemic disorders.
- A PH specialist should be consulted for patients who require initiation or any adjustment to pulmonary vasodilator therapy.
- PH is associated with an increased surgical risk.

References

1. Simonneau G, Montani D, Celermajer DS, Denton CP, Gatzoulis MA, Krowka M, et al. Haemodynamic definitions and updated clinical classification of pulmonary hypertension. Eur Respir J. 2019;53(1). Available from: https://doi.org/10.1183/13993003.01913-2018.
2. Galie N, Humbert M, Vachiery J-L, Gibbs S, Lang I, Torbicki A, et al. ESC/ERS guidelines for the diagnosis and treatment of pulmonary hypertension: web addenda. Eur Respir J. 2015;. Available from: https://orbi.uliege.be/bitstream/2268/188918/1/Web_Addenda_ESC-ERS_PH_Guidelines_ERJ-2015.pdf
3. Frost A, Badesch D, Gibbs JSR, Gopalan D, Khanna D, Manes A, et al. Diagnosis of pulmonary hypertension. Eur Respir J. 2019;53(1). Available from: https://doi.org/10.1183/13993003.01904-2018.
4. Rich S, editor. Primary pulmonary hypertension : exective summary from the World Symposium – Primary Pulmonary

Hypertension. http://www.who.int/ncd/cvd/pph.html [Internet]. 1998 [cited 2019 Jul 21]; Available from: https://ci.nii.ac.jp/naid/10008042523/.

5. van de Veerdonk MC, Kind T, Marcus JT, Mauritz G-J, Heymans MW, Bogaard H-J, et al. Progressive right ventricular dysfunction in patients with pulmonary arterial hypertension responding to therapy. J Am Coll Cardiol. 2011;58(24):2511–9.
6. Ventetuolo CE, Klinger JR. Management of acute right ventricular failure in the intensive care unit. Ann Am Thorac Soc. 2014;11(5):811–22.
7. Shen Y, Wan C, Tian P, Wu Y, Li X, Yang T, et al. CT-base pulmonary artery measurementin the detection of pulmonary hypertension [internet]. Medicine. 2014;93:e256. Available from: https://doi.org/10.1097/md.0000000000000256.
8. MRC Working Party. Long-term domiciliary oxygen therapy in chronic hypoxic cor pulmonale complicating chronic bronchitis. Lancet. 1981;1:681–5.
9. Olsson KM, Delcroix M, Ghofrani HA, Tiede H, Huscher D, Speich R, et al. Anticoagulation and survival in pulmonary arterial hypertension: results from the comparative, prospective registry of newly initiated therapies for pulmonary hypertension (COMPERA). Circulation. 2014;129(1):57–65.
10. Preston IR, Roberts KE, Miller DP, Sen GP, Selej M, Benton WW, et al. Effect of warfarin treatment on survival of patients with pulmonary arterial hypertension (PAH) in the registry to evaluate early and Long-term PAH disease management (REVEAL) [internet]. Circulation. 2015;132:2403–11. Available from: https://doi.org/10.1161/circulationaha.115.018435.
11. Sitbon O, Humbert M, Jaïs X, Ioos V, Hamid AM, Provencher S, et al. Long-term response to calcium channel blockers in idiopathic pulmonary arterial hypertension. Circulation. 2005;111(23):3105–11.
12. Galiè N, Ghofrani HA, Torbicki A, Barst RJ, Rubin LJ, Badesch D, et al. Sildenafil citrate therapy for pulmonary arterial hypertension [Internet]. N Engl J Med. 2005;353:2148–57. Available from: https://doi.org/10.1056/nejmoa050010.
13. Galiè N, Brundage BH, Ghofrani HA, Oudiz RJ, Simonneau G, Safdar Z, et al. Tadalafil therapy for pulmonary arterial hypertension [internet]. Circulation. 2009;119:2894–903. Available from: https://doi.org/10.1161/circulationaha.108.839274.
14. Ghofrani H-A, D'Armini AM, Grimminger F, Hoeper MM, Jansa P, Kim NH, et al. Riociguat for the treatment of chronic

thromboembolic pulmonary hypertension. N Engl J Med. 2013;369(4):319–29.
15. Ghofrani H-A, Grimminger F, Grünig E, Huang Y, Jansa P, Jing Z-C, et al. Predictors of long-term outcomes in patients treated with riociguat for pulmonary arterial hypertension: data from the PATENT-2 open-label, randomised, long-term extension trial. Lancet Respir Med. 2016;4(5):361–71.
16. Rubin LJ, Badesch DB, Barst RJ, Galie N, Black CM, Keogh A, et al. Bosentan therapy for pulmonary arterial hypertension. N Engl J Med. 2002;346(12):896–903.
17. Pulido T, Adzerikho I, Channick RN, Delcroix M, Galiè N, Ghofrani H-A, et al. Macitentan and morbidity and mortality in pulmonary arterial hypertension. N Engl J Med. 2013;369(9):809–18.
18. Ghofrani H-A, Simonneau G, D'Armini AM, Fedullo P, Howard LS, Jaïs X, et al. Macitentan for the treatment of inoperable chronic thromboembolic pulmonary hypertension (MERIT-1): results from the multicentre, phase 2, randomised, double-blind, placebo-controlled study. Lancet Respir Med. 2017;5(10):785–94.
19. Galiè N, Olschewski H, Oudiz RJ, Torres F, Frost A, Ghofrani HA, et al. Ambrisentan for the treatment of pulmonary arterial hypertension [internet]. Circulation. 2008;117:3010–9. Available from: https://doi.org/10.1161/circulationaha.107.742510.
20. Barst RJ, Rubin LJ, Long WA, McGoon MD, Rich S, Badesch DB, et al. A comparison of continuous intravenous epoprostenol (prostacyclin) with conventional therapy for primary pulmonary hypertension. N Engl J Med. 1996;334(5):296–301.
21. McLaughlin VV. Compassionate use of continuous prostacyclin in the Management of Secondary Pulmonary Hypertension: a case series [internet]. Ann Intern Med. 1999;130:740. Available from: https://doi.org/10.7326/0003-4819-130-9-199905040-00014.
22. Jing Z-C, Parikh K, Pulido T, Jerjes-Sanchez C, White RJ, Allen R, et al. Efficacy and safety of oral treprostinil monotherapy for the treatment of pulmonary arterial hypertension: a randomized, controlled trial. Circulation. 2013;127(5):624–33.
23. Olschewski H, Simonneau G, Galiè N, Higenbottam T, Naeije R, Rubin LJ, et al. Inhaled iloprost for severe pulmonary hypertension. N Engl J Med. 2002;347(5):322–9.
24. Sitbon O, Channick R, Chin K, Frey A, Galiè N, Ghofrani H-A, et al. Effect of selexipag on long-term outcomes in key subgroups of patients with pulmonary arterial hypertension (PAH): GRIPHON Study results [internet]. 43 Pulm Circ Pulm Vasc Dis. 2015. Available from: https://doi.org/10.1183/13993003.congress-2015.oa4995.

Chapter 11
Acquired Cardiomyopathies

Nikoloz Shekiladze, Appesh Mohandas, and Priya Kohli

Abbreviations

ACEI	Angiotensin converting enzyme inhibitor
AF	Atrial fibrillation
AF-CM	Atrial fibrillation induced cardiomyopathy
AICM	Arrhythmia-induced cardiomyopathy
AIDS	Autoimmune deficiency syndrome
AL	Amyloid light chain
ARB	Aldosterone receptor blocker
ARNI	Angiotensin receptor neprolysin inhibitor
ASA	Acetyl salicylic acid (Aspirin)
AT	Atrial tachycardia
ATTR	Transthyretin

N. Shekiladze (✉) · A. Mohandas
Department of Cardiology, Emory University School of Medicine, Atlanta, GA, USA
e-mail: nshekil@emory.edu; Mohandasamohand@emory.edu

P. Kohli
Department of Cardiology, Emory University School of Medicine, Atlanta VA Medical Center, Decatur, GA, USA

B. J. Wells et al. (eds.), *Handbook of Inpatient Cardiology*,
https://doi.org/10.1007/978-3-030-47868-1_11

AV	Atrioventricular
BB	Beta blocker
BNP	Brain natriuretic peptide
CABG	Coronary artery bypass surgery
CAD	Coronary artery disease
CCB	Calcium channel blocker
CM	Cardiomyopathy
CMR	Cardiac magnetic resonance
CRT-D	Cardiac resynchronization therapy – defibrillator
CRT-P	Cardiac resynchronization therapy – pacemaker
DCM	Dilated cardiomyopathy
ECG	Electrocardiogram
EMB	Endomyocardial biopsy
ETOH	Ethanol
FDA	Food and drug administration
FDG	Fluorodeoxyglucose
GCM	Giant cell myocarditis
GDMT	Guideline-directed medical therapy
HCM	Hypertrophic cardiomyopathy
HCTZ	Hydrochlorothiazide
HF	Heart failure
HFpEF	Heart failure with preserved ejection fraction
HFrEF	Heart failure with reduced ejection fraction
HIV	Human immunodeficiency virus
HTN	Hypertension
HTN-CM	Hypertension induced cardiomyopathy
ICD	Implantable cardioverter-defibrillator
ICM	Ischemic cardiomyopathy
LV	Left ventricle
LVEF	Left ventricular ejection fraction
LVH	Left ventricular hypertrophy
MRA	Mineralocorticoid receptor antagonist
NYHA	New York Heart Association
PAN	Polyarteritis nodosa
PCI	Percutaneous coronary intervention
PET	Positron emission tomography
PVC	Paroxysmal ventricular contraction

PVC-CM	Paroxysmal ventricular contraction induced cardiomyopathy
RA	Rheumatoid arthritis
RCT	Randomized controlled trial
RFA	Radiofrequency ablation
RVR	Rapid ventricular response
SLE	Systemic lupus erythematosus
SPECT	Single proton emission computer tomography
T-CM	Tachycardia medicated cardiomyopathy
TTE	Transthoracic echocardiography
VEGF	Vascular endothelia growth factors
VT	Ventricular tachycardia
WMA	Wall motion abnormality

Ischemic Cardiomyopathy

- The term ischemic cardiomyopathy (ICM) has been defined as LV systolic dysfunction with one or more of the following criteria:
  - History of prior myocardial revascularization or myocardial infarction
  - More than 75% stenosis in the left main or left anterior descending arteries
  - Two vessels or more with a greater than 75% stenosis [3]
- ICM encompasses a spectrum of pathophysiological states, including myocardial stunning, hibernation, and scarring.
  - Hibernating (also known as "viable") myocardium describes cells that are still alive with some preservation of membrane integrity and metabolic activity.
  - Hibernating myocardium is an adaptation to repetitive ischemia and can only be established by functional recovery following revascularization [4].
  - Myocardial stunning is a state of reversible hypocontractility that persists despite restoration of blood flow following transient or recurrent ischemia [5].

  - Patients with viable myocardium who are treated medically have increased mortality, and the number of viable segments will decrease over time [6].
- Imaging assessing viability: assessment of viability
  - 20–50% of patients with chronic ischemic left ventricular dysfunction have a significant amount of viable myocardium with the potential for clinical important improvement in LV function after revascularization [6].
  - Modalities of viability assessment include SPECT, PET, CMR, and DSE

Clinical Pearl
In a sub-study of the STICH trial, patients with myocardial viability had lower overall mortality, but revascularization was not associated with mortality benefit. Routine viability assessment prior to surgery is not recommended but should be assessed on case by case basis [7].

Treatment

- GDMT: ASA, high-intensity statin, BB, ACEI, ARNI, MRA, hydralazine + nitrate in African American, loop diuretic, ivabradine (in selected populations)
- The STICH trial compared surgical revascularization with medical therapy in patients with LVEF of 35% or less and CAD amenable to CABG [8]. Patients with critical left main coronary disease or unstable coronary syndromes were excluded from the trial.
- At 56 months, medical therapy plus CABG resulted in trend toward improvement in the primary outcome of all-cause mortality. In extended follow-up (9.8 years), all-cause mortality was lower in the CABG group (STITCHES 2016) [8].
- *Device therapy*:

- Cardiac resynchronization therapy: QRS > 140 msec, LBBB
- Implantable cardioverter-defibrillator (ICD): EF < 35%

Arrhythmia-Induced CMP (AICM)

- Common types: Tachycardia-medicated CM (T-CM), atrial fibrillation-induced CM (AF-CM), and premature ventricular contraction (PVC)-induced CM (PVC-CM).
  - T-CM: reversible LV dysfunction due to increase in ventricular rates regardless of origin of tachycardia [9].

    T-CM can manifest in the setting of either an incessant or paroxysmal tachycardia.

    Supraventricular arrhythmias are the most common etiology (AF and atrial flutter with RVR).

    Other arrhythmias are less common causes: incessant or very frequent paroxysmal AT, persistent atrioventricular (AV)-reciprocating tachycardia and AV nodal re-entrant tachycardia, sustained sinus tachycardia, frequent ventricular tachycardias (idiopathic, bundle branch, and fascicular), and pacemaker-mediated tachycardia.

    T-CM has been reported to present weeks, months, or years after the onset of tachycardia [10].

> **Clinical Pearl**
> Cessation of tachycardia results in normalization of right atrial and arterial pressure with significant recovery of LVEF and cardiac output by 48 h, and full normalization after 1–2 weeks, although some changes such as fibrosis appear to persist despite elimination of the tachycardia and normalization of LV function [11].

An ambulatory ECG monitor for at least a 2-week period is important to confirm or exclude T-CM. TTE or cardiac MRI can assist in excluding other etiologies.

Final diagnosis of T-CM can be only confirmed after recovery or improvement of LV systolic function within 1–6 months after elimination of the tachyarrhythmia.

In addition to optimization of medical therapy for LV systolic dysfunction, treatment consists of suppression of tachycardia based on the culprit arrhythmia (antiarrhythmics (AAs)) and/or RFA.

The recovery of T-CM is not always complete, although treatment should not be discouraged as it may have small yet significant benefits.

- AF-CM: Distinguishing whether AF is the cause or the result of a cardiomyopathy can be a clinical challenge.

  Restoration of sinus rhythm should be considered if AF-CM is suspected.

  AF ablation has been reported to achieve sinus rhythm from 50% to 88% in both paroxysmal and persistent AF patients with HF and CM.
- PVC-CM: The minimum PVC burden that appears to result in cardiomyopathy is 10% [13].

  The proposed mechanisms underlying PVC-induced cardiomyopathy include ventricular dyssynchrony and increased myocardial oxygen demand.

  Patients with PVC-CM are typically young and healthy with no prior cardiac history and have >10,000 to >20,000 PVCs per 24 hours.

  The PVCs have an outflow tract or fascicular morphology.

  LV function improves with PVC suppression or radiofrequency ablation [10].

  Ablation is often considered if the PVC burden is >25%.

Giant Cell Myocarditis (GCM)

- Aggressive, noninfectious autoimmune disorder that is rapidly fatal without advanced HF treatment and multidrug immunosuppression.
- Requires histological or immunohistological confirmation by EMB, surgical heart specimens, or an autopsy.

- Clinical course in GCM usually characterized by acute or fulminant deterioration in left ventricular systolic function (75% of cases), frequent ventricular arrhythmias (14%), and heart block (5%) [12].
- It is attributed to a T-lymphocyte-mediated inflammation of the heart muscle and is associated with systemic autoimmune diseases (20%) [13].
- Prognosis is poor. The median survival from onset of symptoms is 5.5 months [14].
- Treatment with immunosuppressive agents may improve prognosis.

Loeffler's Endocarditis

- Loeffler endocarditis is characterized by eosinophilia, myocardial fibrosis, systemic thromboembolism, and acute HF.
- Occurs when overproduction of eosinophils leads to myocardial damage through infiltration and release of inflammatory cytokines [15].
- Hypereosinophilia may occur because of a primary process (hypereosinophilic syndrome) or it may be secondary to an allergy (particularly drug or vaccination), neoplastic process, or parasitic infection.
- Diagnosis of hypereosinophilic syndrome is made in the presence of eosinophils >1500/μL.
- Echocardiography and MRI can be helpful in the diagnosis of eosinophilic myocarditis.
- Corticosteroid therapy is generally considered primary therapy for eosinophilic myocarditis, but its efficacy is not well supported.

Autoimmune Cardiomyopathy

- These are rare causes of cardiomyopathy and HF.
- Proposed mechanisms: immune-mediated myocarditis, progressive fibrosis, and apoptosis with resultant restric-

tive and dilated phenotypes, and progressive atherosclerosis with subsequent ischemic cardiomyopathy [16].

- Most common associations: systemic lupus erythematosus (SLE), scleroderma, RA, dermatomyositis, and polyarteritis nodosa (PAN)
- There are three main mechanisms for SLE-induced HF:
  - Atherosclerosis
  - Myocarditis/inflammation
  - Drug-induced impairments from SLE treatment
- SLE leads to a 2- to 10-fold higher risk of MI and CAD than for age-matched control subjects, with greater risk among younger patients [17].
- Standard workup for cardiomyopathy does not help delineate SLE as the cause, but echocardiography, ECG, and coronary angiography are still recommended. EMB is nonspecific, with an increase in interstitial connective tissue and myocardial scarring.
- Treatment of SLE-HF is dependent on the underlying cause:
  - Myocarditis: pulse-dose steroids followed by high-dose prednisone [18].
  - Atherosclerosis: standard PCI vs. medical management.

Scleroderma

- Pulmonary hypertension and restrictive physiology are more common.
- Possibly due to intermittent vascular spasm with intramyocardial Raynaud's phenomenon.
- Progressive systemic sclerosis can lead to conduction abnormalities, arrhythmias, HF, angina pectoris with normal coronary arteries, myocardial fibrosis, pericarditis, and sudden death.
- Late-contrast enhancement with gadolinium can be used to characterize patchy fibrosis and myocardial edema interspersed with normal myocardium in scleroderma [19].
- Diagnosis is often based on a high clinical suspicion.

- An EMB can be useful if there is suspicion of acute myocarditis, given reports of favorable response to intravenous methylprednisolone.
- No specific treatments are available for scleroderma-induced HF.
- Cardiac transplantation can be considered if the systemic burden of scleroderma is low [20].

Chagas

- 50,000 people die of Chagas disease each year [21].
- *Trypanosoma cruzi*, the causative organism, is transmitted by insects common in Latin America. Symptomatic chronic Chagas disease develops in approximately 10%–30% of infected people. DCM is a late manifestation of the disease and is generally seen during the chronic phase.
- Acute Chagas disease is usually a mild illness with a low case-fatality rate.
  - Heart is often heavily parasitized.
  - Severe myocarditis develops in a small proportion of patients.
- Widespread lymphocytic infiltration is often seen in cardiac tissue, as well as diffuse interstitial fibrosis of myocardial cells.
- The conduction system is often affected: RBBB, LAFB, or complete AV block can be seen.
- Death usually results from rhythm disturbances or progressive HF.
- Efficacy of pharmacologic therapy targeted to *T. cruzii* is limited [21].

HIV

- In the pre-highly active antiretroviral therapy era, 40% of initially asymptomatic HIV-positive patients were diagnosed with DCM with significantly depressed LVEF during the 5-year follow-up.

- The incidence of DCM was higher among patients with AIDS or low CD4 counts [22].
- Symptomatic HF is seen in approximately one-half of these patients with myocardial involvement.
- Other than the treatment for HIV, the treatment of HF in patients with symptomatic HIV cardiomyopathy is the same as the conventional treatment for patients with DCM.
- The prognosis of HIV cardiomyopathy when untreated remains poor, with a >50% mortality rate in 2–3 years [23]

HTN

- HTN causes diastolic dysfunction via increased LV wall thickness, ischemia, and hypertrophy [24].
- Some patients progress from HFpEF to HFrEF. MI can propagate this transition [25].
- TTE is integral to diagnosis [24].
  - LVH (40% hypertensive patients)
  - Diastolic dysfunction (50%)
- If LV wall thickness is ≥15 mm, other etiologies of LVH, such as amyloid or hypertrophic cardiomyopathy, should also be considered [33].
- MRI with and without contrast may be useful in distinguishing HTN-CM from HCM or amyloidosis [26].
- Treatment: In addition to GDMT, anti-hypertensives (ACEI and HCTZ, for example) reduce LV mass and reverse remodeling. Weight loss and sodium restriction should also be counseled [24].

Amyloid

- Most commonly due to AL or ATTR (transthyretin) proteins [27].
  - Distinction between these is crucial as it affects treatment and prognosis [28].

- Typically presents as diastolic dysfunction first; systolic dysfunction can occur later. May present with arrhythmias: atrial fibrillation, heart block [29].
- ECG: rather than low voltage, consider whether voltage on ECG is less than expected for the degree of LVH. If so, this may be consistent with cardiac amyloidosis [30] (See Fig. 11.1).
- Labs: skewed serum-free light chains and characteristic serum and urine immunofixation suggest AL amyloidosis in the correct context. These labs are normal in ATTR amyloidosis [31]. BNP and troponin can be elevated in either case and are prognostic [32].
- TTE: LVH, often >1.4 cm especially in ATTR; relative apical sparing on TTE strain imaging [33]. See Figs. 11.2, 11.3, and 11.4.

Clinical Pearl

Nuclear imaging: Tc99 pyrophosphate scan is highly sensitive and specific for ATTR amyloidosis [38]. This test is noninvasive and relatively inexpensive

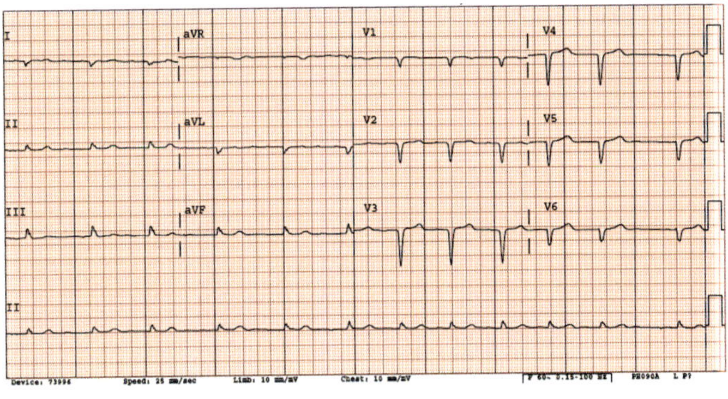

FIGURE 11.1 ECG demonstrates atrial fibrillation, low voltage in limb leads, left posterior fascicular block, poor R wave progression ("pseudo-infarct pattern")

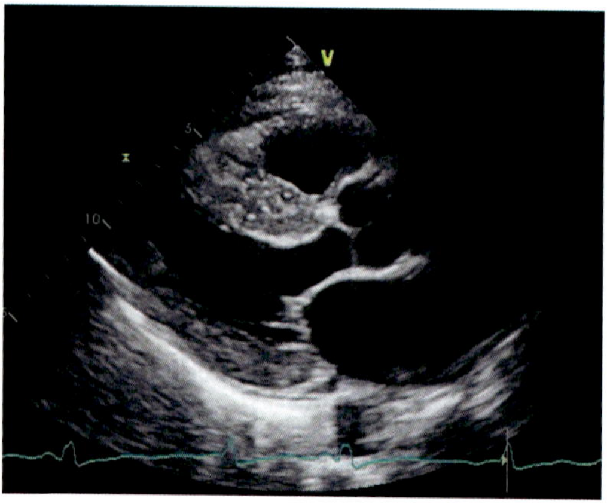

FIGURE 11.2 Parasternal long axis view of the heart demonstrating left ventricular hypertrophy and speckled pattern of myocardium "classic" for cardiac amyloidosis

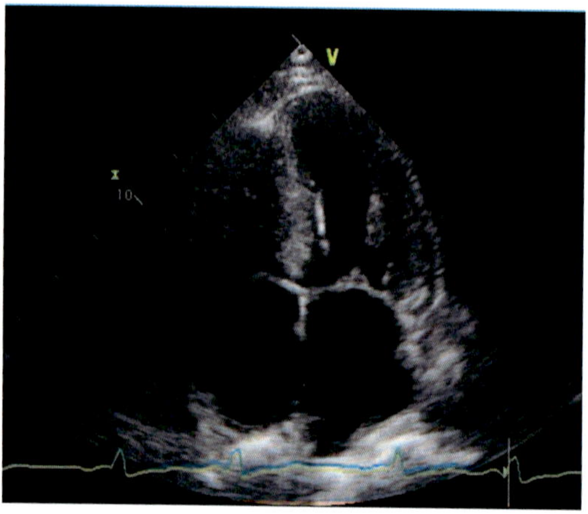

FIGURE 11.3 Apical 4 chamber view of the heart demonstrating thick left ventricle and biatrial enlargement

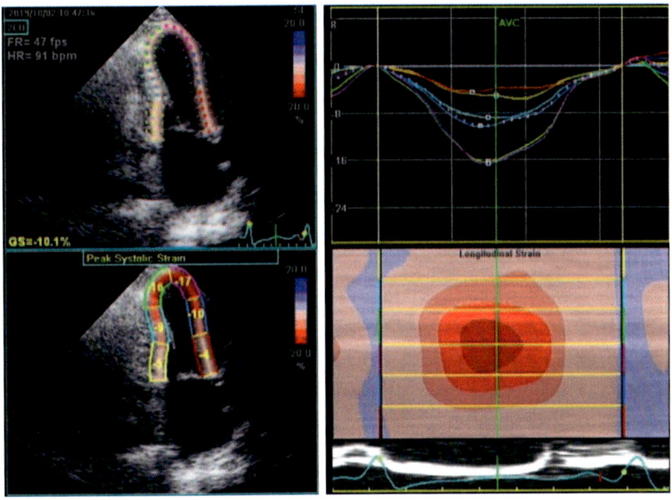

FIGURE 11.4 Longitudinal strain bull's eye plot pattern with relative apical sparing in patient with cardiac amyloidosis

- Endomyocardial biopsy is still the gold-standard of diagnosis.
- MRI may suggest cardiac amyloidosis (delayed gadolinium enhancement, "failure to null") but may not differentiate subtype [34].
- AL has a prognosis of months even with chemotherapy and less once cardiac symptoms develop. ATTR has a prognosis of close to 6 years [28]. ATTR may masquerade as HFpEF [30]
- Treatment [35]
  - Both subtypes: Diuretics are mainstay. Aldosterone antagonists may be tolerated. CCB, BB, and high-dose ACEI/ARB may not be well tolerated. Digoxin may have further increased toxicity.
  - AF is common as are intracardiac thrombi.
  - AL: referral to hematologist for chemotherapy.

ATTR Clinical Pearl
Tafamidis is FDA approved; can decrease symptoms and prolong survival in NYHA I–III patients.

Sarcoidosis

- More common in African Americans and those <55 years old [15].
- Up to 25% of patients with systemic sarcoidosis may have cardiac disease as confirmed by MRI, but only 2–5% are symptomatic [36].
- Characterized by the presence of noncaseating granulomas [15].
- Clinical features vary by the location and activity of granulomas [37]: asymptomatic to sudden cardiac death.
- Arrhythmia (especially atrial but also VT), heart block (with syncope) and HF are common presentations.
- ACE levels elevated in 60% of patients with active sarcoidosis but not sensitive or specific for diagnosis or activity.
- TTE usually abnormal in active symptomatic disease: systolic or diastolic dysfunction, WMA.
- Cardiac biopsy: negative result does not rule it out due to patchy involvement.
- MRI is the test of choice: Late gadolinium enhancement, early granuloma enhancement on T2.
- FDG PET may be able to detect metabolically active granulomas [15, 36, 37].
- Treatment with corticosteroids: 40–60 mg prednisone tapered slowly over months [15, 37].
  - 5-year survival is ~50%.
  - Treat HF with GDMT.
  - ICD may be reasonable in patients with cardiac sarcoidosis.

ETOH/Toxin/Drug [15, 38]

- Alcoholic CM is one of the most common etiologies of acquired CM.
- Usually patients have been heavy drinkers for >10 years with >100 g/day.
- Development of alcoholic CM depends on total intake and can be influenced by genetics.
- Abstinence and initiation of HF GDMT are recommended treatment and recovery of EF is not uncommon, but prognosis remains poor.
- Thiamine and folate should be supplemented in appropriate patients.
- Cocaine-related CM can be present in the absence of CAD. Standard HFrEF therapy can be used (including beta blockers) in patients with >6 months abstinence.
- In active or relapsed cocaine users, using non-selective beta-blockers may be safer.
- Methamphetamines can cause cardiomyopathy. Abstinence and GDMT may lead to recovery.

Chemotherapeutic Agents [15, 39]

- All patients should have robust screening and optimization of underlying cardiac disease prior to initiating chemotherapy.
- Anthracycline agents were initially thought to cause cardiotoxicity only at high doses, but recent data suggests any dose can cause cardiomyopathy.
  - Risk is greater with doses >500 mg/m^2.
  - Early recognition and initiation of HF therapy can reverse cardiomyopathy.
- Trastuzumab, VEGF inhibitors, bortezomib, and carfilzomib can cause cardiomyopathy in some patients
  - Reversal of HF is likely with HF GDMT.

Clinical Pearl
Cardiotoxicity due to chemotherapy is defined as a decline in LVEF of at least 5–10% to a level < 55% with symptoms of HF

Stress-Induced Cardiomyopathy (Takotsubo Cardiomyopathy)

- Transient LV dysfunction due to an emotional trigger.
- Typically seen in women over age 50.
- Presentation tends to mimic acute MI including ST elevation and troponin leak.
- Diagnosis [15]
  - Apical ballooning of the left ventricle is often seen on imaging.
  - Regional wall motion abnormalities involve more than one epicardial coronary artery.
  - Angiography rules out coronary obstruction or plaque rupture.
  - Pheochromocytoma or myocarditis are ruled out.
- In-hospital mortality can be as high as 4.5% [40].
- Recovery is often rapid, with many patients having resolution of LVEF in about 7 days.
- Treatment is generally supportive with little evidence for HF GDMT.

Iron-Overload CM [41]

- Genetic: hereditary hemochromatosis (White Americans, Northern Europeans)
- Acquired: transfusions in beta-thalassemia major (people of Mediterranean descent)
- Diagnose iron overload

- Transferrin saturation > 45% and ferritin >200–300 μg/L in men or 150–200 μg/L in women
- Cardiac MRI: T2 signal correlates with iron infiltration

- Treatment
  - HF should be treated with GDMT
  - Phlebotomy is used when possible, and chelation is used when anemia is present

Peripartum cardiomyopathy: Please see Chap. 22: Pregnancy and Heart Disease

Key Learning Points

- An accurate diagnosis is crucial to, and may dramatically impact, success of treatment.
- With early detection and initiation of treatment, many cardiomyopathies can be reversed or improved.
- ATTR amyloidosis is emerging as a previously underappreciated cause of HFpEF and can be mistaken for hypertensive CM. FDA-approved treatments are now available.

References

1. Zipes D. In: Falk R, editor. Braunwald's Heart disease. Philadelphia: Elsevier; 2019.
2. Knowlton KU. Dilated cardiomyopathy. Circulation. 2019;139(20): 2339–41.
3. Briceno N, Schuster A, Lumley M, Perera D. Ischaemic cardiomyopathy: pathophysiology, assessment and the role of revascularisation. Heart. 2016;102(5):397–406.
4. Camici PG, Prasad SK, Rimoldi OE. Stunning, hibernation, and assessment of myocardial viability. Circulation. 2008;117(1):103–14.
5. Bolli R. Oxygen-derived free radicals and postischemic myocardial dysfunction ("stunned myocardium"). J Am Coll Cardiol. 1988;12(1):239–49.

6. Allman KC, Shaw LJ, Hachamovitch R, Udelson JE. Myocardial viability testing and impact of revascularization on prognosis in patients with coronary artery disease and left ventricular dysfunction: a meta-analysis. J Am Coll Cardiol. 2002;39(7):1151–8.
7. Bonow RO, Maurer G, Lee KL, Holly TA, Binkley PF, Desvigne-Nickens P, et al. Myocardial viability and survival in ischemic left ventricular dysfunction. N Engl J Med. 2011;364(17):1617–25.
8. Velazquez EJ, Lee KL, Deja MA, Jain A, Sopko G, Marchenko A, et al. Coronary-artery bypass surgery in patients with left ventricular dysfunction. N Engl J Med. 2011;364(17):1607–16.
9. Huizar JF, Ellenbogen KA, Tan AY, Kaszala K. Arrhythmia-induced cardiomyopathy: JACC state-of-the-art review. J Am Coll Cardiol. 2019;73(18):2328–44.
10. Watanabe H, Okamura K, Chinushi M, Furushima H, Tanabe Y, Kodama M, et al. Clinical characteristics, treatment, and outcome of tachycardia induced cardiomyopathy. Int Heart J. 2008;49(1):39–47.
11. Ling LH, Kalman JM, Ellims AH, Iles LM, Medi C, Sherratt C, et al. Diffuse ventricular fibrosis is a late outcome of tachycardia-mediated cardiomyopathy after successful ablation. Circ Arrhythm Electrophysiol. 2013;6(4):697–704.
12. Cooper LT Jr, Berry GJ, Shabetai R. Idiopathic giant-cell myocarditis--natural history and treatment. Multicenter Giant cell myocarditis study group investigators. N Engl J Med. 1997;336(26):1860–6.
13. Rosenstein ED, Zucker MJ, Kramer N. Giant cell myocarditis: most fatal of autoimmune diseases. Semin Arthritis Rheum. 2000;30(1):1–16.
14. Mason JW, O'Connell JB, Herskowitz A, Rose NR, McManus BM, Billingham ME, et al. A clinical trial of immunosuppressive therapy for myocarditis. The myocarditis treatment trial investigators. N Engl J Med. 1995;333(5):269–75.
15. Bozkurt B, Colvin M, Cook J, Cooper LT, Deswal A, Fonarow GC, et al. Current diagnostic and treatment strategies for specific dilated cardiomyopathies: a scientific statement from the American Heart Association. Circulation. 2016;134(23):e579–646.
16. Hollan I, Meroni PL, Ahearn JM, Cohen Tervaert JW, Curran S, Goodyear CS, et al. Cardiovascular disease in autoimmune rheumatic diseases. Autoimmun Rev. 2013;12(10):1004–15.
17. Schoenfeld SR, Kasturi S, Costenbader KH. The epidemiology of atherosclerotic cardiovascular disease among patients with SLE: a systematic review. Semin Arthritis Rheum. 2013;43(1):77–95.

18. Doherty NE, Siegel RJ. Cardiovascular manifestations of systemic lupus erythematosus. Am Heart J. 1985;110(6):1257–65.
19. Tzelepis GE, Kelekis NL, Plastiras SC, Mitseas P, Economopoulos N, Kampolis C, et al. Pattern and distribution of myocardial fibrosis in systemic sclerosis: a delayed enhanced magnetic resonance imaging study. Arthritis Rheum. 2007;56(11):3827–36.
20. Martens E, Lange P, Pohl T, Nickel T, Juchem G, Kaczmarek I, et al. Heart transplantation in a 36-year-old experiencing terminal heart failure caused by systemic sclerosis. Transplantation. 2012;94(2):e13–5.
21. Rossi MA, Bestetti RB. The challenge of chagasic cardiomyopathy. The pathologic roles of autonomic abnormalities, autoimmune mechanisms and microvascular changes, and therapeutic implications. Cardiology. 1995;86(1):1–7.
22. Barbaro G, Di Lorenzo G, Grisorio B, Barbarini G. Incidence of dilated cardiomyopathy and detection of HIV in myocardial cells of HIV-positive patients. Gruppo Italiano per lo studio Cardiologico Dei Pazienti Affetti da AIDS. N Engl J Med. 1998;339(16):1093–9.
23. Grody WW, Cheng L, Lewis W. Infection of the heart by the human immunodeficiency virus. Am J Cardiol. 1990;66(2):203–6.
24. Kuroda K, Kato TS, Amano A. Hypertensive cardiomyopathy: a clinical approach and literature review. World J Hypertens. 2015;5(2):41–52.
25. Weintraub RG, Semsarian C, Macdonald P. Dilated cardiomyopathy. Lancet. 2017;390(10092):400–14.
26. Takeda M, Amano Y, Tachi M, Tani H, Mizuno K, Kumita S. MRI differentiation of cardiomyopathy showing left ventricular hypertrophy and heart failure: differentiation between cardiac amyloidosis, hypertrophic cardiomyopathy, and hypertensive heart disease. Jpn J Radiol. 2013;31(10):693–700.
27. Lee S-P, Park J-B, Kim H-K, Kim Y-J, Grogan M, Sohn D-W. Contemporary imaging diagnosis of cardiac amyloidosis. J Cardiovasc Imaging. 2019;27(1):1–10.
28. Pinney JH, Whelan CJ, Petrie A, Dungu J, Banypersad SM, Sattianayagam P, et al. Senile systemic amyloidosis: clinical features at presentation and outcome. J Am Heart Assoc. 2013;2(2):e000098.
29. Lane T, Fontana M, Martinez-Naharro A, Quarta CC, Whelan CJ, Petrie A, et al. Natural history, quality of life, and outcome in cardiac transthyretin amyloidosis. Circulation. 2019;140(1):16–26.

30. González-López E, Gallego-Delgado M, Guzzo-Merello G, de Haro-del Moral FJ, Cobo-Marcos M, Robles C, et al. Wild-type transthyretin amyloidosis as a cause of heart failure with preserved ejection fraction. Eur Heart J. 2015;36(38):2585–94.
31. Gillmore JD, Maurer MS, Falk RH, Merlini G, Damy T, Dispenzieri A, et al. Nonbiopsy diagnosis of cardiac transthyretin amyloidosis. Circulation. 2016;133(24):2404–12.
32. Pereira NL, Grogan M, Dec GW. Spectrum of restrictive and infiltrative cardiomyopathies: part 1 of a 2-part series. J Am Coll Cardiol. 2018;71(10):1130–48.
33. Pagourelias ED, Mirea O, Duchenne J, Van Cleemput J, Delforge M, Bogaert J, et al. Echo parameters for differential diagnosis in cardiac amyloidosis: a head-to-head comparison of deformation and nondeformation parameters. Circ Cardiovasc Imaging. 2017;10(3):e005588.
34. Gertz MA, Benson MD, Dyck PJ, Grogan M, Coelho T, Cruz M, et al. Diagnosis, prognosis, and therapy of transthyretin amyloidosis. J Am Coll Cardiol. 2015;66(21):2451–66.
35. Emdin M, Aimo A, Rapezzi C, Fontana M, Perfetto F, Seferović PM, et al. Treatment of cardiac transthyretin amyloidosis: an update. Eur Heart J. 2019:40(45):ehz298.
36. Youssef G, Beanlands RSB, Birnie DH, Nery PB. Cardiac sarcoidosis: applications of imaging in diagnosis and directing treatment. Heart. 2011;97(24):2078–87.
37. Doughan AR. Cardiac sarcoidosis. Heart. 2006;92(2):282–8.
38. Fernández-Solà J. Cardiovascular risks and benefits of moderate and heavy alcohol consumption. Nat Rev Cardiol. 2015;12(10):576–87.
39. Lenneman CG, Sawyer DB. Cardio-oncology: an update on cardiotoxicity of cancer-related treatment. Circ Res. 2016;118(6):1008–20.
40. Singh K, Carson K, Shah R, Sawhney G, Singh B, Parsaik A, et al. Meta-analysis of clinical correlates of acute mortality in Takotsubo cardiomyopathy. Am J Cardiol. 2014;113(8):1420–8.
41. Díez-López C, Comín-Colet J, González-Costello J. Iron overload cardiomyopathy: from diagnosis to management. Curr Opin Cardiol. 2018;33(3):334–40.

Chapter 12
Cardiogenic Shock and Advanced Heart Failure Therapies

Mohsin Chowdhury and Pablo A. Quintero

Introduction

- Cardiogenic shock (CS) is a state of cellular and tissue hypoxia due to hypoperfusion mediated by a low-cardiac-output state.
- Hemodynamic definition of CS includes persistent hypotension (systolic blood pressure <90 mm Hg or mean arterial pressure 30 mm Hg lower than baseline) with severe reduction in cardiac index (<2.2 L/min/m^2) and elevated filling pressures [1].
- CS is often associated with multisystem organ failure and has a high mortality rate (in-hospital mortality 27–51%).
- Patients present with signs of clinical hypoperfusion including cold extremities, oliguria, mental confusion, dizziness, and a narrow pulse pressure and often have labora-

M. Chowdhury (✉) · P. A. Quintero
Cardiovascular Medicine, Beth Israel Deaconess Medical Center/Harvard Medical School, Boston, MA, USA
e-mail: mchowdhu@bidmc.harvard.edu

B. J. Wells et al. (eds.), *Handbook of Inpatient Cardiology*,
https://doi.org/10.1007/978-3-030-47868-1_12

tory signs of hypoperfusion (metabolic acidosis, elevated serum lactate, elevated serum creatinine, and elevated transaminases).

Hemodynamics

See Chap. 32 for details on right heart catheterization.

- Patients with CS are characterized by low cardiac output (CO)/cardiac index (CI), elevated systemic vascular resistance (SVR), and high filling pressures (↑ central venous pressure and/or ↑ pulmonary capillary wedge pressure (PCWP))
- As summarized in Table 12.1, there are several phenotypes of CS, with "cold and wet" being the most common.

Clinical Pearl
Among the three phenotypes of cardiogenic shock, "cold and wet" is the most common.

TABLE 12.1 Phenotypes of cardiogenic shock

		Volume status	
		Wet	Dry
Afterload	Cold	Classic cardiogenic shock (↓CI, ↑SVR, ↑CVP/PCWP)	Euvolemic cardiogenic shock (↓CO/CI, ↑SVR, ↔CVP/PCWP)
	Warm	Vasodilatory cardiogenic shock ("mixed" shock) (↓CI, ↓/↔SVR, ↑CVP/PCWP)	Non-cardiogenic shock (↑CI, ↓SVR, ↓CVP/PCWP)

CI cardiac index, *SVR* systemic vascular resistance, *CVP* central venous pressure, *PCWP* pulmonary capillary wedge pressure

Etiologies

- Most common cause of CS is acute coronary syndrome (ACS) (as many as 81% of patients presenting with CS had underlying ACS [2]). Other common causes are summarized in Table 12.2.

> **Clinical Pearl**
> Acute coronary syndrome is the most common cause of cardiogenic shock (CS). Unless another underlying etiology has been identified, all patients presenting with CS should undergo evaluation for coronary artery disease.

Table 12.2 Etiologies of cardiogenic shock

Complications of acute myocardial infarction	Papillary muscle rupture
	Ventricular septal rupture
	Free wall rupture
Acute decompensated heart failure	Chronic heart failure (known etiology) with acute decompensation
	Dilated cardiomyopathy
	Myocarditis
	Stress-induced cardiomyopathy (Takotsubo)
	Peripartum cardiomyopathy
	Coronary artery dissection
	Post-cardiotomy shock

(continued)

TABLE 12.2 (continued)

Valvular heart disease	Stenosis
	Acute regurgitation
	Valvular obstruction
	Mechanical failure of prosthetic valves
Arrhythmia	Atrial arrhythmia with rapid ventricular rate
	Bradycardia
	Ventricular tachycardia
Extracardiac/obstructive	Cardiac tamponade
	Constriction
	Pulmonary embolism
Other	Aortic dissection
	Toxidromes
	Hypothermic myocardial depression
	Hypo-/hyperthyroidism
	Pheochromocytoma
	Myocardial depression in setting of septic shock
	Myocardial contusion
	Post-cardiac arrest stunning

Evaluation

After or concurrent to initial hemodynamic resuscitation and stabilization, comprehensive work-up should be pursued to identify the underlying etiology.

- CBC (with differential), comprehensive metabolic panel, TSH, lactic acid, atrial blood gas, troponin, NT-proBNP (or BNP).
- Resting 12-lead ECG.
- Chest X-ray (provides information on cardiac size, pulmonary congestion, and may suggest alternative pathology).
- Comprehensive transthoracic echocardiogram (TTE). Consider transesophageal echocardiogram if TTE images are inadequate or diagnosis remains uncertain.
- Although studies on benefit of pulmonary artery catheter (PAC) in CS are mixed, PAC remains an important diagnostic and management tool especially for patients with diagnostic or therapeutic uncertainty and those being considered for advanced therapies. PAC can confirm the presence and severity of CS, RV involvement, and pulmonary pressures and offer real-time, objective feedback on response to interventions.

Clinical Pearl
Consider early right heart catheterization and placement of leave-in PAC in patients with diagnostic or therapeutic uncertainty

Management

- Goal of therapy should focus on addressing the underlying cause and restoring and maintaining satisfactory tissue perfusion.
- If acute MI is the underlying cause, baring contraindications, coronary reperfusion should be pursued emergently (see Chap. 1). There is improved 6-month mortality with emergency revascularization (vs initial medical stabilization and delayed revascularization) for acute MI complicated by CS (SHOCK, *NEJM* 1999 [3]).

- Avoid β-blockers and renin-angiotensin-aldosterone system (RAAS) antagonists.
- Inotropes and vasopressors are frequently used for the management of CS, although outcome data is sparse. Typical target mean arterial blood pressure goal should be >65 mm Hg. Table 12.3 summarizes the mechanism of action, usual infusion dose, hemodynamic effects, and special considerations for commonly used vasopressors and inotropes. Efforts should be made to minimize the number of agents and their dose.
- Patients on monoamine oxidase inhibitors are extremely sensitive to vasopressors and therefore require lower than usual dose.
- Although there is paucity of high-quality evidence to support the routine use of mechanical circulatory support (MCS) devices, patients with persistent CS should undergo evaluation by multidisciplinary team for considerations for MCS [4]. Figure 12.1 summarizes potential management pathway for CS. Palliation should be considered during each of these steps.
- Temporary MCS can be used as a bridge to recovery, bridge to decision, bridge to durable ventricular assist device (VAD), or bridge to transplant (BTT) in appropriately selected patients with CS, whereas durable VAD is used as BTT or as destination VAD.
- Table 12.4 summarizes the relative merits of currently available MCS devices. MCS device selection should be based on availability, multidisciplinary team familiarity, and patient-specific needs.

Clinical Pearl

Although inotropes and vasopressors remain a cornerstone of management of CS, due to their deleterious effects, the number of agents and dose should be minimized.

Table 12.3 Mechanism of action, usual infusion dose, hemodynamic effects, and special considerations for commonly used vasopressors and inotropes

Drug	Usual dose	Receptor binding				Hemodynamic effects	Special considerations
		α_1	β_1	β_2	Dopaminergic		
Phenylephrine	0.1–10 μg/kg/min	+++	–	–	–	↑↑SVR	Preferred over other vasopressors in patients with aortic stenosis, mitral stenosis, and dynamic LVOT obstruction
Vasopressin	0.02–0.04 units/min	Stimulates V_1 receptors in vascular smooth muscle				↑↑SVR, ↔PVR	
Norepinephrine	0.05–0.4 μg/kg/min	++++	++	+	–	↑CO, ↑SVR	
Epinephrine	0.01–0.5 μg/kg/min	++++	++++	+++	–	↑↑CO, ↑↑SVR	
Dopamine	0.5–2 μg/kg/min	–	+	–	+++	↑CO	Dysrhythmias occur commonly Subgroup analysis showed increased mortality (compared to norepinephrine) with use in CS (SOAP II, *NEJM* 2010 [5]).
	2–5 μg/kg/min	Variable				Variable	
	5–10 μg/kg/min	+	+++	+	++	↑↑CO, ↑SVR	
	10–20 μg/kg/min	+++	++	–	++	↑CO, ↑↑SVR	

(continued)

Table 12.3 (continued)

Drug	Usual dose	Receptor binding				Hemodynamic effects	Special considerations
		α_1	β_1	β_2	Dopaminergic		
Dobutamine	2.5–20 μg/kg/min	+	++++	++	–	↑↑CO, ↓SVR, ↓PVR	Contraindicated in idiopathic hypertrophic subaortic stenosis
Milrinone	0.125–0.75 μg/kg/min	PDE-3 inhibitor				↑CO, ↓SVR, ↓PVR	Conservative initial dose and cautious uptitration is recommended for patients with renal impairment
Isoproterenol	2–20 μg/min	–	++++	++	–	↑↑CO, ↓SVR, ↓PVR	

SVR systemic vascular resistance, *PVR* peripheral vascular resistance, *CO* cardiac output, *PDE-3* phosphodiesterase-3, *CS* cardiogenic shock

Clinical Pearl
Routine placement of an intra-aortic balloon pump is not beneficial in acute MI with cardiogenic shock.

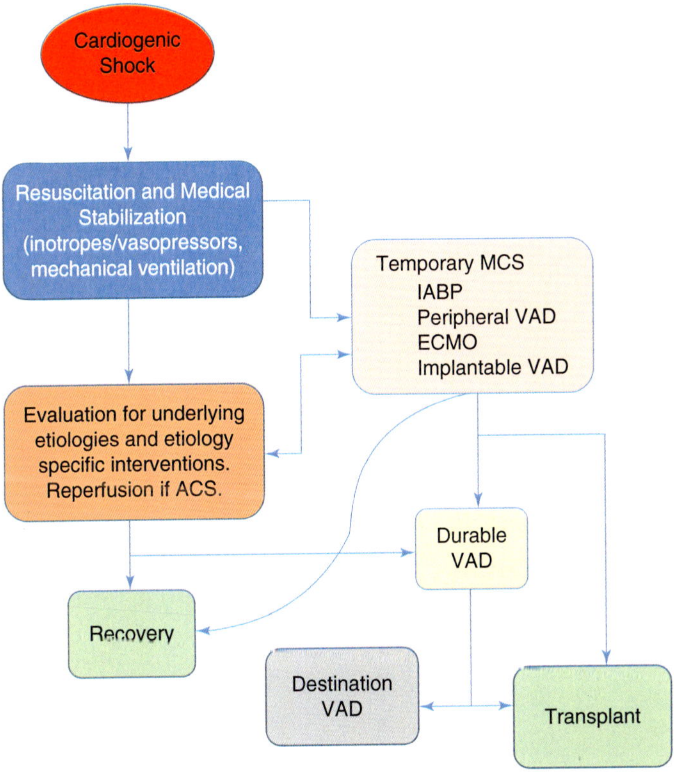

FIGURE 12.1 Potential management pathway for cardiogenic shock. ACS acute coronary syndrome, IABP intra-aortic balloon pump, VAD ventricular assist device, ECMO extracorporeal membrane oxygenation

TABLE 12.4 Contraindications to use and device characteristics of currently available mechanical circulatory devices

Device		Contraindications	Flow	Insertion	Placement	Support provided	Comments
IABP		Common contraindications include Significant AR Severe PAD Bleeding diathesis Intracardiac thrombus Recent CVA or head trauma Uncontrolled sepsis	Pulsatile	Percutaneous	Descending aorta.	0.3–0.5 L/min	Not beneficial in acute MI complicated by CS (IABP-SHOCK II, *NEJM* 2012 [6] and Circulation 2019 [7])
Impella	2.5 CP 5.0 RP		Axial	Percutaneous: 2.5, CP and RP. Percutaneous or surgical cut down: 5.0	LV → Aorta RV → PA (RP)	1–5 L/min Up to 4.0 L/min (RP)	No difference in 30-day mortality or secondary endpoint in acute MI complicated by CS with Impella CP compared to IABP (IMPRESS, *JACC* 2016 [8]).
PHP				Percutaneous	LV → Aorta	1–5.5 L/min	Complex insertion Investigational in the USA
Tandem heart			Centrifugal	Surgical	LA → Aorta	2.5–5.0 L/min	
Protek duo			Centrifugal	Surgical	LA → Aorta (LV) and RA → PA (RV)	Up to 5 L/min	
CentriMag			Centrifugal	Surgical	LA → Aorta (LV) and/or RA → PA (RV)	Up to 10 L/min	RV CentriMag is investigational in the USA
VA ECMO			Centrifugal	Percutaneous	RA → Aorta	3–7 L/min	Does not unload ventricle or decrease MVO_2 May require LV venting for ↑EDV, ↑EDP and ↓EF

Durable VAD		Axial: HM II Centrifugal: HM III, HeartWare	Surgical	LV → Aorta and/or RV → PA	3–10 L/min

IABP intra-aortic balloon pump, *PHP* percutaneous heart pump, *VAD* ventricular assist device, *ECMO* extracorporeal membrane oxygenation, *AR* aortic regurgitation, *CVA* cerebrovascular accident, *PAD* peripheral arterial disease, *LV* left ventricle, *RV* right ventricle, MVO_2 myocardial oxygen consumption, *EDV* end-diastolic volume, *EDP* end-diastolic pressure, *EF* ejection fraction, *HM* HeartMate

Key Learning Points

1. Cardiogenic shock (CS) is a state of tissue hypoperfusion due to low cardiac output which has a spectrum of severity and myriad of cardiac and non-cardiac etiologies.
2. CS has a very high mortality rate thus a prompt recognition, establishment of underlying etiology and appropriate therapy can be life-saving.
3. Goal of treatment is to restore and maintain satisfactory tissue perfusion. Treatment of underlying cause, use of inotropes and vasopressors, and mechanical circulatory support (for appropriate patient) remain the cornerstones of treatment of CS.

References

1. van Diepen S, Katz JN, Albert NM, Henry TD, Jacobs AK, Kapur NK, Kilic A, Menon V, Ohman EM, Sweitzer NK, Thiele H, Washam JB, Cohen MG, American Heart Association Council on Clinical C, Council on C, Stroke N, Council on Quality of C, Outcomes R and Mission L. Contemporary management of cardiogenic shock: a scientific statement from the American Heart Association. Circulation. 2017;136:e232–68.
2. Harjola VP, Lassus J, Sionis A, Kober L, Tarvasmaki T, Spinar J, Parissis J, Banaszewski M, Silva-Cardoso J, Carubelli V, Di Somma S, Tolppanen H, Zeymer U, Thiele H, Nieminen MS, Mebazaa A. CardShock study I and network G. Clinical picture and risk prediction of short-term mortality in cardiogenic shock. Eur J Heart Fail. 2015;17:501–9.
3. Hochman JS, Sleeper LA, Webb JG, Sanborn TA, White HD, Talley JD, Buller CE, Jacobs AK, Slater JN, Col J, McKinlay SM, LeJemtel TH. Early revascularization in acute myocardial infarction complicated by cardiogenic shock. SHOCK Investigators. Should we emergently revascularize occluded coronaries for cardiogenic shock. N Engl J Med. 1999;341:625–34.
4. Vahdatpour C, Collins D, Goldberg S. Cardiogenic shock. J Am Heart Assoc. 2019;8:e011991.

5. De Backer D, Biston P, Devriendt J, Madl C, Chochrad D, Aldecoa C, Brasseur A, Defrance P, Gottignies P, Vincent JL, Investigators SI. Comparison of dopamine and norepinephrine in the treatment of shock. N Engl J Med. 2010;362:779–89.
6. Thiele H, Zeymer U, Neumann FJ, Ferenc M, Olbrich HG, Hausleiter J, Richardt G, Hennersdorf M, Empen K, Fuernau G, Desch S, Eitel I, Hambrecht R, Fuhrmann J, Bohm M, Ebelt H, Schneider S, Schuler G, Werdan K, Investigators I-SIT. Intraaortic balloon support for myocardial infarction with cardiogenic shock. N Engl J Med. 2012;367:1287–96.
7. Thiele H, Zeymer U, Thelemann N, Neumann FJ, Hausleiter J, Abdel-Wahab M, Meyer-Saraei R, Fuernau G, Eitel I, Hambrecht R, Bohm M, Werdan K, Felix SB, Hennersdorf M, Schneider S, Ouarrak T, Desch S, de Waha-Thiele S, Investigators IIT. Intraaortic balloon pump in cardiogenic shock complicating acute myocardial infarction: long-term 6-year outcome of the randomized IABP-SHOCK II trial. Circulation. 2019;139:395–403.
8. Ouweneel DM, Engstrom AE, Sjauw KD, Hirsch A, Hill JM, Gockel B, Tuseth V, van der Schaaf RJ, Henriques JP. Experience from a randomized controlled trial with Impella 2.5 versus IABP in STEMI patients with cardiogenic pre-shock. Lessons learned from the IMPRESS in STEMI trial. Int J Cardiol. 2016;202:894–6.

Chapter 13
Native Valve Disease

John C. Lisko and Vasilis C. Babaliaros

Abbreviations

ATC	Anticoagulation
AR	Aortic regurgitation
AS	Aortic stenosis
AVA	Aortic valve area
CT	Cardiac computed tomography
CHF	Congestive heart failure
EROA	Effective regurgitant orifice area
EF	Ejection fraction
ESD	End systolic diameter
GDMT	Guideline-directed medical therapy
HTN	Hypertension
LV	Left ventricular
MR	Mitral regurgitation
MS	Mitral stenosis
PBMC	Percutaneous balloon mitral commissurotomy
STS-PROM	Society for Thoracic Surgeons Predicted Risk of Mortality Score
SAVR	Surgical aortic valve replacement

J. C. Lisko · V. C. Babaliaros (✉)
Cardiology, Emory University Hospital, Atlanta, GA, USA
e-mail: vbabali@emory.edu

B. J. Wells et al. (eds.), *Handbook of Inpatient Cardiology*,
https://doi.org/10.1007/978-3-030-47868-1_13

SVi	Stroke volume index
TEE	Transesophageal echocardiography
TAVR	Transcatheter aortic valve replacement

Aortic Stenosis (AS)

Background

- Aortic stenosis is the most common cause of left ventricular (LV) outflow obstruction.
- Typically diagnosed by calculated aortic valve area (AVA) and measured gradients on echocardiography or cardiac catheterization.

> **Clinical Pearl**
> The transthoracic echocardiogram is a simple, noninvasive, radiation-free modality for evaluating native valve disease.

- Pathophysiology: Progressive narrowing of the aortic valve leads to LV pressure overload
- AVA is the first step in assessment [1, 2]
  - Mild aortic stenosis: AVA > 1.5 cm^2
  - Moderate aortic stenosis: AVA 1.0–1.5 cm^2
  - Severe aortic stenosis: AVA < 1.0 cm^2

> **Clinical Pearl**
> An aortic valve gradient >40 mmHg, velocity >4 m/s, or area <1 cm^2 indicates severe aortic stenosis.

- Aortic valve gradients are influenced by LV stroke volume [3].
  - *Classic, high-flow, high-gradient aortic stenosis* meets all of the following criteria (Fig. 13.1):

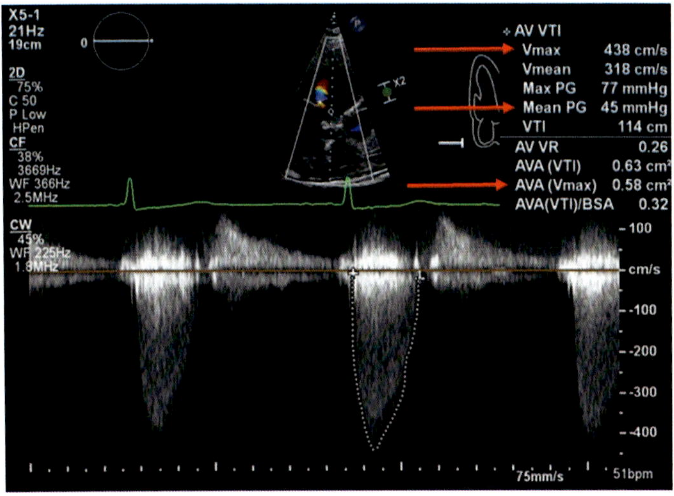

FIGURE 13.1 Echocardiographic diagnosis of severe aortic stenosis. Above, a continuous wave Doppler tracing through the aortic valve. The red arrows illustrate the key diagnostic requirements for severe AS (Vmax > 4 m/s, mean gradient> 40 mmHg, an AVA <1.0 cm^2)

Mean aortic valve gradient: >40 mmHg or peak velocity across the aortic valve >4 m/s
Aortic valve area < 1.0 cm^2
Stroke volume index: (SVi) >35 mL/m^2

– *Low-flow, low-gradient aortic stenosis*: Meets all of the following criteria:
  Mean aortic valve gradient: <40 mmHg or peak velocity across the aortic valve <4 m/s
  Aortic valve area < 1.0 cm^2
  Svi: <35 mL/m^2
  Left ventricular ejection fraction: LVEF <50%
– *Paradoxical low-flow, low-gradient aortic stenosis* meets all of the following criteria:
  Mean aortic valve gradient: <40 mmHg or peak velocity across the aortic valve <4 m/s
  Aortic valve area < 1.0 cm^2

Svi: <35 mL/m^2
LVEF: >50%

- Pseudo-severe AS: In patients with low stroke volume (e.g., low LVEF), AVA may appear falsely low due to reduced valve opening from low-flow state.

  To distinguish pseudo-stenosis from low-flow low-gradient AS, use *dobutamine stress echo*. At peak stress, calculated AVA > 1.0 cm^2 for pseudo-stenosis. For true low-flow low-gradient severe AS, AVA will remain <1 cm^2 while gradients increase to severe range.

Evaluation and Management

- Presentation
  - Physical exam: Harsh, systolic, crescendo-decrescendo murmur best heard over the right upper sternal border. Late-peaking murmurs suggest more severe disease. May have loss of second heart sound. Delayed and blunted carotid upstroke (*parvus et tardus*).
  - Most patients are asymptomatic until AS is severe.
  - The classic symptom progression is angina → syncope → congestive heart failure (CHF) [4].
  - The most common presentation: dyspnea on exertion, exertional pre-syncope, and exertional angina.
- Differential diagnosis:
  - Aortic sclerosis without stenosis
  - Subvalvular stenosis
  - Supravalvular stenosis
  - Hypertrophic obstructive cardiomyopathy
- Prognosis: correlates with symptoms [4]
  - Angina: average survival—5 years
  - Syncope: average survival—3 years
  - CHF: average survival—2 years
- Treatment
  - Mechanical correction is the only therapy shown to improve symptoms and survival.

- The optimal treatment strategy should be based on the patient's operative risk, calculated using the Society for Thoracic Surgeons (STS) Predicted Risk of Mortality (PROM) score.
- The STS-PROM score does not account for frailty, liver disease, or tricuspid valve disease, all of which increase operative risk.
  - Low-risk patients: STS-PROM < 4.0% [5, 6]
  - Intermediate-risk patients: STS-PROM ≥ 4% but ≤ 10% [7]
  - High-risk patients: STS-PROM ≥ 10%
- Surgical aortic valve replacement
  - Requires adequate aortic anatomy for cardiopulmonary bypass, median sternotomy, and general anesthesia.
  - Class I recommendation for patients at low-, intermediate-, and high-surgical risk [1, 2].
  - Mechanical aortic valve: should be considered in young patients (<55 years of age), in those with another indication for anticoagulation, and in those at high risk for a second aortic intervention.
    - Advantages: Low rate of valve failure, excellent hemodynamics.
    - Disadvantages: Requires lifelong anticoagulation (ATC), often audible, no role for TAVR in cases of valve degeneration.
- Bioprosthetic aortic valve
  - Advantages: No role for lifelong ATC, amenable to TAVR.
  - Disadvantages: Less durable. Patients may need another valve replacement.
- Transcatheter aortic valve replacement
  - Allows for a fully percutaneous aortic valve replacement, without cardiopulmonary bypass, and often without the need for general anesthesia [6,7] (Fig. 13.2).
  - Because of the minimally invasive nature of the technique, many patients can be discharged to home within 24 hours of implantation [8].

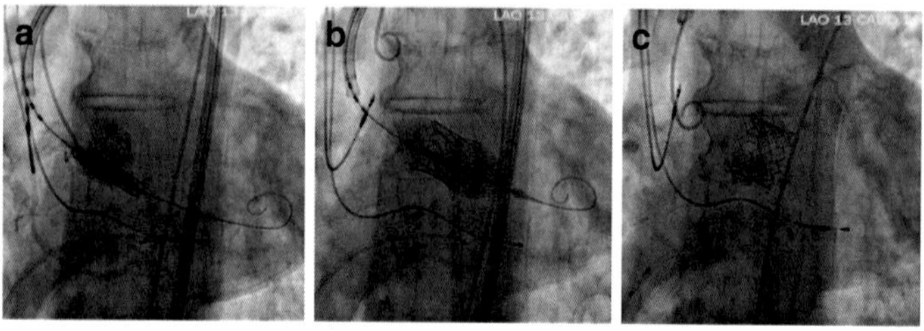

FIGURE 13.2 TAVR implantation. TAVR is a fully percutaneous approach to aortic valve replacement. Panel (**a**) demonstrates transcatheter heart valve before deployment. Panel (**b**) demonstrates that valve during expansion. Panel (**c**) shows the valve post deployment. Note that this technique does not require cardiopulmonary bypass

Approved for severe, symptomatic, non-rheumatic AS [1, 2].

There is a lack of data for the use of TAVR in patients with bicuspid aortic stenosis.

Registry data suggest a higher rate of stroke and pacemaker implantation for bicuspid AS compared to tricuspid AS [9].

Guideline recommendations [1, 2]:

- Class I for patients at prohibitive and high surgical risk.
- Class IIa recommendation for patients at intermediate surgical risk.
- Currently, FDA has approved this guidelines for patients at low-surgical risk, but the guidelines have not been updated since completion of the low-risk trials.

Valve selection

- Sizing is determined using gated cardiac computed tomography (CT) and/or transesophageal echocardiography (TEE).

Aortic Regurgitation (AR)

Background

- Unlike AS, aortic regurgitation can be acute or chronic
- Acute causes:
  - Endocarditis
  - Trauma
  - Aortic dissection
- Chronic causes:
  - Bicuspid aortic valve degeneration
  - Calcific degeneration
  - Rheumatic disease
  - Dilation of the aortic root from:
    - Congenital causes
    - Hypertension (HTN)
    - Vasculitis
- In most patients, only severe AR will be clinically relevant during hospital admission
- Pathophysiology: regurgitation leads to LV volume overload → LV dilation → congestive heart failure
- Prognosis
  - Asymptomatic patients with chronic aortic regurgitation, LVEF > 50%, and a LV end-systolic dimension ≤45–50 mm have a low risk of death.
  - In patients with severe aortic regurgitation and LV dysfunction with HF symptoms, risk of death approaches 6–25% per year.

> **Clinical Pearl**
> Changes in ventricular size or function in patients with valvular heart disease should prompt cardiology consultation.

Evaluation and Management

- Physical exam:
  - Early diastolic murmur (starting immediately after A2), wide pulse pressure, water hammer (Corrigan) pulse. Other findings best seen in chronic AR: head bob with each heartbeat (de Musset's sign), capillary pulsations in fingertips (Quincke's pulses), systolic/diastolic bruit over femoral artery with partial compression (Duroziez's sign).
- Presentation
  - Acute: Sudden onset dyspnea or congestive heart failure.
  - Chronic: Incidentally discovered dilated aortic sinuses/ascending aorta or dyspnea on exertion.
- Diagnosis is based on echocardiography [10].
  - Severe AR
    - Flail leaflets on qualitative analysis
    - Pressure ½ time < 200
    - Diastolic blood flow reversal in descending aorta
    - Regurgitant volume of >60 mL/beat
- Treatment
  - The role of medical therapy for aortic regurgitation has not been well established.
  - There are no data to support routine vasodilatory therapy in patients with severe AR and preserved ventricular function [11].
  - Aortic valve replacement is recommended for the following patients with severe AR [1, 2]:
    - Symptoms attributable to AR
    - Asymptomatic but with an EF <50%
    - Asymptomatic but with an end systolic diameter (ESD) >50 mm
    - Asymptomatic but with an ESD >65 mm and low surgical risk
    - Another indication for cardiac surgery
      - Replacement is also suggested for patients with moderate AR undergoing another cardiac surgery

- The standard therapy for aortic regurgitation remains SAVR
  - TAVR has been performed "off-label" in this population [12]
  - There are no commercially available TAVR devices for AR

Mitral Stenosis (MS)

Background

- MS is relatively uncommon in the United States
  - Often related to rheumatic valvular changes or severe mitral calcification
    - History should include a detailed evaluation for prior rheumatic fever, chest radiation, or significant renal disease.
- Pathophysiology: Narrowing of the mitral valve → left atrial pressure overload → pulmonary hypertension
- Prognosis:
  - Rheumatic MS is a progressive disease. The prognosis worsens once a patient becomes symptomatic.
  - 44% 5-year survival in symptomatic patients without correction [13].
- Diagnosis is primarily based on echocardiography [14]
  - Planimetered mitral valve area ≤ 1.5 cm^2
  - Diastolic pressure half-time ≥ 150 ms (narrowed orifice → delayed filling)
  - Gradient:
    - The gradient across the mitral valve is directly related to the patient's heart rate
    - Mild MS: Mean gradient <5 mm Hg
    - Moderate MS: Mean gradient 5–10 mm Hg
    - Severe MS: Mean gradient >10 mm Hg

Presentation and Management

- Presentation: Decreased exercise tolerance, dyspnea on exertion/congestive heart failure
- Physical exam: Opening snap following S2 with diastolic rumble, heard best at apex. S2-to-opening snap interval is *inversely* correlated with MS severity. Often difficult to auscultate, especially in setting of atrial fibrillation, which is commonly associated.
- Treatment [1, 2]
  - Medical therapy

    Rate-controlling medications to reduce heart rate to the lowest tolerated rate (increased diastolic filling time) in patients with (1) atrial fibrillation with a rapid ventricular response or (2) normal sinus rhythm and exercise-induced symptoms.

    Anticoagulation in patients with concomitant atrial fibrillation. Use warfarin only for valvular atrial fibrillation, no novel oral anticoagulants.
  - Mechanical correction

    Percutaneous balloon mitral commissurotomy (PBMC) in symptomatic patients with suitable anatomy.

    - TEE is necessary to determine a patient's anatomic suitability for valvuloplasty.

    Mitral valve surgery for severely symptomatic patients who are not candidates for PBMC.

Mitral Regurgitation (MR)

Background

- Definition
  - Correctly defining the etiology of MR is essential to optimizing treatment [15]

MR is classified as *primary* (degenerative) MR when the etiology of the MR is attributable to a problem with the mitral valve.

MR is classified as *secondary* (functional) when the etiology of the MR is attributable to myocardial disease. Echocardiography is the main imaging modality for assessing the mitral valve [10].

- Severe MR is defined by:
  - Vena contracta width ≥ 0.7 cm
  - Effective regurgitant orifice area (EROA) ≥ 0.40 cm
  - Regurgitant volume ≥ 60 mL
  - Regurgitant fraction ≥ 50%
- TEE is often useful to better define the severity and etiology of MR.
- Cardiac MRI is useful to accurately quantify the degree of mitral regurgitation and for patients with suboptimal echo windows.

- Pathophysiology
  - MR leads to chronic LV volume overload → compensatory LV dilation → congestive heart failure.
- Prognosis
  - Primary MR: 66% of asymptomatic patients require surgery within 5 years because of LV dysfunction, pulmonary HTN, or atrial fibrillation [16].
  - Secondary MR: 23.5% mortality rate at 24 months in the COAPT Trial [17].

Presentation and Management

- Presentation
  - The severity of a patient's symptoms is related to the severity of MR, associated pressure in the pulmonary artery, and associated arrhythmias (MR → atrial dilatation → atrial fibrillation).

- Patients commonly present with symptoms of poor forward cardiac output (fatigue) and dyspnea on exertion.
- Acute MR may present as sudden onset dyspnea, flash pulmonary edema, and significant hemodynamic compromise: this raises the concern for a papillary muscle rupture, ruptured mitral chordae, or leaflet rupture from endocarditis.

• Physical exam: Holosystolic murmur best heard at the LV apex, radiating to axillae. May hear mid-systolic click with mitral valve prolapse. In acute MR, there may be little-to-no murmur.
• Treatment
  - The complexity of the mitral valve and available therapies requires a heart team approach to patient care [1, 2, 17, 18].
  - Mechanical correction has shown survival benefit in patients with MR.
• Treatment of *primary* mitral regurgitation
  - Surgery remains the gold standard of treatment [1, 2].
  - Mitral valve repair is preferred to replacement in the following conditions:
    When the MR is limited to the posterior leaflet
    When the MR involves the anterior or both leaflets *and* durable repair can be accomplished
  - Class I recommendations for surgery are to be followed in the following groups with chronic, severe, primary MR:
    Symptomatic patients with MR and an LVEF >30%
    Asymptomatic patients with an EF of 30–60%
  - The MitraClip (Abbott Vascular) is a fully percutaneous edge-to-edge repair system that has shown efficacy in patients with severe primary MR at prohibited surgical risk [19].

• Treatment of *secondary* mitral regurgitation [1, 2, 15, 17, 18]
  - The mainstays of therapy for secondary mitral regurgitation treat underlying myocardial disease.
  - Prior to considering any mechanical correction to secondary MR, it is essential to:
    Evaluate for reversible ischemia and pursue revascularization if possible

Optimize guideline-directed medical therapy (GDMT) for congestive heart failure

Consider cardiac resynchronization therapy (typically reserved for patients with an underlying left bundle branch block and QRS duration >150 ms)

Consider consultation with advanced heart failure services

- Surgical repair is a Class IIB recommendation in patients with NYHA III-IV CHF symptoms if it is felt the degree of MR rather then left ventricular dysfunction causes symptoms
- The MitraClip has been studied in patients with secondary MR
- Results from the two largest studies are conflicting

The COAPT Trial demonstrated a significant reduction in HF hospitalization and all-cause death at 24 months in patients undergoing MitraClip + GMDT compared to GDMT alone [17].

The Mitra-FR Trial failed to show significant outcomes in patients undergoing MitraClip + GMDT compared to GDMT alone [18].

These differences may be attributable to patient selection, operator experience, or titration of medical therapy [20].

Patients should be evaluated by patients with expertise in heart failure management prior to undergoing MitraClip for SMR.

Pulmonary and Tricuspid Valves

- Background: Right-sided valvular heart disease is much less common than left-sided disease. Trace to mild disease is a common incidental echo finding [1, 2, 10, 14, 21].
- Common etiologies of tricuspid disease
  - Stenosis: Rheumatic heart disease, carcinoid syndrome, congenital abnormalities, pacemaker endocarditis, pacemaker-induced adhesions, lupus, mechanical obstruction secondary to tumor.

  - Regurgitation: The most common cause is due to annular dilation. The most common primary cause is myxomatous degeneration.
- Common etiologies of pulmonic disease
  - Stenosis: Congenital >>> acquired causes.
  - Regurgitation: Most likely to be from congenital disease or post-percutaneous valvuloplasty. Acquired disease occurs in <1% of patients.
- See Table 13.1 for evaluation of right-sided valve disease.

TABLE 13.1 Evaluation of right-sided valve disease

Valve	Severe stenosis criteria	Severe regurgitation criteria	Class I indications for surgery
Tricuspid	Mean gradient >5 mmHg Pressure ½ time ≥ 190 ms Valve area ≤ 1 cm²	RA/RV dilatation IVC diameter: >2.5 cm Color flow: Large central jet Systolic flow reversal in hepatic vein EROA (cm²) ≥ 0.40	Stenosis Severe stenosis at the time of left-sided surgery Isolated, symptomatic severe stenosis Regurgitation Functional severe regurgitation at the time of left-sided surgery
Pulmonic	Peak velocity: >4 m/s Peak gradient: >64 mm Hg	RV size: dilated Deceleration time < 260 ms Pressure ½ time < 100 ms Prominent diastolic flow reversal in PA RF >40%	Stenosis Moderate to severe stenosis and unexplained heart failure, cyanosis, or exercise intolerance → balloon valvuloplasty, followed by surgical repair if failed valvuloplasty

Criteria reflect select criteria that may be commonly reported in echo reports

RA right atrium, *RV* right ventricle, *IVC* inferior vena cava, *EROA* effective regurgitant orifice area, *RF* regurgitant fraction

Key Learning Points

1. A multidisciplinary heart team is essential to providing high-quality valve care
2. Echocardiographic findings always warrant correlation with clinical symptoms.
3. Medical therapy, surgery, and transcatheter therapy play a complementary role in the care of patients with native valve disease.

References

1. Nishimura RA, et al. 2017 AHA/ACC focused update of the 2014 AHA/ACC guideline for the management of patients with valvular heart disease: a report of the American College of Cardiology/American Heart Association Task Force on Clinical Practice Guidelines. Circulation. 2017;135(25):e1159–95.
2. Nishimura RA, et al. 2014 AHA/ACC guideline for the management of patients with valvular heart disease: executive summary: a report of the American College of Cardiology/American Heart Association Task Force on Practice Guidelines. Circulation. 2014;129(23):2440–92.
3. Pibarot P, Dumesnil JG. Low-flow, low-gradient aortic stenosis with normal and depressed left ventricular ejection fraction. J Am Coll Cardiol. 2012;60(19):1845–53.
4. Braunwald E. Aortic stenosis: then and now. Circulation. 2018;137(20):2099–100.
5. Mack MJ, et al. Transcatheter aortic-valve replacement with a balloon-expandable valve in low-risk patients. N Engl J Med. 2019;380(18):1695–705.
6. Adams DH, et al. Transcatheter aortic-valve replacement with a self-expanding prosthesis. N Engl J Med. 2014;370(19):1790–8.
7. Leon MB, et al. Transcatheter or surgical aortic-valve replacement in intermediate-risk patients. N Engl J Med. 2016;374(17):1609–20.
8. Kamioka N, et al. Predictors and clinical outcomes of next-day discharge after minimalist transfemoral transcatheter aortic valve replacement. JACC Cardiovasc Interv. 2018;11(2):107–15.

9. Yoon SH, et al. Outcomes in transcatheter aortic valve replacement for bicuspid versus tricuspid aortic valve stenosis. J Am Coll Cardiol. 2017;69(21):2579–89.
10. Zoghbi WA, et al. Recommendations for noninvasive evaluation of native valvular regurgitation: a report from the American Society of Echocardiography Developed in Collaboration with the Society for Cardiovascular Magnetic Resonance. J Am Soc Echocardiogr. 2017;30(4):303–71.
11. Shen W, et al. Noninvasive assessment of acute effects of nifedipine on rest and exercise hemodynamics and cardiac function in patients with aortic regurgitation. J Am Coll Cardiol. 1984;4(5):902.
12. Yoon SH, et al. Transcatheter aortic valve replacement in pure native aortic valve regurgitation. J Am Coll Cardiol. 2017;70(22):2752–63.
13. Munoz S, et al. Influence of surgery on the natural history of rheumatic mitral and aortic valve disease. Am J Cardiol. 1975;35:234–42.
14. Baumgartner H, et al. Echocardiographic assessment of valve stenosis: EAE/ASE recommendations for clinical practice. J Am Soc Echocardiogr. 2009;22(1):1–23; quiz 101-2.
15. Grayburn PA, Sannino A, Packer M. Proportionate and disproportionate functional mitral regurgitation: a new conceptual framework that reconciles the results of the MITRA-FR and COAPT Trials. JACC Cardiovasc Imaging. 2019;12(2):353–62.
16. David TE, et al. Late outcomes of mitral valve repair for mitral regurgitation due to degenerative disease. Circulation. 2013;127(14):1485–92.
17. Stone GW, et al. Transcatheter mitral-valve repair in patients with heart failure. N Engl J Med. 2018;379(24):2307–18.
18. Obadia JF, et al. Percutaneous repair or medical treatment for secondary mitral regurgitation. N Engl J Med. 2018;379(24):2297–306.
19. Feldman T, et al. Randomized comparison of percutaneous repair and surgery for mitral regurgitation: 5-year results of EVEREST II. J Am Coll Cardiol. 2015;66(25):2844–54.

20. Mauricio R, Kumbhani DJ. MitraClip: how do we reconcile the inconsistent findings of MITRA-FR and COAPT? Curr Cardiol Rep. 2019;21(12):150.
21. Stout KK, et al. 2018 AHA/ACC guideline for the management of adults with congenital heart disease: a report of the American College of Cardiology/American Heart Association Task Force on Clinical Practice Guidelines. Circulation. 2019;139(14):e698–800.

Chapter 14
Prosthetic Valve Disease

Ankit Ajay Bhargava and Allen L. Dollar

Abbreviations

ASA	Aspirin
CBC	Complete blood count
CT	Computed tomography
DOAC	Direct oral anticoagulant
FFP	Fresh frozen plasma
INR	International normalized ratio
LDH	Lactate dehydrogenase
PCC	Prothrombin complex concentrate
PPM	Patient prosthesis mismatch
PVL	Paravalvular leak
TAVR	Transcatheter aortic valve replacement
TEE	Transesophageal echocardiogram
TTE	Transthoracic echocardiogram
UFH	Unfractionated heparin
VKA	Vitamin K antagonist
VTE	Venothromboembolism

A. A. Bhargava (✉) · A. L. Dollar
Department of Cardiovascular Medicine, Emory University Hospital School of Medicine, Atlanta, GA, USA
e-mail: aabharg@emory.edu

B. J. Wells et al. (eds.), *Handbook of Inpatient Cardiology*,
https://doi.org/10.1007/978-3-030-47868-1_14

Valve Types

There are two varieties of prosthetic valves: mechanical valves and bioprosthetic valves. Examples are pictured in Fig. 14.1.

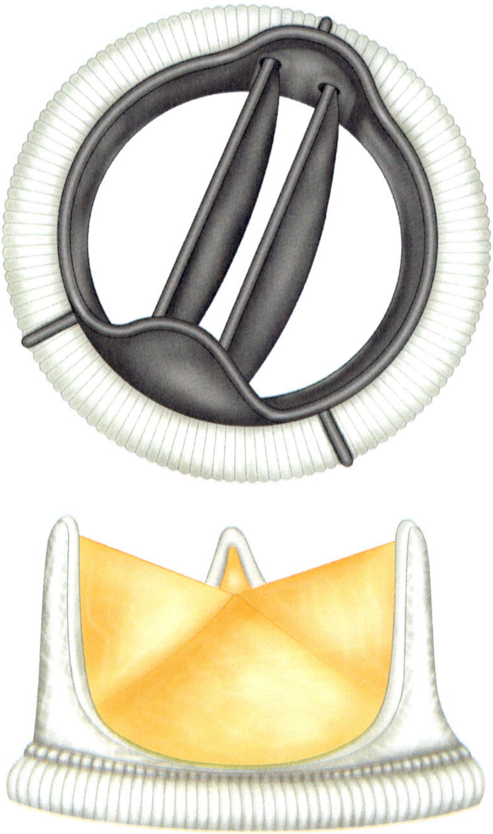

FIGURE 14.1 St. Jude bileaflet mechanical aortic valve (left) and Carpentier-Edwards bioprosthetic aortic valve (right)

- *Mechanical valves* – Designs include the caged ball, single tilting disc, and bileaflet tilting disc. Essentially all contemporary mechanical valves utilize the bileaflet tilting disc design [1, 2].
  - Increased durability
  - Increased thrombogenicity
- *Bioprosthetic valves* – Typically xenografts (collected from animal tissue such as bovine pericardium or porcine valves) and rarely autografts/homografts (derived from human valve tissue) [1].
  - Decreased durability
  - Decreased thrombogenicity
- *Transcatheter valves* – All available forms derived from biological tissue.
  - To allow endovascular delivery, the valve is crimped and delivered via a stent frame that then expands once in the appropriate position. These stents can be either balloon-expandable or self-expanding [1].

Choice of Valve Prosthesis

The choice between pursuing valve replacement with either a mechanical or prosthetic valve is dependent on multiple factors and summarized in Table 14.1.

Patients are stratified into three groups for prosthetic valve candidacy based on age and risk of bleeding:

1. Patients who are *less than 50 years of age* without a contraindication for anticoagulation → mechanical valve [4].
   - Patients in this demographic generally have a lower bleeding risk profile and a greater chance of going through life without needing reintervention.
2. Patients who are *greater than 70 years of age* or those at any age who are unable or unwilling to receive lifelong anticoagulation with a vitamin K antagonist (VKA) → bioprosthetic valve [4].
   - Older age is associated with a higher risk of bleeding.
   - Higher likelihood for other procedures or surgeries in this subset of the population that would otherwise require interruption in anticoagulation.

TABLE 14.1 Factors that favor mechanical versus bioprosthetic valves [3]

		Mechanical	Bioprosthetic
Age	<50 years	✓	
	50–70 years	✓	✓
	>70 years		✓
Shorter expected life span			✓
Anticoagulation for another reason (atrial fibrillation, VTE)		✓	
High bleeding risk/contraindication to anticoagulation			✓
Higher morbidity/mortality with reintervention (e.g., porcelain aorta)		✓	

3. Patients that fall in the range of *50–70 years of age* will have similar outcomes for both mechanical and bioprosthetic valves [4, 5].
   - From the standpoint of valve durability, the use of valve-in-valve techniques for bioprosthetic valve replacement has decreased the need for surgical replacement, thereby reducing the risk of reoperation.
   - While these techniques have predominantly been used in aortic valves, they have been successfully used in mitral valves as well [6].

Anticoagulation

Mechanical Valves

- Require lifelong anticoagulation in order to prevent valve thrombosis and thromboembolism [3, 4].

- Combination of thrombogenic valve material, abnormal flow conditions, and high shear stress leads to an environment of increased platelet activation → higher rates of thrombosis in the absence of anticoagulation [3, 4].
- The anticoagulant of choice remains VKAs such as warfarin, with heparin (unfractionated or low molecular weight) used as a bridging agent until the INR is at the designated therapeutic target [3, 4].
- *Direct oral anticoagulants (DOACs) are contraindicated* and have been associated with both increased bleeding and thromboembolic events in patients with mechanical valves [7].

Bioprosthetic Valves

- Managed with aspirin therapy alone in the long term [3, 4].
- Recommended to have a period of anticoagulation with a VKA in the first 3–6 months following valve replacement [4].

The INR goal for prosthetic valves is dependent on the *type of valve* (bioprosthetic vs. mechanical), *position of the valve* (aortic vs. mitral), and *presence of other risk factors for thromboembolism*.

Antiplatelet and anticoagulation therapies with INR goals are summarized in Table 14.2.

Clinical Pearl

- Aspirin 75–100 mg per day is indicated in *all* prosthetic valves, including mechanical valves with VKA [3, 4].
- Mechanical *mitral* valves have even higher thrombogenic potential than mechanical *aortic* valves. Anticoagulation goal for mechanical mitral valves is therefore an INR between 2.5 and 3.5, not 2.0 and 3.0 [4, 5].

Table 14.2 Antiplatelet and anticoagulation goals by valve type [4]

Type	Position	Antiplatelet/anticoagulation goals	
Mechanical	Aortic	Without risk factors[a]	VKA (INR = 2.5) ASA 75–100 mg QD
		With risk factors[a]	VKA (INR = 3.0) ASA 75–100 mg QD
		On-X valve[b]	VKA (INR 1.5–2.0) ASA 75–100 mg QD
	Mitral	VKA (INR 3.0) ASA 75–100 mg QD	
Bioprosthetic	Aortic	VKA (INR = 2.5) for first 3–6 months ASA 75–100 mg QD	
	Mitral	VKA (INR = 2.5) for first 3–6 months ASA 75–100 mg QD	
	TAVR	±VKA for first 3 months after implantation Clopidogrel 75 mg QD for first 6 months ASA 75–100 mg QD lifelong	

[a]*Risk factors*: atrial fibrillation/flutter, prior thromboembolism, severe left ventricular dysfunction (ejection fraction <30%), or hypercoagulable state

[b]In patients without risk factors who receive a *mechanical On-X aortic valve*, an even lower target INR of 1.5–2.0 may be reasonable starting 3 months after implantation

Prosthetic Valve Complications

The frequencies and types of complications depend on the prosthetic valve and are summarized in Table 14.3.

Table 14.3 Summary of valve complications, diagnostic modalities, and management [4, 8–10]

Complication	Diagnostic orders	Management
Bleeding or supratherapeutic INR	CBC, INR	If INR 5–10 without bleed → hold VKA If INR > 10 without bleed → hold VKA and give vitamin K PO 1–2.5 mg If bleeding needs to be reversed urgently → hold VKA and give PCC or FFP with vitamin K PO
Thromboembolism	TTE, TEE	Adjust anticoagulation regimen: Mechanical – increase INR goal by 0.5 Bioprosthetic – add VKA to ASA
Valve thrombosis/ pannus formation	TTE, TEE, fluoroscopy, CT	Mechanical – surgery (pannus/thrombus) vs. fibrinolysis (thrombus only) Bioprosthetic – UFH bridge to VKA
Patient prosthesis mismatch	TTE, TEE	Surgical consultation
Prosthetic valve stenosis	TTE, TEE, ±blood cultures	Re-do surgery Valve-in-valve procedure if bioprosthetic valve
Prosthetic valve regurgitation	TTE, TEE, ±blood cultures, LDH if concerned for hemolysis	Re-do surgery Percutaneous paravalvular intervention

(continued)

Table 14.3 (continued)

Complication	Diagnostic orders	Management
Infective endocarditis	TTE, TEE, blood cultures	IV antibiotics tailored to organism ± surgical intervention

TTE transthoracic echocardiogram, *TEE* transesophageal echocardiogram, *LDH* lactate dehydrogenase, *VKA* vitamin K antagonist, *PCC* prothrombin complex concentrate, *FFP* fresh frozen plasma, *ASA* aspirin, *UFH* unfractionated heparin

In this section, we will highlight these issues and the necessary considerations to manage these complications as they arise.

Bleeding and Supratherapeutic INR

- Bleeding complications are among the most common adverse events seen in prosthetic valve recipients. This is of particular concern with mechanical heart valves due to the absolute need for lifelong anticoagulation.
- When the INR > 5, the risk of hemorrhage increases significantly [8, 9].
- If the INR is between 5 and 10, hold the VKA [8, 9].
- If INR >10 and not bleeding, administer a small dose of *oral vitamin K* (1–2.5 mg) [8, 9].
  - Oral vitamin K is preferred over the intravenous route as they are equally efficacious, and the intravenous route is associated with anaphylaxis and potential transient hypercoagulability.
  - Oral vitamin K offers a more gradual decline in INR and avoids overshooting the therapeutic range and putting the patient at increased risk of thrombosis.

Clinical Pearl
In *emergency situations* where bleeding must be controlled or is life threatening (such as with intracranial hemorrhage), intravenous prothrombin complex concentrate (PCC) is the agent of choice, though fresh frozen plasma (FFP) may be used if PCC is not available. The half-life of PCC is relatively short. Its administration should be combined with vitamin K to hasten longer lasting reductions in the INR [9].

Thromboembolism

- The annual risk of a thromboembolic event occurring is 1–2% for mechanical valves and 0.7% for bioprosthetic valves [3].
- On average, patients are only in therapeutic INR range about 60–70% of the time [3, 4].
- The initial assessment for suspected prosthetic valve thromboembolism starts with a transthoracic echocardiogram (TTE) to evaluate valve hemodynamics compared to prior studies.
- A transesophageal echocardiogram (TEE) is often needed for further characterization of the valve.
- Fluoroscopic valve cineradiography is also useful to assess valve leaflet motion in mechanical prostheses.

Clinical Pearl
If thromboembolism has occurred despite having a therapeutic INR:

- For patients on VKA, the INR goal is to shift up by 0.5 (for example, the target INR for a mechanical aortic valve goes from 2.5 to 3.0, with a range of 2.5–3.5, [3]).
- For patients with a bioprosthetic valve who are only on aspirin, adding a VKA would be reasonable [3].

Prosthetic Valve Thrombosis and Pannus Formation

- Valve thrombosis should be suspected in any patient with a prosthetic valve, particularly mechanical valve, who presents with recent onset of dyspnea or thromboembolic event, especially if anticoagulation is subtherapeutic.
- Assessment of valve motion, leaflet opening, and the extent of thrombus should be performed *urgently* as these patients have the potential of deteriorating rapidly.
- Multimodality imaging with TTE, TEE, fluoroscopy, and computed tomography (CT) are all options for investigating potential thrombosis [3].
- Obstruction of the valve is usually caused by *either thrombus or pannus ingrowth (fibrous ingrowth into the valve orifice),* though both can certainly occur simultaneously [2].
  - Clinically, valve thrombosis is more likely than pannus ingrowth when there is a history of:
    - Inadequate anticoagulation
    - Acute onset of symptoms
    - Shorter time interval between surgical implantation and onset of symptoms
  - Valve thrombosis can potentially be treated with fibrinolysis, whereas pannus ingrowth requires surgical or transcatheter (if bioprosthetic valve) intervention [3].
  - The decision to pursue fibrinolytic therapy versus surgical intervention for mechanical valve thrombosis is complex. Consultation of cardiology and cardiothoracic surgery services is needed to guide decision-making.
- Bioprosthetic valve thrombosis is less common → *treatment with VKA or unfractionated heparin (UFH) is the first-line treatment* [3].

Patient-Prosthesis Mismatch

- Patient-prosthesis mismatch (PPM) occurs when the size of the prosthetic valve does not allow for adequate flow to meet the metabolic demands of the patient, despite the valve itself functioning properly [2].

- While planning of surgical valve implantation takes into account the size of the patient and native annulus size, sometimes the native annular geometry and presence of calcium limit the ability to place the optimally sized valve [2].
- Aortic root enlargement may be considered at the time of surgery to accommodate a larger-sized valve [2].

Prosthetic Valve Stenosis

- Valve stenosis can arise from multiple etiologies.
  - *For mechanical valves,* chronic thrombus or pannus formation causing obstruction of normal leaflet motion is a common scenario [3].
  - *For bioprosthetic valves*, leaflet fibrosis and calcification from chronic wear-and-tear are the most common reasons for stenosis; mechanical valves rarely have this problem due to their superior durability [3].

    For severely symptomatic patients, *a transcatheter valve-in-valve procedure* may be a reasonable option in those with prohibitive surgical risk.

    This approach has largely been used in the aortic valve position, and has also been successfully tried in the pulmonic, mitral, and tricuspid valve positions [3, 6].
  - In both valve types, infective endocarditis is an important etiology for stenosis that must be considered.

Prosthetic Valve Regurgitation

- Prosthetic valve regurgitation can be either transvalvular (through the valve) or paravalvular (gap between prosthetic valve and native annular tissue).
- In both cases, the initial evaluation begins with a TTE, though TEE is often necessary for full evaluation of the valve and the etiology of regurgitation.

- For *mechanical valves*, the regurgitation is often due to either a paravalvular leak (PVL) or pannus formation that blocks the normal closing of the prosthetic valve.
  - *Intervention*: patients with intractable hemolysis or symptomatic heart failure that is due to severe regurgitation or PVL → require *surgical* intervention, no catheter-based options [3, 4].
- For *bioprosthetic valves*, the regurgitation is usually a result of either leaflet degeneration or calcification.
  - *Intervention*: both asymptomatic and symptomatic patients with severe regurgitation → *surgery or transcatheter* interventions are options in patients with bioprosthetic valves [3, 4].
- Paravalvular leaks may result in heart failure symptoms or hemolytic anemia (anemia typically mild).
  - Percutaneous paravalvular repair is an option in patients who have intractable hemolysis or New York Heart Association (NYHA) class III–IV symptoms and at high risk for surgery [3, 4].
- As in the case of valve stenosis, infective endocarditis is another etiology that must be investigated in new onset regurgitation or PVL [2, 3].

Infective Endocarditis of the Prosthetic Valve

- Patients with prosthetic heart valves are among those with the highest risk of an adverse outcome from infective endocarditis. Risk of developing infective endocarditis is 50 times that of the general population [3].
- In patients with unexplained fevers or new symptoms of heart failure attributable to prosthetic valve dysfunction (such as stenosis or valvular regurgitation), at least two sets of blood cultures should be obtained [3].
- Antibiotic therapy is tailored to the organism cultured and often requires several weeks of intravenous antibiotics for treatment [3].

- Diagnostic evaluation is often initiated with TTE for expediency; however, a TEE is almost always necessary due to the high risk nature of prosthetic valves and the need to assess for complications, such as a perivalvular abscess [3].
- Multidisciplinary consultation with infectious disease, cardiothoracic surgery, and cardiology heart valve teams is essential due to the complexity and morbidity associated with prosthetic valve endocarditis.
- In many cases, surgery may be indicated in addition to antibiotic therapy. The decision to pursue surgery is complex and individualized, though some factors that favor surgical intervention include [10] the following:
  - Persistent bacteremia despite proper antibiotic therapy
  - Perivalvular abscess
  - Development of heart block
  - Recurrent emboli despite proper antibiotic therapy
  - Severe valvular insufficiency
  - Large (>10 mm in diameter), mobile vegetation.

Key Learning Points

1. Mechanical valves are more durable and more thrombogenic when comparezd to bioprosthetic valves. Mechanical valves therefore require both aspirin and a VKA for anticoagulation lifelong, whereas bioprosthetic valves will typically only need aspirin lifelong.
2. Patients with a prosthetic valve who present with new onset heart failure symptoms should be evaluated for a prosthetic valve complication (prosthetic valve regurgitation, stenosis, thrombus, paravalvular leak, endocarditis).
3. Diagnostic investigation for prosthetic valve complications often starts with a TTE. However, multimodality imaging with TEE, CT, or fluoroscopy can all be utilized to come to the correct diagnosis.

References

1. Russo M, Taramasso M, Guidotti A, Pozzoli A, Nietilspach F, Segesser LK, et al. The evolution of surgical valves. Cardiovasc Med. 2017;20(12):285–92.
2. Dangas GD, Weitz JI, Giustino G, Makkar R, Mehran R. Prosthetic heart valve thrombosis. J Am Coll Cardiol. 2016;68(24):2670–89.
3. Nishimura RA, Otto CM, Bonow RO, Carabello BA, Erwin JP 3rd, Guyton RA, et al. 2014 AHA/ACC guideline for the management of patients with valvular heart disease: a report of the American College of Cardiology/American Heart Association Task Force on Practice Guidelines. J Am Coll Cardiol. 2014;63(22):e57–185.
4. Nishimura RA, Otto CM, Bonow RO, Carabello BA, Erwin JP 3rd, Fleisher LA, et al. 2017 AHA/ACC focused update of the 2014 AHA/ACC guideline for the management of patients with valvular heart disease: a report of the American College of Cardiology/American Heart Association Task Force on Clinical Practice Guidelines. Circulation. 2017;135(25):e1159–e95.
5. Chikwe J, Chiang YP, Egorova NN, Itagaki S, Adams DH. Survival and outcomes following bioprosthetic vs mechanical mitral valve replacement in patients aged 50 to 69 years. JAMA. 2015;313(14):1435–42.
6. Kamioka N, Babaliaros V, Morse MA, Frisoli T, Lerakis S, Iturbe JM, et al. Comparison of clinical and echocardiographic outcomes after surgical redo mitral valve replacement and transcatheter mitral valve-in-valve therapy. JACC Cardiovasc Interv. 2018;11(12):1131–8.
7. Eikelboom JW, Connolly SJ, Brueckmann M, Granger CB, Kappetein AP, Mack MJ, et al. Dabigatran versus warfarin in patients with mechanical heart valves. N Engl J Med. 2013;369(13):1206–14.
8. Baumgartner H, Falk V, Bax JJ, De Bonis M, Hamm C, Holm PJ, et al. 2017 ESC/EACTS guidelines for the management of valvular heart disease. Eur Heart J. 2017;38(36):2739–91.

9. Pernod G, Godier A, Gozalo C, Tremey B, Sie P. French clinical practice guidelines on the management of patients on vitamin K antagonists in at-risk situations (overdose, risk of bleeding, and active bleeding). Thromb Res. 2010;126(3):e167–74.
10. Baddour LM, Wilson WR, Bayer AS, Fowler VG Jr, Tleyjeh IM, Rybak MJ, et al. Infective endocarditis in adults: diagnosis, antimicrobial therapy, and management of complications: a scientific statement for healthcare professionals from the American Heart Association. Circulation. 2015;132(15):1435–86.

Chapter 15
Infective Endocarditis

John Ricketts and Jesse T. Jacob

Introduction

- Infective endocarditis (IE), though relatively infrequent (incidence: 3–7 cases per 100,000 person-years) can be a life-threatening infection.
- Historically, IE occurred in
  - Younger patients with injection drug use (IDU) and rheumatic valvular disease
  - Older patients with prosthetic materials including valves and implanted cardiac devices
- Most commonly due to *Staphylococcus aureus*, streptococci, coagulase-negative staphylococci, and gram-negative organisms [1].

J. Ricketts (✉)
Division of Cardiovascular Disease, Emory University Hospital, Atlanta, GA, USA
e-mail: Jricke2@emory.edu

J. T. Jacob
Division of Infectious Diseases, Emory University School of Medicine, Atlanta, GA, USA
e-mail: jtjacob@emory.edu

B. J. Wells et al. (eds.), *Handbook of Inpatient Cardiology*,
https://doi.org/10.1007/978-3-030-47868-1_15

Clinical Presentation/Initial Workup

- Few patients with classic left-sided (mitral/aortic) IE will present with acute valvular dysfunction or systemic embolization and vascular phenomena such as Janeway lesions and Osler nodes.
  - Non-specific symptoms such as persistent fevers, malaise, weight loss, and joint pain are more common.
- Right-sided (tricuspid/pulmonic valve) endocarditis more common in IDU.
  - Can be complicated by septic pulmonary emboli to the lungs.
- Patients suspected of having IE should be clinically evaluated using the modified Duke criteria as the primary diagnostic schema per the Infectious Disease Society of America (IDSA) guidelines (Table 15.1).
  - Concordance between the Duke criteria and clinical assessment by infectious disease experts is high (72–90%) [2].
- For suspected IE, *before starting empiric antibiotic therapy (see below), obtain three sets of blood cultures* from different venipuncture sites, with the first and last samples drawn at least 1 h apart [3] (Class 1; Level of Evidence as per IDSA guidelines) (*Clinical Pearl*).
  - A leading cause of "culture-negative endocarditis" is the administration of antibiotic therapy prior to obtaining blood cultures.
- The most common bacteria are staphylococci (*S. aureus* and coagulase-negative staphylococci), followed by streptococci and enterococci [3].
  - *S. aureus* IE not associated with IDU primarily affects the left side of the heart and is associated with a mortality rate of 25–40%.
  - *S. aureus* IE associated with IDU frequently involves the tricuspid valve with cure rates as high as >85% and can be treated with short courses of antibiotics of 2–4 weeks [3].

TABLE 15.1 Modified Duke criteria

The modified Duke criteria for the diagnosis of IE
Major criteria
Blood cultures positive for IE
Typical microorganisms consistent with IE from two separate blood cultures:
Viridans streptococci, *Streptococcus bovis*, HACEK group, *S. aureus*, or community-acquired enterococci in the absence of a primary focus, or microorganisms consistent with IE from persistently positive blood cultures defined as follows: At least 2 positive cultures of blood samples drawn >12 h apart or all 3 or a majority of ≥4 separate cultures of blood (with first and last sample drawn at least 1 h apart)
Single positive blood culture for *Coxiella burnetii* or anti-phase 1 IgG antibody titer ≥1:800
Evidence of endocardial involvement
Echocardiogram positive for IE
Minor criteria
Predisposition, predisposing heart condition, or IVDU
Fever, temperature > 38 °C
Vascular phenomena, major arterial emboli, septic pulmonary infarcts, mycotic aneurysm, intracranial hemorrhage, conjunctival hemorrhages, and Janeway lesions
Immunological phenomena: glomerulonephritis, Osler nodes, Roth spots, and rheumatoid factor
Microbiological evidence: positive blood culture but does not meet a major criterion as noted above (excludes single positive cultures for coagulase-negative staphylococci and organisms that do not cause endocarditis) or serological evidence of active infection with organism consistent with IE

- Coagulase-negative staphylococci are frequently associated with prosthetic heart valves.
  S. lugdunensis can mimic *S. aureus*, with a high rate of perivalvular extension and metastatic infection [3].
- *Streptococcal IE often originates from oral (dental disease) or gut sources.*
- Enterococcal IE more often occurs in patients who are older and more debilitated and in those who have pre-existing renal failure, underlying co-morbidities, and more healthcare-associated infections when compared to other patients with endocarditis [3].
- Gram-negative bacilli, including the HACEK (*Haemophilus*, *Aggregatibacter* (formerly *Actinobacillus*), *Cardiobacterium*, *Eikenella*, *Kingella*) organisms, account for ~5–10% of all community-acquired native valve endocarditis in non-IDU patients [4].
- Fungal endocarditis is rare but has survival rates <20%.
- Common risk factors include patients with devices such as pacemakers/defibrillators, central venous catheters, and prosthetic valves.
- A "stand-alone indication" for surgical valvular replacement [3].
- Multiple studies have placed the frequency of true culture-negative endocarditis at 5–10% [5, 6].
- True culture-negative endocarditis is caused by rare pathogens that do not grow in routine blood culture systems. The most common of these organisms are *Bartonella*, *C. burnetii*, and *Brucella*.
- Non-infectious valvular vegetations, whether relatively asymptomatic or clinical IE, can be due to the following:
- Neoplasia (atrial myxoma, neoplastic disease, carcinoid)
- Autoimmune diseases (rheumatic disease, systemic lupus erythematosus, polyarteritis nodosa, and Behcet's disease)
- Post-valvular surgical changes
- Miscellaneous (eosinophilic heart disease, ruptured chordae, myxomatous degeneration).

- Echocardiography
  - Echocardiography should be performed expeditiously in patients suspected of having IE [3] (Class 1; Level of Evidence as per IDSA guidelines) (Fig. 15.1).
  - While IE can be diagnosed at the bedside, echocardiography is an essential diagnostic (presence of vegetation/valvular dysfunction) and prognostic (surgical planning) tool.
  - Transthoracic echocardiogram (TTE) should be done initially in all cases of suspected endocarditis. Discuss concerns about factors that might limit utility of TTE such as patient body habitus, with your cardiology consultant.

    When TTE is negative and clinical suspicion is low, then other causes of illness should be considered.

    When TTE is negative and clinical suspicion remains high or the patient has a high risk of complications (e.g., prosthetic valve, new heart block), then transesophageal echocardiogram (TEE) should be obtained (Fig. 15.2).

    In patients with a positive TTE, a subsequent TEE should almost always be performed, except in cases where the likelihood of complications is low or subsequent imaging is unlikely to change management such as small vegetation size and lack of valvular dysfunction (Clinical Pearl).
  - Potential exists for both false positives and false negatives with echocardiography.

    Preexisting valve abnormalities, previous scarring, or normal anatomic structures can mimic changes of endocarditis.

    If the vegetation has already embolized, study may be negative.
  - Echo also helps in delineating which patients might benefit more from surgical intervention.

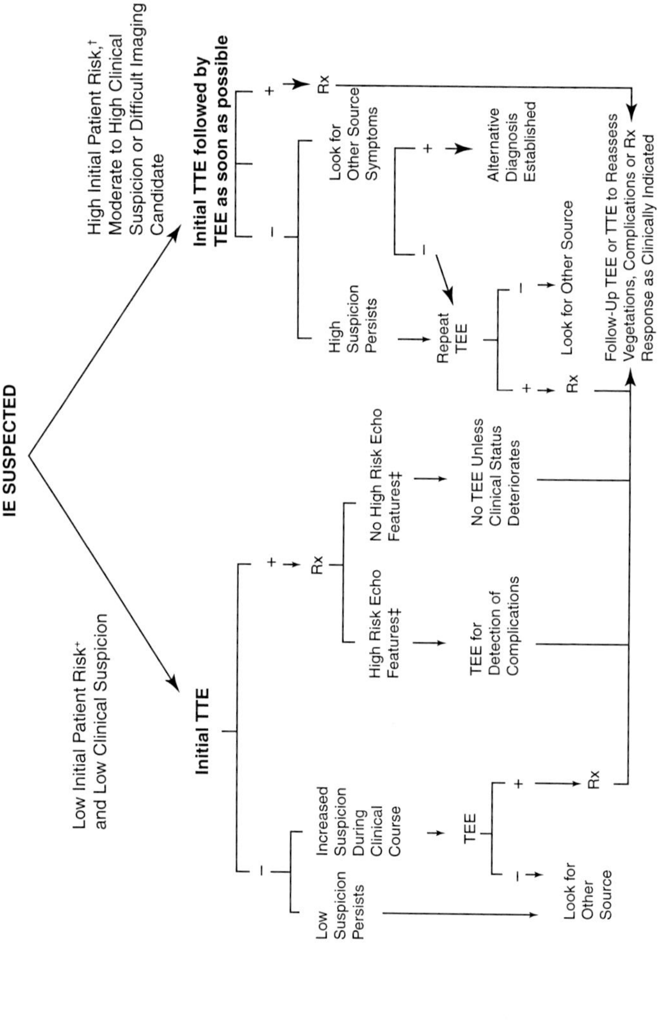

FIGURE 15.1 Echo decision tree for suspected endocarditis. (IDSA guidelines, courtesy of AHA, 2005)

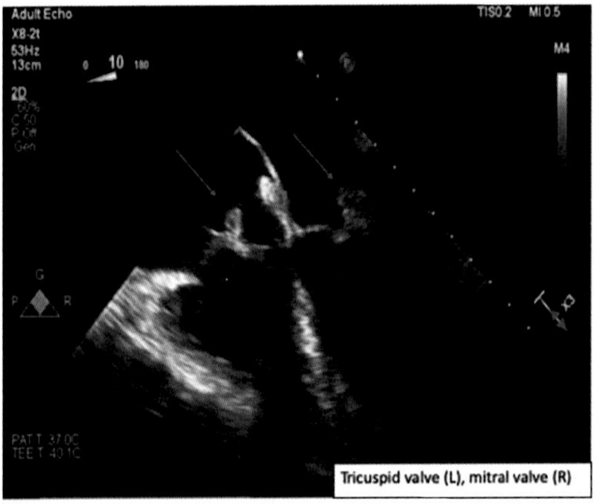

FIGURE 15.2 TEE image showing combined TV and MV vegetations. (Recorded 4/10/2019 by John Ricketts, MD)

Treatment

General

- In clinically stable patients, obtain blood cultures before initiating therapy.
  - *Administration of antibiotics prior to blood cultures is a common cause of "culture-negative" endocarditis and reduces rates of recovery of bacteria via blood culture by 35–40%* [7] *(Clinical Pearl).*
- The goal is to eliminate infection and sterilize vegetations using antibiotic therapy targeted at the relevant organisms and may require both medical (infectious diseases consultation) and surgical (cardiac surgery consultation) approaches.
- High bacterial density, slow rate of growth, and low metabolic activity necessitate prolonged courses (4–6 weeks) of antibiotics, though can be shorter for right-sided IE [8].
- Days of therapy should be counted from the first day of negative blood cultures.

Early/Empiric

- Initial antibiotic therapy in endocarditis is nearly always empirical and should be based on factors that relate to patient characteristics, prior antimicrobial exposures and microbiological findings, and epidemiologic features (see Table 6 of IDSA guidelines [3]).
  - Vancomycin and ceftriaxone are reasonable first-line agents in most scenarios
- Infectious disease consultation should accompany the selection of an empiric regimen to help guide therapy.
- Obtain two sets of blood cultures every 24–48 h until negative.

Directed

- Common pathogens are listed below but therapy should be tailored to the patient, in consultation with an infectious disease specialist.
- Staphylococci
  - Most common strains in IE are *S. aureus* and coagulase-negative staphylococci.
  - For methicillin-susceptible staphylococci, beta-lactam therapy (nafcillin or cefazolin) is preferred.

    Vancomycin should only be used for severe penicillin allergy in consultation with infectious diseases.
  - For methicillin-resistant staphylococci, vancomycin (alternative: daptomycin) remains the agent of choice.
  - Gentamicin and rifampin should not be routinely used for native valve IE [3].
  - Six weeks is recommended for most patients with left-sided IE, though 4 weeks can be used for right-sided IE.

    Some data support oral therapy for 4 weeks in right-sided IE in the setting of IDU [9, 10].
- Streptococci
  - Most commonly from the viridans group (such as *S. mitis, S. salivarius,* and *S. mutans*) and *S. gallolyticus* (formerly *S. bovis*).

In native valves, both penicillin G and ceftriaxone can be used as monotherapy for 4 weeks with highly penicillin-susceptible strains. In some patients with uncomplicated endocarditis, rapid response to therapy, and no underlying renal dysfunction, a 2-week course of gentamicin in addition to penicillin G or ceftriaxone is reasonable. If the strain is penicillin resistant, then vancomycin plus gentamicin should be used for 4 weeks [2].

In patients allergic to penicillin and ceftriaxone, a 4-week course of vancomycin IV is used.

- Organisms such as *S. pneumoniae*, *S. pyogenes*, and groups B, C, F, and G β-hemolytic streptococci are uncommon.

  Some, such as group B streptococci, may benefit from early surgical intervention [11].

- Enterococci
  - Enterococci are the third leading cause of endocarditis, with *E. faecalis* (~97%) and *E. faecium* (~1–2%) being the most common organisms [3].
  - Typical antibiotic regimens consist of ampicillin or aqueous penicillin G plus gentamicin or ampicillin plus ceftriaxone. Both of these regimens have recommended durations of 4–6 weeks for native valve disease and at least 6 weeks for prosthetic valve disease. If a patient is unable to tolerate, or resistant to penicillin or ampicillin, vancomycin should be used instead in combination with gentamicin [3].
  - Vancomycin-resistant enterococcus (VRE) endocarditis should be managed in conjunction with infectious disease specialists, but either linezolid or daptomycin is frequently used.
- Other organisms
  - HACEK organisms are usually treated with ceftriaxone IV for 4–6 weeks.
  - For-culture negative IE, vancomycin plus ceftriaxone is often used, though treatment should be targeted for the most likely organisms.
  - Fungal endocarditis is usually treated with amphotericin B.

Surgery

- Surgery has become a vital part of treatment for patients with IE, with about 50% of both native and prosthetic valve endocarditis patients undergoing valve surgery during their initial hospitalization [3].
- Early surgery is indicated in patients who present with signs or symptoms of heart failure, patients with fungal or multidrug-resistant bacterial pathogens, patients with new-onset heart block or abscess, and patients who do not respond appropriately to antibiotic therapy (complete list in Table 15.2).

TABLE 15.2 Indications for potential surgical intervention in endocarditis

Indications for potential surgical intervention
Vegetation
Persistent vegetation after systemic embolization
Anterior mitral leaflet vegetation with size >10 mm
≥1 embolic events during the first 2 weeks of antimicrobial therapy
Increase in vegetation size despite appropriate antimicrobial therapy
Valvular dysfunction
Acute aortic or mitral insufficiency with signs of ventricular failure
Heart failure unresponsive to medical therapy
Valve perforation or rupture
Perivalvular extension
Valvular dehiscence, rupture, or fistula
New heart block
Large abscess or extension of abscess despite appropriate antimicrobial therapy

Modified from Baddour et al. [2]

- Involve cardiac surgery early if potential surgical intervention may be needed.

Post-discharge Therapy

- Should be arranged in conjunction with your infectious disease consultant.
  - Most patients will be discharged with home IV antibiotics.
  - Selected patients may be managed with an oral regimen including those with IDU.
- The timing for transition from inpatient to outpatient antibiotic therapy is based on the local availability of medical care in the outpatient setting, risk factors, and timing of potential adverse outcomes [12].

Monitoring/Adverse Events/Complications

Embolization

- Systemic embolization occurs in 22–50% of cases of endocarditis and can affect a variety of body systems, such as cerebral, coronary, pulmonary, and peripheral emboli [13].
  - Up to 65% of embolic events involve the central nervous system, and 90% of these involve the middle cerebral arteries [14].
  - Highest incidence of emboli is seen with mitral valve disease (anterior more than posterior leaflet) and in infections with *S. aureus*, *Candida*, and HACEK organisms [3].
  - Most emboli will occur within the first 2–4 weeks of antibiotic therapy [15].
  - *Neurologic imaging should be performed in all patients with endocarditis who develop severe, localized headache, neurologic deficits, or meningeal signs* [3] *(Clinical Pearl)*.

Asymptomatic patients may have positive MRI. MRI findings should be interpreted with neurology consultants to determine the time of surgery to avoid hemorrhagic conversion of emboli.

Perivalvular Abscess

- Extension of infection beyond the valve annulus leads to a higher mortality rate, higher likelihood of developing heart failure, and more frequent need for cardiac surgery [3].
- Occurs in 10–40% of native valve disease and 56–100% of prosthetic valve disease [16], and most commonly on the aortic valve, where it spreads near the membranous septum and AV node, frequently causing AV block.
  – New AV block has a positive predictive value of 88% for abscess formation, but a sensitivity of only 45% [17].
- TEE has high sensitivity (76–100%) and specificity (95%) for detecting perivalvular abscess, with a positive predictive value of 87% and a negative predictive value of 89% [18].
- Evaluation by surgery should be obtained early for all patients with perivalvular abscess.

Anticoagulation

- The optimal role of anticoagulation in patients with infective endocarditis, especially those with mechanical valves, remains controversial.
- Decisions on anticoagulation should be made in conjunction with your cardiology consultant based on the patient's risk of thrombosis versus their risk of bleeding, as well as any concurrent thrombotic or hemorrhagic complications.

Key Learning Points

1. Always obtain three sets of blood cultures prior to initiating empiric antibiotic coverage for infective endocarditis.
2. Empiric antibiotic coverage should be broad initially and then narrowed once blood culture results for specific organisms are available.
3. Start with a transthoracic echocardiogram and then proceed to transesophageal echocardiogram with the assistance of your cardiology team.
4. Have a low threshold to involve surgery for evaluation for surgical intervention, as almost 50% of patients undergo valve surgery during their initial hospitalization.
5. Have a high suspicion for embolic complications in patients who exhibit new neurologic complications early in their treatment course.

References

1. Duval X, Delahaye F, Alla F, Tattevin P, Obadia JF, Le Moing V, Doco-Lecompte T, Celard M, Poyart C, Strady C, Chirouze C, Bes M, Cambau E, Iung B, Selton-Suty C, Hoen B, AEPEI Study Group. Temporal trends in infective endocarditis in the context of prophylaxis guideline modifications: three successive population-based surveys. J Am Coll Cardiol. 2012;59:1968–76. https://doi.org/10.1016/j.jacc.2012.02.029.
2. Fowler VG Jr, Sanders LL, Kong LK, McClelland RS, Gottlieb GS, Li J, Ryan T, Sexton DJ, Roussakis G, Harrell LJ, Corey GR. Infective endocarditis due to S. aureus: 59 prospectively identified cases with follow-up. Clin Infect Dis. 1999;28:106–14. https://doi.org/10.1086/515076.
3. Baddour LM, Wilson WR, Bayer AS, et al. Infective endocarditis in adults: diagnosis, antimicrobial therapy, and management of complications: a scientific statement for healthcare profes-

sionals from the American Heart Association. Circulation. 2015;132(15):1435–86.

4. Werner M, Andersson R, Olaison L, Hogevik H. A clinical study of culture-negative endocarditis. Medicine (Baltimore). 2003;82:263–73. https://doi.org/10.1097/01.md.0000085056.63483.d2.
5. Hoen B, Selton-Suty C, Lacassin F, Etienne J, Briançon S, Leport C, Canton P. Infective endocarditis in patients with negative blood cultures: analysis of 88 cases from a one-year nationwide survey in France. Clin Infect Dis. 1995;20:501–6.
6. Pazin GJ, Saul S, Thompson ME. Blood culture positivity: suppression by outpatient antibiotic therapy in patients with bacterial endocarditis. Arch Intern Med. 1982;142:263–8.
7. Andrews MM, von Reyn CF. Patient selection criteria and management guidelines for outpatient parenteral antibiotic therapy for native valve infective endocarditis. Clin Infect Dis. 33:203–9. https://doi.org/10.1086/321814.
8. Durack DT, Beeson PB. Experimental bacterial endocarditis, II: survival of a bacteria in endocardial vegetations. Br J Exp Pathol. 1972;53:50–3.
9. Dworkin RJ, Lee BL, Sande MA, Chambers HF. Treatment of right-sided S. aureus endocarditis in intravenous drug users with ciprofloxacin and rifampicin. Lancet. 1989;2:1071–3.
10. Lefort A, Mainardi JL, Selton-Suty C, Casassus P, Guillevin L, Lortholary O. Streptococcus pneumoniae endocarditis in adults: a multicenter study in France in the era of penicillin resistance (1991-1998): the Pneumococcal Endocarditis Study Group. Medicine (Baltimore). 2000;79:327–37.
11. Geraci JE, Wilson WR. Symposium on infective endocarditis, III: endocarditis due to Gram-negative bacteria: report of 56 cases. Mayo Clin Proc. 1982;57:145–8.
12. Sanfilippo AJ, Picard MH, Newell JB, Rosas E, Davidoff R, Thomas JD, Weyman AE. Echocardiographic assessment of patients with infectious endocarditis: prediction of risk for complications. J Am Coll Cardiol. 1991;18:1191–9.
13. Heiro M, Nikoskelainen J, Engblom E, Kotilainen E, Marttila R, Kotilainen P. Neurologic manifestations of infective endocarditis: a 17-year experience in a teaching hospital in Finland. Arch Intern Med. 2000;160:2781–7.
14. Steckelberg JM, Murphy JG, Ballard D, Bailey K, Tajik AJ, Taliercio CP, Giuliani ER, Wilson WR. Emboli in infective endocarditis:

the prognostic value of echocardiography. Ann Intern Med. 1991;114:635–40. https://doi.org/10.7326/0003-4819-114-8-635.
15. Hess A, Klein I, Iung B, et al. Brain MRI findings in neurologically asymptomatic patients with infective endocarditis. AJNR Am J Neuroradiol. 2013;34:1579–84.
16. Carpenter JL. Perivalvular extension of infection in patients with infectious endocarditis. Rev Infect Dis. 1991;13:127–38.
17. Blumberg EA, Karalis DA, Chandrasekaran K, Wahl JM, Vilaro J, Covalesky VA, Mintz GS. Endocarditis-associated paravalvular abscesses: do clinical parameters predict the presence of abscess? Chest. 1995;107:898–903.
18. Daniel WG, Mügge A, Martin RP, Lindert O, Hausmann D, Nonnast-Daniel B, Laas J, Lichtlen PR. Improvement in the diagnosis of abscesses associated with endocarditis by transesophageal echocardiography. N Engl J Med. 1991;324:795–800. https://doi.org/10.1056/NEJM199103213241203.

Chapter 16
Peripheral Artery Disease, Carotid Artery Disease, and Renal Artery Disease

Dandan Chen and Bryan J. Wells

Abbreviations

ABI	Ankle-brachial index
ALI	Acute limb ischemia
CAS	Carotid artery stent
CEA	Carotid endarterectomy
CLI	Chronic limb ischemia
CTA	Computed tomography angiography
DM	Diabetes mellitus
DUS	Duplex ultrasound
FMD	Fibromuscular dysplasia
HLD	Hyperlipidemia

D. Chen (✉)
Department of Medicine, Division of Cardiology, Emory University, Atlanta, GA, USA
e-mail: dchen50@emory.edu

B. J. Wells
Department of Medicine, Division of Cardiology, Emory University Hospital Midtown, Atlanta, GA, USA
e-mail: bjwells@emory.edu

B. J. Wells et al. (eds.), *Handbook of Inpatient Cardiology*,
https://doi.org/10.1007/978-3-030-47868-1_16

HTN	Hypertension
IC	Intermittent claudication
ICA	Internal carotid artery
MRA	Magnetic resonance angiography
PAD	Peripheral arterial disease
TBI	Toe-branchial index
TIA	Transient ischemic attack
TSPG	Translesional systolic pressure gradient

Peripheral Artery Disease

Introduction and Risk Factors

- Peripheral arterial disease (PAD) is defined as narrowing and obstruction of blood flow of major systemic arteries other than those of the cerebral and coronary circulations. The most common etiology is atherosclerosis; however, there are many causes of PAD including vasculitis (Takayasu and giant cell arteritis), dysplastic syndromes, fibromuscular dysplasia (FMD), degenerative conditions, thrombosis, and thromboembolism [2, 4, 7].
- Risk factors: Age ≥ 65 years, smoking, hypertension (HTN), hyperlipidemia (HLD), diabetes mellitus (DM), obesity, with known atherosclerotic disease in another vascular beds, family history of vascular disease, ionizing radiation, repetitive injury (commonly associated with upper extremity PAD). *Smoking and DM are the strongest predictors of morbidity and mortality* [2, 10].

Clinical Manifestations of PAD

- *Lower extremity PAD.*
  - *Asymptomatic PAD*: Over 50% of patients.
  - *Intermittent claudication (IC)*: Exertional aching pain typically in the calves and/or buttocks and relived by rest.

- *Chronic limb ischemia (CLI)*: Resting pain or nonhealing wounds or ulceration with or without tissue necrosis (gangrene). Need early surgical consult and angiography.
- *Acute limb ischemia (ALI)*: "*Six P's*": pain, pallor, paralysis, pulselessness, poikilothermia, and paranesthesia. It is a medical emergency and requires prompt revascularization. The Rutherford classifications for ALI are shown in Table 16.1.

• *Upper extremity PAD*. Arm and hand claudication, digital ulceration, and neurologic symptoms caused by vertebral-subclavian steal.

Table 16.1 The Rutherford classifications for acute limb ischemia [13]

	Viable (I)	**Marginally threatened (IIa)**	**Immediately threatened (IIb)**	**Nonviable (III)**
Pain	Mild	Moderate	Severe	Variable
Capillary refill	Intact	Delayed	Delayed	Absent
Muscle weakness	None	None	Mild-to-moderate	Complete, paralysis (rigor)
Sensory loss	None	None or minimal (toes only)	More than toes; rest pain in feet	Complete, anesthetic
Arterial Doppler	Audible	Inaudible	Inaudible	Inaudible
Venous Doppler	Audible	Audible	Audible	Inaudible
Treatment	Urgent evaluation	Urgent revascularization	Emergency revascularization	Amputation

Clinical Pearl
If patients present with the "six P's" – pain, pallor, paralysis, pulselessness, poikilothermia, and paresthesia – then it is a medical emergency and requires prompt revascularization for acute limb ischemia (ALI).

Physical Examination

- *Lower extremity PAD.* Skin appearance (positive Burger's test), temperature, palpation of all peripheral pulses (branchial, radial, femoral, popliteal, dorsalis, pedis, and posterior tibial arteries), auscultation for bruits (aortic, renal, femoral), and extremity neurologic examination.
- *Upper extremity PAD.* Besides the above physical findings, the simplest and excellent screening test is to check blood pressure in both arms. A brachial blood pressure difference of >15–20 mm Hg is abnormal and suggestive of subclavian (or innominate) artery stenosis.

Diagnosis

- *Ankle-brachial index (ABI).* The initial diagnostic tests for diagnosing and assessing the severity of PAD as well as monitoring the progress of existing disease and response to treatment are given in Table 16.2. ABI ≤ 0.9 suggests PAD and ABI > 1.4 indicates that arteries are not compressible,

TABLE 16.2 Ankle-brachial index (ABI) to assess the severity of PAD

Severity	Normal	Borderline	Mild	Moderate	Severe	Non-compressible
ABI	1.00–1.40	0.91–0.99	0.71–0.90	0.41–0.70	<0.40	>1.40

which may be due to end-stage renal disease and long-standing DM. *Toe-branchial index (TBI) is an alternative approach for these patients. Exercise ABI testing* is useful when resting ABI is normal or borderline [2, 8, 10].

- *Duplex ultrasound (DUS), computed tomography angiography (CTA),* and *magnetic resonance angiography (MRA)* are useful noninvasive tests to evaluate anatomy and surveillance after revascularization. *But they should NOT be performed for the anatomic assessment in patients with asymptomatic PAD* [2, 8, 10].
- *Catheter-based angiography* is recommended for the evaluation of patient for whom revascularization procedures are planned or for whom noninvasive techniques are inconclusive [2, 8, 10].

Differential Diagnosis

Symptomatic baker's cyst, venous claudication, acute/chronic compartment syndrome, nerve root compression, hip arthritis, foot/ankle arthritis.

Treatment

- *Aggressive modification of risk factors*: Supervised exercise therapy is the first-line therapy for claudication (CLEVER trial) [17]. Lifestyle modification including smoking cessation, weight loss, and dietary intervention. Aggressive managements for HTN, DM, and HLD
- *Pharmacological therapies*:
  - Antiplatelet therapy: *Aspirin alone* (75–325 mg daily) or *clopidogrel alone* (75 mg daily). *Dual antiplatelet therapy (aspirin and clopidogrel)* may be reasonable to reduce the risk of limb-related events in patients with symptomatic PAD after revascularization [2, 8].
  - Symptomatic relief therapy: *Cilostazol* (100 mg orally twice daily) is a phosphodiesterase-3 enzyme inhibitor,

which can improve walking distance in patients with claudication. If symptoms remain unimproved after 3 months, it should be discontinued. *Cilostazol is contraindicated in heart failure of any severity* [2, 8].
  - Anticoagulation: The combination of low-dose rivaroxaban 2.5 mg twice a day and aspirin significantly lower the incident of major adverse limb events and the related complications but increase the major bleeding risk (COMPASS trial) [18].
- *Revascularization.* Patients with lifestyle-limiting claudication with an inadequate response to medical therapy and exercise should be considered for revascularization. Percutaneous angioplasty with or without stenting is the first option. *Urgent or emergent vascular surgical consult and revascularization are required for ALI* [2, 6, 8].

Carotid Artery Disease

Introduction and Risk Factors

- The atherosclerotic carotid disease usually develops at branch points and bends especially at the bifurcation of the common carotid artery and origin of the internal carotid artery (ICA). The progression of carotid plaques results in carotid stenosis, obstruction, or plaque rupture, which can cause ischemic stroke or transient ischemic attack from embolization thrombosis or hemodynamic compromise. There is a linear increase in the risk of stroke while the stenosis increases to >70% [2, 3].
- Risk factors: smoking, age, gender (men $\gg$ women if age $<$ 75 years; women $\gg$ men if age $>$ 75 years), HTN, HLD, DM, other vascular diseases (e.g., CAD, PAD).

Clinical Manifestations

- *Asymptomatic* carotid atherosclerosis is a marker of increased risk for ischemic stroke, myocardial infarction, and vascular death.
- *Symptomatic* carotid disease is defined as focal neurologic symptoms (e.g., amaurosis fugax, contralateral weakness or numbness, dysarthria or aphasia, spatial neglect, homonymous visual loss) in the distribution of a carotid artery with a significant stenosis. *All patients with a recent stroke or a transient ischemic attack (TIA) should be evaluated for carotid artery disease* [2, 3].

Diagnosis

NOT recommended to screen asymptomatic individual. However, it is reasonable to screen with DUS in asymptomatic individuals with carotid bruit and in patients who have symptomatic atherosclerotic disease in another vascular bed (i.e., PAD, CAD, or aortic aneurysm), or have two or more risk factors for atherosclerotic disease.

- *Noninvasive studies* (Table 16.3): *DUS*: the first-line screening test. *CTA:* high sensitivity, reproducibility, and ability to visualize the entire carotid artery including extracranial and intracranial portions. It also provides information about adjacent bony and soft tissue structures. *Contrast-enhanced MRA:* higher quality images and less artifact when compared with CTA.
- *Contrast angiography*: The gold standard for assessment of carotid atherosclerosis. Typically, only needed for diagnostic uncertainty or if intervention is considered.

TABLE 16.3 Noninvasive studies for carotid artery disease

	Sensitivity	Specificity
DUS	80–95%	80–95%
CTA	75–100%	63–95%
MRA	91–95%	88–92%

DUS duplex ultrasound, *CTA* computed tomography angiography, *MRA* magnetic resonance angiography

Clinical Pearl
All patients with a recent stroke or a transient ischemic attack (TIA) should be evaluated for the carotid artery disease.

Treatment

- *Aggressive cardiovascular risk factor modifications* as discussed in the PAD section.
- *Antiplatelet therapy*:
  - *Aspirin (75–325 mg daily)* in all patients with extracranial carotid or vertebral atherosclerosis to reduce ischemic cardiovascular events.
  - *Clopidogrel (75 mg daily)* may be used as an alternative to aspirin without increasing bleeding risk, when there is contraindication to aspirin therapy, aspirin allergy, or resistance (CAPRIE trial) [17].
  - *Low-dose aspirin (50 mg daily) plus dipyridamole (200 mg twice daily)* may be superior to aspirin alone or dipyridamole alone in the prevention of ischemic stroke, or vascular death (ESPS-2 study) [16].
  - *DAPT* is *NOT* routinely used in patients with carotid atherosclerosis in the absence of an endovascular intervention or alternative indication (e.g., coronary stenting).

- *Anticoagulation*: *NOT* recommended unless there is an alternate indication for anticoagulation (i.e., mechanical heart valve, atrial fibrillation).
- *Invasive interventions: Carotid endarterectomy (CEA)* and *carotid artery stent (CAS)* with embolic protection device (EPD) have similar safety and efficacy. *Both should only be performed at institutions where the perioperative stroke and death rate is at the most <3% in asymptomatic patients and <6% in symptomatic patients* [3, 13].
  - CAS superior to CEA if difficult surgical anatomy, prior neck irradiation, restenosis after CEA, and significant comorbidities that may increase surgical risk].
  - CEA superior to CAS if older patients, anatomic difficulty for stenting.
  - *Indications for invasive interventions:* Symptomatic, and low or average surgical risk, and the ipsilateral ICA stenosis >50% as documented by noninvasive imaging, and the anticipated rate of perioperative stroke or mortality is <6%. It is reasonable to perform CEA in asymptomatic patients who have >70% of stenosis in the ICA if the risk of perioperative stroke, MI, and death is low. A full assessment of comorbid conditions, life expectancy, and a thorough discussion of the risks and benefits of the procedure should be performed prior to the procedure. Prophylactic CAS might be considered in highly selected patients with asymptomatic carotid stenosis (minimum 60% of stenosis by catheter angiography and 70% by validated DUS). But its effectiveness may not be superior to medical therapy alone [2, 3, 11].
- *Complications and postprocedural management*:
  - *Periprocedural cerebrovascular events* (MI, TIA/stroke): Adequate procedural anticoagulation during PCI, and preloading with antiplatelet is helpful to minimize stroke risk [2, 3].
  - *Bradycardia and hypotension*: Usually occur within 24 hours after intervention because of stretching of the carotid sinus baroreceptors.

  - *Management*: fluid resuscitation, atropine administration, and/or a low-dose vasopressor infusion (i.e., dopamine or phenylephrine). *Unless the patient is hypertensive, antihypertensive and negative inotropic medications are usually withheld perioperation* [2].
- *Hyperperfusion syndrome*: Presented with ipsilateral headache with or without focal neurologic symptoms due to the rapid return of flow to a chronically underperfused cerebral vascular bed with resultant disordered autoregulation. Severe HTN, critical carotid stenosis, and contralateral carotid occlusion are the most common risk factors. Thus, *strict blood pressure control (SBP < 150 mm Hg) is critical in patients following carotid stenting.*
- *Antiplatelet therapy*: Patients undergoing CAS should be preloaded with DAPT (aspirin and clopidogrel) at least 2 days prior to the procedure if possible. Patient undergoing CEA should be preloaded at least with aspirin or clopidogrel. After the procedure, lifelong aspirin therapy should be continued, and clopidogrel should be continued for at least 6 weeks. If patients have recurrent symptoms or a history of neck irradiation, clopidogrel should be continued indefinitely.
- *Wound care*: Antibiotics are limited to perioperative prophylaxis (Cefozolin).
- *Duplex surveillance*: Repeat DUS should be obtained 3–6 weeks following procedures to establish a new baseline for future comparison. Duplex surveillance is performed at 6 months and then annually.

Renal Arterial Disease

Introduction

- The most common causes of renal artery stenosis (RAS) are atherosclerosis and fibromuscular dysplasia (FMD). Atherosclerosis counting for 90% of RAS primarily affects over the age of 45 years and usually involves the ostium or the proximal main renal artery. This disorder is particularly common in patients with diffuse atherosclerosis. FMD accounts for <10% and most often affects women under the age of 50 years and typically involves the distal main renal artery or the segmental branches.

Clinical Manifestations and Physical Findings

- *HTN*: abrupt onset of HTN (age < 30 years, often secondary to FMD; age > 55 years, often due to atherosclerotic disease) or previously well-controlled chronic hypertension becoming resistant to medical therapy (three-drug regimen including a diuretic).
- *Azotemia*: unexplained or an acute rise in serum creatinine following the administration of ACEIs or ARBs.
- *Recurrent flash pulmonary edema* often with normal left ventricular function.
- Epigastric bruits, evidence of atherosclerosis in other vascular beds (e.g., carotid or femoral bruits and diminished pedal pulses)
- Unilateral *atrophic kidney* or *a size discrepancy between the two kidneys*. If bilateral RAS exists, there may be no size discrepancy between kidneys.

Diagnosis

- *Laboratory study*: Acute elevation of creatinine; rapid decline of estimated glomerular filtration rate (eGFR) and measured GFR.
- *Imaging studies*: Comparison of sensitivity and specificity with angiography is shown in Table 16.4. *DUS*: it is highly useful for surveillance of renal arteries after stenting. A peak systolic velocity >200 cm/second if diagnosed by duplex Doppler ultrasonography. *MRA*: noninvasive and

Table 16.4 Imaging studies for renal artery stenosis

	Sensitivity	Specificity
DUS	84–98%	62–99%
MRA	90–100%	76–94%
CTA	59–96%	82–99%

DUS duplex ultrasound, *CTA* computed tomography angiography, *MRA* magnetic resonance angiography

has ability to generate 3D reconstructions. *CTA*: can be used to detect in-stent restenosis because of no significant imaging artifact with metal clips or stents. Luminal narrowing >75% if diagnosed with magnetic resonance angiography or computerized tomography angiography (or >70% with additional evidence of renal ischemia; or >50% with post-stenotic dilation) [6].

- *Renal angiogram*:the gold standard for the diagnosis of RAS. It can visualize the main renal and accessory renal arteries and their branches. Luminal narrowing >60% if diagnosed with conventional angiography, followed by measurement of translesional systolic pressure gradients (TSPG >20 mmHg defined as a significant RAS) [6].

Treatment

Despite antihypertensive therapy, RAS tends to progress and may be associated with renal ischemia and loss of renal function.

- *Medical therapy*: management for HTN: ACEIs and ARBs are preferred for unilateral RAS. ACEIs and ARBs should not be used in patients with bilateral RAS or a solitary kidney with RAS [1].
- *Percutaneous revascularization*: Early restoration of renal artery patency may improve hypertension management and minimize progressive renal dysfunction. *Cure of hypertension after revascularization is most likely in patients*

who have been hypertensive for less than 5 years. Significant proteinuria (>1 g/d), renal atrophy, parenchymal renal disease, and diffuse renal arterial disease are also predictors of poor outcomes with RAS interventions. *Indications: severe RAS (>70% stenosis or 50–70% stenosis with peak pressure gradient > 20 mmHg or mean gradient > 10 mmHg) PLUS* progressive renal dysfunction, or poorly controlled HTN, or recurrent episodes of unstable angina, or recurrent unexplained flash pulmonary edema [15].

- *Surgical revascularization*: Including surgical bypass (aortorenal, celiac-renal, or mesenteric-renal) and endarterectomy. *Indications*: Patients with RAS and aortic diseases (either aneurysmal or occlusive). Patients with significant atherosclerotic RAS and clinical indications for intervention with multiple renal arteries or early branching main renal artery. Patient with FMD associated with microaneurysms or complex disease involving segmental renal arteries [10, 14].

Clinical Pearl

ACEIs and ARBs should not be used in patients with bilateral renal artery stenosis (RAS) or a solitary kidney with RAS. Cure of hypertension after revascularization for RAS is most likely in patients who have been hypertensive for less than 5 years.

Key Learning Points

1. Careful history and exam skills are important for the recognition and evaluation of PAD.
2. The ankle brachial index (ABI) is the initial diagnostic test of choice diagnosis and assessment of PAD severity and response to treatment.
3. Invasive management of PAD is generally reserved for patients who are symptomatic or with end-organ damage.

References

1. ASTRAL Investigators, Wheatley K, Ives N, et al. Revascularization versus medical therapy for renal-artery stenosis. N Engl J Med. 2009;361:1953–62.
2. Griffin BP. Manual of cardiovascular medicine. 5th ed. Philadelphia: Wolters Kluwer; 2019. p. 407–19.
3. Brott TG, Halperin JL, Abbara S, Bacharach JM, Barr JD, Bush RL, Cates CU, Creager MA, Fowler SB, Friday G, Hertzberg VS, EB MI, Moore WS, Panagos PD, Riles TS, Rosenwasser RH, Taylor AJ. 2011 ASA/ACCF/AHA/AANN/AANS/ACR/ASNR/CNS/SAIP/SCAI/SIR/SNIS/SVM/SVS guideline on the management of patients with extracranial carotid and vertebral artery disease: executive summary. A report of the American College of Cardiology Foundation/American Heart Association Task Force on Practice Guidelines, and the American Stroke Association, American Association of Neuroscience Nurses, American Association of Neurological Surgeons, American College of Radiology, American Society of Neuroradiology, Congress of Neurological Surgeons, Society of Atherosclerosis Imaging and Prevention, Society for Cardiovascular Angiography and Interventions, Society of Interventional Radiology, Society of NeuroInterventional Surgery, Society for Vascular Medicine, and Society for Vascular Surgery. Circulation. 2011;124(4):489–532.
4. Campia U, Gerhard-Herman M, Piazza G, Goldhaber SZ. Peripheral artery disease: past, present, and future. Am J Med. 2019;132(10):1133–41.
5. CAPRIES Steering Committee. A randomised, blinded, trial of clopidogrel versus aspirin in patients at risk of ischaemic events (CAPRIE). Lancet. 1996;348(9038):1329–39.
6. Chonchol M, Linas S. Diagnosis and management of ischemic nephropathy. Clin J Am Soc Nephrol. 2006;1(2):172–81.
7. Conte SM, Vale PR. Peripheral arterial disease. Heart Lung Circ. 2018;27(4):427–32.
8. Gerhard-Herman MD, Gornik HL, Barrett C, Barshes NR, Corriere MA, Drachman DE, Fleisher LA, Fowkes FGR, Hamburg NM, Kinlay S, Lookstein R, Misra S, Mureebe L, Olin JW, Patel RAG, Regensteiner JG, Schanzer A, Shishehbor MH, Stewart KJ, Treat-Jacobson D, Walsh ME. 2016 AHA/ACC guideline on the management of patients with lower extremity peripheral artery disease: executive summary: a report of the

American College of Cardiology/American Heart Association Task Force on Clinical Practice Guidelines. J Am Coll Cardiol. 2017;69(11):1465–508.

9. Hughes JS, Dove HG, Gifford RW Jr, Feinstein AR. Duration of blood pressure elevation in accurately predicting surgical cure of renovascular hypertension. Am Heart J. 1981;101(4):408–13.
10. Levin SR, Arinze N, Siracuse JJ. Lower extremity critical limb ischemia: a review of clinical features and management. Trends Cardiovasc Med. 2019;30(3):125.
11. MRC European Carotid Surgery Trial: interim results for symptomatic patients with severe (70-99%) or with mild (0-29%) carotid stenosis. European Carotid Surgery Trialists' Collaborative Group. Lancet. 1991;337:1235–43.
12. North American Symptomatic Carotid Endarterectomy Trial. Methods, patient characteristics, and progress. Stroke. 1991;22:711–20.
13. Rutherford RB, Baker JD, Ernst C, et al. Recommended standards for reports dealing with lower extremity ischemia: revised version. J Vasc Surg. 1997;26:517–38.
14. Rundback JH, Sacks D, Kent KC, AHA Councils on Cardiovascular Radiology, High Blood Pressure Research, Kidney in Cardiovascular Disease, Cardio-Thoracic and Vascular Surgery, and Clinical Cardiology, and the Society of Interventional Radiology FDA Device Forum Committee, et al. Guidelines for the reporting of renal artery revascularization in clinical trials. American Heart Association. Circulation. 2002;106(12):1572–85.
15. Textor SC, Misra S, Oderich GS. Percutaneous revascularization for ischemic nephropathy: the past, present, and future. Kidney Int. 2013;83:28–40.
16. Murphy TP, Cutlip DE, Regensteiner JG, et al. CLEVER Study Investigators. Supervised Exercise Versus Primary Stenting for Claudication Resulting From Aortoiliac Peripheral Artery DiseaseCirculation. 2012; 125(1):130–9.
17. Diener HC, Cunha L, Forbes C, et al. European Stroke Prevention Study 2: dipyridamole and acetylsalicylic acid ithe secondary prevention of stroke. J Neurol Sci. 1996;143(1-2):1–13.
18. Branch KR, Probstfield JL, Eikelboom JW, et al. Rivaroxaban With or Without Aspirin in Patients With Heart Failure and Chronic Coronary or Peripheral Artery Disease. Circulation. 2019;140(7):529–537.

Chapter 17
Aortic Disease

Marvin Louis Roy Lu and Rebecca LeLeiko

Abbreviations

AAS	Acute aortic syndrome
ACE	Angiotensin converting enzyme
ACR	American College of Rheumatology
BB	Beta blockers
BPM	Beats per minute
CCB	Calcium channel blockers
CRP	C-reactive protein
CT	Computed tomography
CTA	Computed tomography angiogram
CXR	Chest X-ray
ECG	Electrocardiogram
ESR	Erythrocyte sedimentation rate
ICD	Implantable cardiac defibrillator
IMH	Intramural hematoma
IV	Intravenous

M. L. R. Lu (✉)
Cardiovascular Disease, Emory University School of Medicine, Atlanta, GA, USA
e-mail: mylu2@emory.edu

R. LeLeiko
Department of Internal Medicine, Division of Cardiology, Emory University Hospital, Atlanta, GA, USA

B. J. Wells et al. (eds.), *Handbook of Inpatient Cardiology*,
https://doi.org/10.1007/978-3-030-47868-1_17

MRA	Magnetic resonance angiogram
MRI	Magnetic resonance imaging
PAU	Penetrating aortic ulcer
SBP	Systolic blood pressure
TEE	Transesophageal echocardiogram
TNF	Tumor necrosis factor

Acute Aortic Syndrome

Acute Aortic Syndrome (AAS)

A general term that includes acute aortic dissection, intramural hematoma, and symptomatic penetrating aortic ulcer.

- Acute aortic dissection – rupture or tear of the aortic intima that spreads anterograde or retrograde causing the formation of an intimal flap and creating a false lumen.
  - Due to mechanisms that cause weakening of the medial layers, and degeneration of the tunica media such as elastic fiber disruption, loss of vascular smooth muscle cells and increased proteoglycan deposition are found.
- Aortic intramural hematoma (IMH) – hematoma confined within the medial wall layers without any intimal tear.
- A penetrating aortic ulcer (PAU) – focal ulceration of an atherosclerotic plaque that extends into the internal elastic lamina and forms a hematoma within the tunica media layer.

Risk Factors

- Long-standing hypertension – most common predisposing factor, occurring in 72% of patients [1]. Patients with pre-existing aortic aneurysm, dyslipidemia, smoking, and cocaine use are also at risk.
- Connective tissue disorders such as Marfan syndrome, Loeys-Dietz syndrome (EDS), vascular type of Ehlers-

Danlos syndrome (EDS), and bicuspid aortic valve-related aortopathies have a genetic predisposition to AAS.

- Trauma and medical procedures such as cardiac catheterization and vascular interventions can also be associated with AAS.

Classification (Table 17.1)

> **Clinical Pearl**
> Stanford A or Debakey I or II dissections are surgical emergencies – call the surgeon stat!

Clinical Presentation

- Over 90% of patients present with pain in either the chest or back, described as sharp, severe, and sudden in onset [1].
- A pulse deficit may be appreciated (weak or absent pulse compared to heart sounds) in the brachial, femoral, or carotid area. This is caused by the intimal flap or compression of the true lumen by a hematoma.
- Signs of acute aortic regurgitation – may be difficult to appreciate because of its short duration caused by the rapid equilibration of aortic and left ventricular diastolic pressures.

TABLE 17.1 Aortic dissection classifications

Stanford classification		**Debakey classification**	
	Location of the dissection flap		**Location of the dissection flap**
Type A	Ascending aorta ± descending aorta	Type I	Ascending and descending aorta
Type B	Descending aorta only	Type II	Ascending aorta
		Type III	Descending aorta

- Diastolic decrescendo murmur
- Widened pulse pressure
- Hypotension
- Heart failure symptoms

- Syncope – may indicate development of cardiac tamponade, or stroke secondary to obstruction of the great vessels.
- Signs of ischemia
  - Spinal cord ischemia – acute onset paraplegia
  - Mesenteric ischemia – severe abdominal pain out of proportion to physical exam
  - Renal ischemia – oliguria and rising serum creatinine level
- Signs of compression
  - Horner's syndrome – compression of the cervical sympathetic ganglion
  - Hoarseness – compression of the recurrent laryngeal nerve

> **Clinical Pearl**
> Acute onset severe chest pain in the presence of a pulse deficit and a new diastolic murmur should make you suspect an acute aortic syndrome.

Diagnosis

- ECG to rule out acute coronary syndrome.
- Chest X-ray (CXR) will show a widened mediastinum in 60–90% of cases, but data from the International Registry of Acute Aortic Dissection (IRAD) show that >20% of AAS patients will present without any mediastinal or aortic abnormalities [1].
- The choice of imaging modality largely depends on equipment availability, with computed tomography (CT) scan being the most widely available in the emergency department [2] (Table 17.2).

TABLE 17.2 Imaging modalities for the detection of aortic dissection

Imaging modality	Sensitivity (%)	Specificity (%)
Computed tomography	100	98
Transesophageal echocardiogram (TEE)	99	90
Magnetic resonance imaging (MRI)	100	98

Management

- Medical therapy is aimed at (1) lowering heart rate to <60 beats per minute (bpm) and (2) lowering systolic blood pressure (SBP) to 100–120 mmHg [3, 4].
  - *Intravenous (IV) Beta Blockers (BB)* – first-line therapy.

    If BB naïve – esmolol preferred (titratable, short half-life).

    Labetalol – reduces both heart rate and blood pressure control from beta and alpha adrenergic blockade, respectively.

    Other IV infusions – propranolol and metoprolol.
  - If BB are contraindicated – non-dihydropyridine calcium channel blockers (CCB) such as diltiazem or verapamil can be used.
  - *Vasodilators* such as nitroprusside and nicardipine are added if SBP is still >120 mmHg after adequate rate control with BB/CCB. *DO NOT USE* prior to rate control as it may cause reflex tachycardia and can increase left ventricular contraction, leading to an increase in aortic wall stress.
  - Provide adequate pain control.
- Surgical therapy generally indicated for ascending aortic involvement or with associated high-risk features (Fig. 17.1).

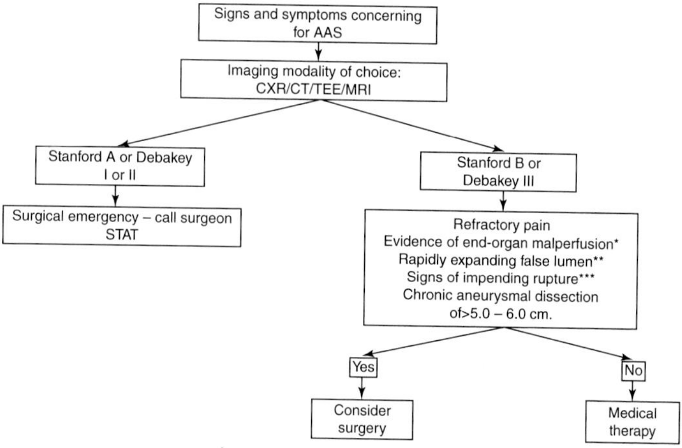

FIGURE 17.1 Management algorithm for acute aortic syndrome (AAS). *Visceral ischemia (mesenteric, renal, hepatosplenic), spinal ischemia, or limb ischemia. **>5 mm expansion in 6 months or >1 cm in 1 year. ***Hemorrhagic pleural effusion or expanding periaortic hematoma

Clinical Pearl
The first line of therapy for aortic dissection is IV beta blocker therapy. Add vasodilators only if SBP is still >120 mmHg after maximizing rate control with BB or CCB.

Aortic Aneurysm

Definition

- True aneurysm – permanent localized dilatation (at least 50% increase in diameter) of the artery that involves all three layers, although the intima and media may be too attenuated and difficult to visualize. For dilatation <50%, this is termed *ectasia*.
- Pseudoaneurysm – collection of blood contained by peri-arterial connective tissue and not by arterial wall layers.

Diagnosis

- Usually found incidentally through various imaging modalities.
- Ultrasound screening for abdominal aortic aneurysm is indicated in men of ages 65–74 who have ever smoked [5].
- Selection of the appropriate diagnostics depend on patient-related factors (allergy to contrast, claustrophobia, renal function, ICD placement) and institution-related factors such as availability of equipment and specialist.

> **Clinical Pearl**
> Aortic aneurysm is usually asymptomatic and found incidentally. Ultrasound screening is only indicated in men of ages 65–74 who have ever smoked. There is not enough evidence to support screening in other populations except in those with concomitant connective tissue disorders such as Marfan syndrome, LDS, and vascular EDS.

Management

- Blood pressure control
  - Drugs of choice are *beta blockers*, and *angiotensin converting enzyme (ACE) inhibitors or angiotensin receptor blockers (ARB)*.
- Surgical repair is reasonable for the following:
  - Thoracic aortic aneurysm
  - Chronic aortic dissection, intramural hematoma, or a penetrating aortic ulcer with an ascending aortic or aortic sinus diameter of ≥5.5 cm or a rate of growth of ≥0.5 cm/year even in the absence of symptoms
- In patients undergoing surgical aortic valve intervention, concomitant repair or replacement of the ascending aorta is indicated if the diameter is ≥4.5 cm.

Clinical Pearl
Surgical repair should be considered in AAS with a ≥5.5 cm diameter or a rate of growth of ≥0.5 cm/year even in the absence of symptoms. Patients with connective tissue disorders such as Marfan syndrome have a lower cut-off.

Special Populations with Associated Aortic Disease

Marfan Syndrome

- *FBN1* gene mutation is seen which encodes fibrillin-1, and to a lesser extent MFS2 gene.
- Usually present with a dilated aortic root and/or ascending aorta and are predisposed to ascending aortic dissection.
- Annual imaging is recommended to measure aortic diameter. More frequent imaging if the maximal aortic diameter is ≥4.5 cm or shows significant growth from baseline.
- Surgical repair is indicated if the external diameter of the root or the ascending aorta reaches ≥5.0 cm or less if the following are present:
  - Family history of aortic dissection at a diameter ≤5.0 cm
  - Severe aortic regurgitation
  - Rapid growth of ≥0.5 cm/year
- Women should be advised against pregnancy. Otherwise surgical replacement can be considered if the diameter reaches ≥4.0 cm in women who want to get pregnant.

Loeys-Dietz Syndrome

- *TGFBR1, TGFBR2, SMAD3, TGFB2*, or *TGFB3* autosomal gene mutation. These are associated with LDS types 1–5, respectively [6].

- Hypertelorism, bifid uvula and arterial ectasias, tortuosity, and aneurysm.
- The arterial disease is very aggressive and widespread in these patients, with a mean age of death at 26 years old noted in LDS types 1 and 2.
- Diagnosis made through a combination of diffuse arterial aneurysms, a family history of LDS, and confirmed by molecular testing.
- Cardiovascular care of these patients include the following:
  - Annual echocardiography to assess aortic root and ascending aorta
  - Strict blood pressure control
  - Avoid contact or competitive sports and isometric exercises
  - Avoid stimulant medications (such as decongestants) and vasoconstrictors (such as triptans)
  - Baseline head to pelvis MRA or CTA; with repeat imaging every 2 years or sooner in the presence of arterial aneurysms
- Aortic surgery is indicated if the maximal aortic diameter is >4.0 cm, or a rapidly expanding aortic root (>0.5 cm/year).

Vascular Type of Ehlers-Danlos Syndrome

- *COL3A1* autosomal dominant gene mutation which causes a defect in the collagen III synthesis.
- Arterial ruptures including aortic dissection and intestinal and uterine ruptures. Tissue fragility and hemorrhagic tendencies complicate surgery.
- Similar indications for surgical repair as with Marfan syndrome.

Turner Syndrome

- Partial or complete absence of one sex chromosome in a female phenotype, termed 45 XO.

- Bicuspid aortic valve (10–25%), coarctation of the aorta (8%), and dilation of the ascending aorta. These patients should undergo imaging to evaluate for these complications and repeat imaging done in 5–10 years if the initial results are within normal limits. If abnormalities exist then annual follow-up imaging is recommended.
- Similar indications for surgical repair as with Marfan syndrome.

Vasculitis

Takayasu Arteritis

- Idiopathic vasculitis of the elastic arteries involving the aorta and its branches.
- Female predominant 10:1, <40 years of age. Crosses racial and ethnic lines.
- Acute symptoms include fatigue, night sweats, weight loss, and generalized malaise. Once the vascular inflammation sets, the patients may have organ dysfunction, particularly cerebrovascular insufficiency (vision disturbances, stroke-like symptoms).
- 1990 American College of Rheumatology (ACR) criteria:
  - Age of onset younger than 40 years
  - Intermittent claudication
  - Diminished brachial artery pulse
  - Subclavian artery or aortic bruit
  - Systolic blood pressure variation of greater than 10 mmHg between arms
  - Angiographic (CT, MR) evidence of aorta or aortic branch vessel stenosis
  - Elevated ESR and CRP [7]
- The most common aneurysmal formation is in the descending aorta, although stenosis occurs more commonly than aneurysms.
- Management

- High-dose corticosteroids (prednisone 40–60 mg or equivalent dosages); steroids may be required for 1–2 years.
- Second-line therapies include methotrexate, azathioprine, and anti-TNF agents.

Clinical Pearl
Takayasu arteritis is a disease of young women (<40 years of age). Giant cell arteritis is a disease of old men and women (>50 years of age).

Giant Cell Arteritis

- Idiopathic vasculitis affecting the aorta and its branches.
- Female predominant 3:2, age > 50. Mostly affects northern Europeans.
- Symptoms include typical B symptoms acutely such as weight loss, night sweats, and fever. Scalp tenderness, headache, and jaw claudication are common as well as neurologic symptoms such as visual disturbances and various neuropathies.
- Polymyalgia rheumatica occurs 50% of the time – inflammation of proximal muscles and present as pain and stiffness, particularly with initiation of movement.
- 1990 ACR criteria for diagnosis:
  - Age older than 50 years
  - Recent-onset localized headache
  - Temporal artery pulse attenuation or tenderness
  - Erythrocyte sedimentation rate greater than 50 mm/h
  - Arterial biopsy demonstrating necrotizing vasculitis [8]
- Initial therapy is similar to that of Takayasu arteritis.
- *DO NOT DELAY* initiation of glucocorticoid therapy while waiting for biopsy result. The biopsy result does not get affected if it is done within 2 weeks of therapy [9].

Clinical Pearl

Steroids are the first line of therapy for aortic vasculitis. Do not delay the initiation of treatment while waiting for biopsy results.

Key Learning Points

1. Long-standing hypertension is the most common risk factor for acute aortic dissection. Connective tissue disorders such as Marfan syndrome and vascular EDS are also at elevated risk.
2. Over 90% of patients with AAS present with acute chest or back pain. Other signs and symptoms include syncope, a pulse deficit, new diastolic murmur, and signs of organ ischemia such as rising paraplegia, abdominal pain, and oliguria.
3. >20% of AAS will not present with any mediastinal widening on CXR. The initial imaging of choice is CT largely due to its rapid availability in the emergency department.
4. Management depends on the location of the AAS. Proximal AAS involving the ascending aorta and aortic arch are surgical emergencies, while AAS confined to the descending aorta can be medically managed with IV BB/CCB ± vasodilators.
5. Surgical repair is reasonable in patients with a thoracic aortic aneurysm, chronic aortic dissection, intramural hematoma, or a penetrating aortic ulcer with an ascending aortic or aortic sinus diameter of ≥5.5 cm or a rate of growth of ≥0.5 cm/year even in the absence of symptoms.
6. The mainstay of therapy for autoimmune aortopathies is steroids.

References

1. Hagan PG, Nienaber CA, Isselbacher EM, et al. The International Registry of Acute Aortic Dissection (IRAD). JAMA. 2000;283(7):897–903.
2. Mussa FF, Horton JD, Moridzadeh R, et al. Acute aortic dissection and intramural hematoma: a systematic review. JAMA. 2016;316:754–63.
3. Hiratzka LF, Bakris GL, Beckman JA, et al. 2010 ACCF/AHA/AATS/ACR/ASA/SCA/SCAI/SIR/STS/SVM guidelines for the diagnosis and management of patients with thoracic aortic disease. J Am Coll Cardiol. 2010;55(14):e27–e129.
4. Erbel R, Aboyans V, Boileau C, Bossone E, et al. 2014 ESC guidelines on the diagnosis and treatment of aortic diseases. Eur Heart J. 2014;35(41):2873–926.
5. Ashton HA, Buxton MJ, Day NE, Kim LG, Marteau TM, Scott RA, Thompson SG, Walker NM. The Multicentre Aneurysm Screening Study (MASS) into the effect of abdominal aortic aneurysm screening on mortality in men: a randomised controlled trial. Lancet. 2002;360:1531–9.
6. MacCarrick G, Black JH III, Bowdin S, El-Hamamsy I, Frischmeyer-Guerrerio PA, Guerrerio AL, et al. Loeys-Dietz syndrome: a primer for diagnosis and management. Genet Med. 2014;16:576–87.
7. Arend WP, Michel BA, Bloch DA, et al. The American College of Rheumatology 1990 criteria for the classification of Takayasu arteritis. Arthritis Rheum. 1990;33:1129–34.
8. Hunder GG, Bloch DA, Michel BA, et al. The American College of Rheumatology 1990 criteria for the classification of giant cell arteritis. Arthritis Rheum. 1990;33:1122–8.
9. Achkar AA, Lie JT, Hunder GG, et al. How does previous corti costeroid treatment affect the biopsy findings in giant cell (temporal) arteritis? Ann Intern Med. 1994;120:987.

Chapter 18
Pericardial Disease, Myocarditis, and Cardiac Tamponade

Bruno B. Lima, Waddah Malas, and Puja K. Mehta

Abbreviations

ACS	Acute coronary syndrome
BNP	Brain natriuretic peptide
CBC	Complete blood count
CMV	Cytomegalovirus
CPK	Creatine phosphokinase
CRP	C-reactive protein
CXR	Chest X-ray
EBV	Ebstein-Barr virus
ECG	Electrocardiogram
HCV	Hepatitis C virus
HIV	Human immunodeficiency virus
NSAID	Nonsteroidal anti-inflammatory drug
TEE	Transesophageal echocardiogram
TTE	Transthoracic echocardiogram

B. B. Lima · W. Malas · P. K. Mehta (✉)
Emory Clinical Cardiovascular Research Institute, Department of Medicine, Division of Cardiology, Emory University School of Medicine, Atlanta, GA, USA
e-mail: pkmehta@emory.edu

B. J. Wells et al. (eds.), *Handbook of Inpatient Cardiology*,
https://doi.org/10.1007/978-3-030-47868-1_18

Pericardial Disease

- Pericardium is a tough double layered fibroserous sac enclosing the heart consisting of a:
  - Visceral layer of serous pericardium (innermost)
  - Pericardial cavity: space between the visceral and parietal layers of the serous pericardium that contains serous, pericardial fluid
  - Parietal layer of serous pericardium
  - Fibrous pericardium (outermost)

Acute Pericarditis

Definition

- Acute pericarditis is the most common pericardial syndrome caused by inflammation of the pericardium that can be isolated or as a manifestation of an underlying systemic disease [1].
- Symptoms can be relapsing, and further classified as incessant type, where discontinuation of or attempts to wean treatment causes relapse in <6 weeks, versus intermittent type, in which symptom-free intervals last >6 weeks but recur

Etiology

- Infectious
  - Most commonly viral (Coxsackie, Echovirus, Adenovirus, HIV, etc.)
  - Bacterial (e.g., tuberculosis, seen especially in constrictive pericarditis)
  - Fungal
  - Toxoplasmosis
- Myocardial infarction: pericarditis may occur either within 1–3 days as an immediate reaction (i.e., post-infarction fibrinous pericarditis) or weeks to months following an acute myocardial infarction (Dressler syndrome)

- Postoperative (post-pericardiotomy syndrome): blunt or sharp trauma to the pericardium
- Collagen vascular disease: systemic lupus erythematosus, rheumatoid arthritis
- Other causes: renal failure (uremia), tumors (Hodgkin lymphoma), radiation

Clinical Pearls
Most cases of acute pericarditis in developed countries are based on viral infections which are self-limiting, with most patients recovering without complications.

Clinical Features

- Although there are no formal diagnostic criteria, the diagnosis of acute pericarditis includes the absence of life-threatening causes of chest pain (acute coronary syndromes [ACS], pulmonary embolism, etc.) plus at least two of the following:
  - *Typical chest pain*: sudden onset, retrosternal, pleuritic, positional (better with leaning forward or upright); pain can radiate to neck, arms, shoulders similar to ACS
  - *Pericardial friction rub*: high pitched, scratch sound heard best at the left sternal border
  - *Suggestive ECG findings* (see below)
  - *New or worsening pericardial effusion* (with or without tamponade)
- Nonspecific findings like low-grade intermittent fever, tachypnea, dyspnea, nonproductive cough can also be present
- Fevers, chills, shaking, lethargy, malaise, myalgias, or upper respiratory symptoms are commonly in infectious causes
- Arthralgia (including morning stiffness), skin lesions, neuropathy, abdominal pain, and Raynaud phenomenon suggest autoimmune etiology

- Acute pericarditis symptoms can mimic life-threatening diseases including:
  - Acute coronary syndromes (ACS)
  - Aortic dissection
  - Pulmonary embolism
  - Pneumothorax
  - Pneumonia

Clinical Pearls
Chest pain is the presenting symptom in virtually all patients for whom a diagnosis of pericarditis would be considered. Although the differential diagnosis of chest pain is extensive, certain features point strongly to pericarditis, especially pleuritic pain that is relieved by sitting forward and that radiates to the trapezius ridge (the latter feature is virtually pathognomonic).

Diagnostics

- The diagnosis is based primarily on a history of pleuritic chest pain and a friction rub heard on auscultation supported by laboratory, ECG, and imaging findings
- Laboratory findings:
  - Nonspecific markers of inflammation: Leukocytosis, ↑ C-reactive protein (CRP), ↑ erythrocyte sedimentation rate (ESR)
  - Elevated cardiac enzymes (troponins, CK-MB): 30% positive in myopericarditis
  - Abnormal renal parameters (BUN, creatinine, electrolytes) if caused by underlying uremia
  - Consider specific tests depending on the clinical scenario: rheumatoid factor, thyroid function tests, ANA, anti-streptolysin O (ASO), viral panel, cytology
- ECG changes in pericarditis are present in most cases, but its absence does not exclude pericarditis. These changes occur in four stages in about 60% of patients

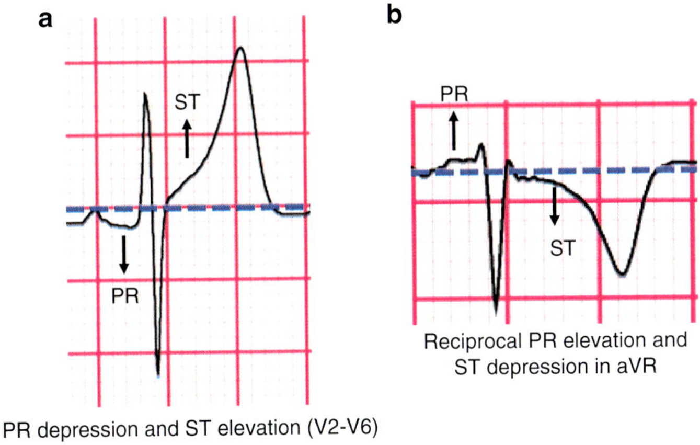

FIGURE 18.1 EKG findings of acute pericarditis. (**a**) Widespread concave ST elevation and PR depression throughout most of the limb leads and precordial leads. (**b**) Reciprocal ST depression and PR elevation in lead aVR (±V1)

- Stage 1: initial diffuse ST elevations, but ST depression in aVR and V1; PR segment depression (Fig. 18.1)
- Stage 2: ST segment normalizes in ~1 week
- Stage 3: inverted T waves
- Stage 4: ECG returns to normal baseline (as prior to onset of pericarditis) after weeks to months
  - Low voltage (QRS amplitude <0.5 mV in limb leads) and electrical alternans suggest effusion

- Imaging findings
  - Chest X-ray (CXR) is usually normal, but can help to rule out other causes of chest pain (e.g., pneumothorax, pneumonia)
  - Echocardiography at presentation and usually 1–2 weeks after treatment initiation to assess for
    - Pericardial effusion
    - Tamponade physiology
    - Focal wall motion abnormalities to rule out ACS
  - Chest CT or cardiac MRI: pericardial thickening/effusion can be often found while looking for other causes of chest pain (e.g., pulmonary embolism, acute aortic syndromes)

Management

- Acute pericarditis is often self-limiting and resolves within approx. 2–6 weeks
- Treat underlying cause (e.g., dialysis for uremia)
- *Anticoagulation increases the risk of hemopericardium thus it should be avoided*
- *NSAIDs (nonsteroidal anti-inflammatory drug)*:
  - Aspirin, ibuprofen, naproxen, and indomethacin are the NSAIDs most commonly used
  - Patients should be treated for a minimum of 2 weeks to minimize scarring [1]
    Aspirin (ASA): 650 mg every 4–6 hours for 2–4 weeks
    Ibuprofen: 600–800 mg every 8 hours
  - Aspirin is the NSAID of choice in patients with post-MI pericarditis or Dressler syndrome

> **Clinical Pearl**
> Glucocorticoids and other NSAIDs relatively contraindicated post-MI due to impaired healing and increase ventricular rupture risk

- *Colchicine*:
  - Colchicine plus conventional therapy with ASA led to a clinically important and statistically significant benefit over conventional treatment, decreasing the recurrence rate in patients with a first episode of acute pericarditis (COPE trial) [2, 3]
  - Colchicine: may be given with or without a loading dose. When a loading dose is chosen, the loading dose is typically 0.6–1.2 mg twice daily on day 1, depending upon the patient's body weight
  - The daily maintenance dose of colchicine is weight-based and is done for 3 months:

    - Patients weighing ≥70 kg should receive 0.6 mg twice daily
    - Patients weighing <70 kg should receive 0.6 mg once daily
  - Gastrointestinal side effects are common: abdominal cramping, abdominal pain, diarrhea, lactose intolerance, nausea, vomiting
  - Other side effects include myotoxicity, hepatotoxicity, and bone marrow suppression
    - Complete blood count (CBC), serum creatinine, transaminases, and creatine phosphokinase (CPK) should be followed
  - If colchicine is administered with drugs that inhibit P-glycoprotein or CYP3A4, the dose of colchicine should be adjusted
  - Colchicine should be avoided in patients with significant hepatic or renal impairment
- *Glucocorticoids*:
  - May be considered when the cause of the acute pericarditis is connective tissue disease, autoimmune conditions, or uremia
  - Prednisone may be prescribed at 1 mg per kg per day with a rapid taper or titrated to a dosage that achieves clinical benefit (0.25 mg per kg per day)
  - Toward the end of the taper (generally 6–8 weeks), NSAIDs or colchicine can be introduced to decrease the risk of recurrence
  - Sometimes it can be challenging to taper steroids in recurrent pericarditis, and a very slow taper over several months may be necessary

Clinical Pearls
Glucocorticoids should not be used as first-line therapy for patients with acute pericarditis since they confer a significant risk of adverse effects and possible recurrence of pericarditis.

- *Surgical Management*:
  - Diagnostic and/or therapeutic pericardiocentesis should be considered in patients with
    - Purulent, tuberculous, or malignant effusions
    - Cardiac tamponade
    - High fever, bacteremia, or signs of sepsis
  - Pericardiectomy or a pericardial window could be considered in patients with recurrent disease who are refractory to intensive medical therapy

Pericardial Effusion and Cardiac Tamponade

Definition

- Pericardial effusion accumulation of fluid in the pericardial space (between the parietal and the visceral pericardium)
- The clinical implications of a pericardial effusion depend on its size, cause and rate of accumulation (Fig. 18.2)

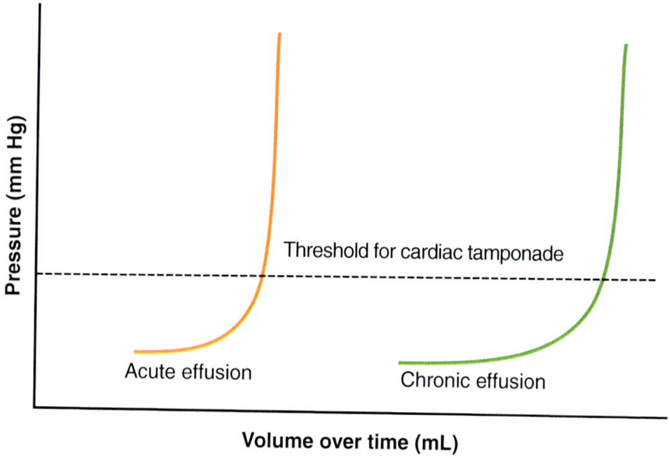

FIGURE 18.2 Relationship between volume and pressure in acute versus chronic cardiac tamponade

- Acute effusions may result in hemodynamic compromise with small amounts of fluid (<250 mL)
- Chronic effusions the pericardium can accommodate more fluid without hemodynamic compromise

- Cardiac tamponade is a medical emergency characterized by hemodynamic instability due to heart compression by a pericardial effusion
  - Fluid accumulation in the pericardial sac leads to increased pericardial pressures that exceed right ventricular filling pressures due to thinner wall
  - The interventricular septum shifts toward the left ventricle leading to decreased diastolic filling, stroke volume, and cardiac output

Etiology

- Hemopericardium
  - Cardiac wall rupture (e.g., complication of myocardial infarction)
  - Chest trauma
  - Aortic dissection
  - Cardiac surgery (e.g., heart valve surgery, coronary artery bypass)
- Serous pericardial effusion
  - Idiopathic
  - Acute pericarditis (especially viral, but also fungal, tuberculous, or bacterial)
  - Malignancy
  - Poststernotomy syndrome
  - Uremic
  - Autoimmune disorders
  - Hypothyroidism

Clinical Features

- Pericardial effusion has a wide range of clinical presentations
  - Most commonly asymptomatic initially

  - Poor exercise tolerance, orthopnea, and peripheral edema
  - Retrosternal chest pain
  - Larger effusions can compress adjacent structures and cause dysphagia, nausea, cough, hoarseness (recurrent laryngeal nerve compression)
- Cardiac tamponade presentation is characterized by the 3 **D**'s of Beck's triad
  - **D**ecreased blood pressure
  - **D**istant heart sounds
  - **D**istended neck veins
- Pulsus paradoxus is another hallmark of cardiac tamponade and is defined as an exaggerated drop in systolic blood pressure. It is done as following
  - Using a sphygmomanometer, inflate the cuff to 20 mm Hg above systolic pressure, then deflate until 1st Korotkoff sound is heard, you should hear it only during expiration (record this number)
  - Next, deflate the cuff until Korotkoff sounds are heard equally during both inspiration and expiration (subtract this number from the first)
  - If the difference between these two numbers is >10 mm Hg, the patient has a pulsus paradoxus of a magnitude equal to the aforementioned difference
  - Differential diagnosis for that phenomenon include, other than cardiac tamponade, constrictive pericarditis, pulmonary embolism, severe asthma/COPD

Diagnostics

- ECG:
  - Low voltage (limb leads <5 mm and precordial limbs <10 mm)
  - Electrical alternans
  - Signs of pericarditis
- TTE should be pursued urgently if tamponade is suspected to look for:
  - Pericardial effusion:

Echo-free space between the two layers of the pericardium

In large effusions, echo may reveal swinging of the heart within the effusion

- Tamponade physiology:

  Late diastolic collapse of the right atrium

  Early diastolic collapse of the right ventricle (RV)

  Collapse of the left atrium (LA)

  Dilated inferior vena cava (IVC) with <50%

  Respiratory-phasic changes in mitral inflow velocity is the echo equivalent of pulsus paradoxus

- Transesophageal echocardiography (TEE) is better suited to evaluate patients with localized/loculated effusions or poor echocardiographic windows

  Postcardiotomy or in cardiac trauma the most common location of the effusion is posterior to the left atrium, thus invisible to TTE

- Diagnostic pericardiocentesis should be considered in patients with large effusions or suspicion for purulent, tuberculous, or neoplastic effusions
- Pericardial biopsy should be considered in patients with effusions of unknown etiology, malignant effusions, or with recurrent effusions despite drainage
- CXR, if effusion >250 mL, shows cardiomegaly with epicardial halo can be present
- Chest CT and MRI can demonstrate pericardial thickening/effusion, calcifications, and ventricular interdependence (real-time cine cardiac MRI) and has the advantage of imaging adjacent structures

Management

- Hemodynamically stable patients with pericardial effusions:
  - Treatment of the underlying cause
  - Hemodynamic monitoring
  - Avoid anticoagulation to prevent hemopericardium until effusion resolves

- Pericardiectomy or pericardial window with an indwelling catheter may be necessary in patients with malignant effusions
- Cardiac tamponade:
  - Urgent drainage of the pericardial effusion either percutaneously or surgically
  - Drainage can be ultrasound guided and can be at the bedside if emergent or in the cath lab under fluoroscopy
  - Pericardial drain is commonly left post procedure to prevent reaccumulation
  - Pericardial window is sometimes needed for patients at risk of reaccumulation – such as cancer patients
  - Aggressive resuscitation with IV fluids ± pressor support if necessary

Myocarditis

Definition

- Myocarditis is an inflammatory disease of the heart usually resulting from viral infections and/or post-viral immune-mediated responses

Etiology

- Infectious
  - Viral: influenzae, Echovirus, EBV, CMV, HIV, HCV, parvovirus B19, human herpesvirus 6
  - Bacterial
    - β-hemolytic *Streptococcus* group A (acute rheumatic fever)
    - *Corynebacterium diphtheriae* (diphtheria, diphtheria toxin)

Borrelia burgdorferi (borreliosis)
Mycobacterium (tuberculosis)
Mycoplasma
  - Fungal (candidiasis, aspergillosis, etc.)
  - Protozoan (Chagas disease)
  - Parasitic (*trichinella*, *echinococcus*)
- Noninfectious
  - Idiopathic (e.g., giant cell myocarditis)
  - Connective tissue diseases
  - Vasculitis syndromes (e.g., Kawasaki disease)
  - Toxic myocarditis
  - Radiation therapy
  - Medication (e.g., sulfonamides)
  - Chemotherapy (e.g., anthracycline, new checkpoint inhibitors/immune modulators used in cancer)
  - Drugs (e.g., alcohol, cocaine)

Clinical Features

- The clinical features of myocarditis are nonspecific, ranging from asymptomatic courses to acute cardiac decompensation
- Typical symptoms are fatigue, weakness, dyspnea, nausea, vomiting
- Flulike symptoms (e.g., fever, arthralgia, myalgia, upper respiratory tract infections) preceding in 1–2 weeks the patient presentation suggest a viral cause
- Cardiac arrhythmias: sinus tachycardia (most common), premature ventricular contractions with palpitations or bradyarrhythmias with syncope
- Chest pain suggests pericardial involvement (perimyocarditis)
- Acute decompensated congestive heart failure with dilated cardiomyopathy or cardiac shock in fulminant cases

Clinical Pearl
Giant-cell myocarditis is aggressive and often fatal, with a rate of death or heart transplantation of 89% and a median survival of only 6 months after symptom onset. Patients typically present in the fourth or fifth decade; the clinical presentation can include congestive heart failure or new-onset cardiomyopathy (in 75% of patients), syncope, palpitations, or sudden death due to ventricular tachycardia (in 15%), and heart block (in 5%).

Diagnostics

- Laboratory findings:
  - Elevated cardiac enzymes
  - Nonspecific markers of inflammation: Leukocytosis, ↑ ESR, and ↑ CRP
  - ↑ Brain natriuretic peptide (BNP)
  - Virus serology
- ECG abnormalities are very nonspecific, but myocarditis should be suspected if the following findings are observed:
  - Sinus tachycardia
  - Arrhythmias: atrial or ventricular ectopic beats, complex ventricular arrhythmia, atrial tachycardia
  - Repolarization abnormalities
  - Heart block: right bundle branch block, complete heart block, AV block
  - Rule out myocardial infarction: loss of R wave and pathological Q wave specific to myocardial infarction
  - Pericardial effusion: low voltage (low R wave with poor progression)
- Imaging findings:
  - CXR: cardiac enlargement, pulmonary congestion, and pleural effusions
  - Cardiac MRI: Involvement of the right ventricular side of the basal interventricular septum is specific for cardiac sarcoidosis, whereas subendocardial involvement is specific for giant-cell myocarditis

- TTE findings are unspecific
  - Decreased ejection fraction, impaired contractility, diffuse hypokinesis, regional wall motion abnormalities
  - Pericardial effusion
  - Rule out possible etiologies of acute decompensated heart failure
- Endomyocardial biopsy:
  - Endomyocardial biopsy is essential for establishing the correct diagnosis of conditions like cardiac sarcoidosis and giant-cell myocarditis that should be considered if high degree of arrhythmias, progressive conduction disease, progressive hemodynamic instability [4]
  - The characteristic pathological features of giant-cell myocarditis include multinucleated giant cells and myocyte necrosis
  - The pathological features of cardiac sarcoidosis also include multinucleated giant cells, but the hallmark features of noncaseating granulomas, fibrosis, and scarring are typically more prominent [5]
  - Immunohistochemical detection of inflammation (with lymphocytic infiltrates in a viral etiology)

Treatment

- If myocarditis is suspected, consider cardiology consultation
- Supportive therapy with cardiac monitoring, oxygen administration, management of fluid status
- Treatment of complications:
  - Acute decompensated heart failure [6]
    - Diuretics
    - Inotropes
    - Mechanical support (e.g., intra-aortic balloon pump, extra-corporeal membrane oxygenation, etc.)
  - Cardiac arrhythmias management: Arrhythmias management with pharmacotherapy (AV nodal agents and anti-arrhythmic medications if needed), and ensure no electrolyte or thyroid abnormalities
  - Heart transplantation

Key Learning Points

- Pericarditis is idiopathic in 80–90% of cases and can be safely managed as an outpatient.
- Features such as fever, high inflammatory markers, a subacute onset, immunosuppression, myocardial involvement (with troponin elevation), and heart failure point to an increased risk of complications and warrant hospitalization for early echocardiography and a full work-up
- Constrictive pericarditis has a long symptom-free period that may take weeks to decades to develop and it is often a clinical diagnosis made with routine investigations
- Myocarditis can have mixed clinical manifestations and should be kept in mind as a possibility in cases presenting with signs and symptoms of myocardial infarction but with normal coronary angiography
- Cardiac MRI offers a noninvasive, reliable tool for diagnosis of myocarditis; additional advantages include repeatability factor, indirect assessment of relative cardiac function, and prognostication

References

1. LeWinter MM. Clinical practice. Acute pericarditis. N Engl J Med. 2014;371(25):2410–6.
2. Imazio M, Bobbio M, Cecchi E, Demarie D, Demichelis B, Pomari F, et al. Colchicine in addition to conventional therapy for acute pericarditis: results of the COlchicine for acute PEricarditis (COPE) trial. Circulation. 2005;112(13):2012–6.
3. Imazio M, Brucato A, Cemin R, Ferrua S, Maggiolini S, Beqaraj F, et al. A randomized trial of colchicine for acute pericarditis. N Engl J Med. 2013;369(16):1522–8.
4. Cooper LT Jr. Myocarditis. N Engl J Med. 2009;360(15):1526–38.
5. Schultz JC, Hilliard AA, Cooper LT Jr, Rihal CS. Diagnosis and treatment of viral myocarditis. Mayo Clin Proc. 2009;84(11):1001–9.
6. Blauwet LA, Cooper LT. Antimicrobial agents for myocarditis: target the pathway, not the pathogen. Heart. 2010;96(7):494–5.

Chapter 19
Pulmonary Embolism and DVT

Stephanie Wang and Michael McDaniel

Abbreviations

aPTT	Activated partial thromboplastin time
CDT	Catheter-directed thrombolysis
CTPA	Computed tomography pulmonary angiogram
CTPH	Chronic thromboembolic pulmonary hypertension
DVT	Deep vein thrombosis
ESC	European Society of Cardiology
IFDVT	Iliofemoral DVT
LMWH	Low molecular weight heparin
NOAC	Novel oral anticoagulants
PE	Pulmonary embolism
PMT	Percutaneous mechanical thrombectomy
PTP	Pre-test probability
PTS	Post thrombotic syndrome
tPA	Alteplase
UFH	Unfractionated heparin
V/Q	Ventilation perfusion scan

S. Wang (✉)
Division of Cardiology, Emory University, Atlanta, GA, USA
e-mail: szwang@emory.edu

M. McDaniel
Division of Cardiology, Emory University School of Medicine, Atlanta, GA, USA

B. J. Wells et al. (eds.), *Handbook of Inpatient Cardiology*,
https://doi.org/10.1007/978-3-030-47868-1_19

VKA Vitamin K antagonists
VTE Venous thromboembolism

Venous Thromboembolism (VTE) Refers to Two Clinical Manifestations: Pulmonary Embolism (PE) and Deep Vein Thrombosis (DVT)

Pulmonary Embolism

- Symptoms include pleuritic chest pain, dyspnea, tachypnea, and tachycardia
- *Initial Workup*
  - Determine pre-test probability (PTP): Wells score, modified Wells score, Geneva score

    Wells score: low <2, intermediate 2–6, high >6
    - Symptoms of DVT (3 points), less likely alternative diagnosis (3), heart rate > 100 (1.5), immobilization for >3 days or surgery in past 4 hours (1.5), prior DVT/PE (1.5), hemoptysis (1), malignancy (1)
  - Based on PTP workup, diagnostic testing as noted below [1, 2]

    Low (~5%): Obtain d-dimer to exclude, followed by computed tomography pulmonary angiogram (CTPA) or ventilation perfusion scan (V/Q) if needed

    Intermediate (~20%): Obtain d-dimer to exclude, followed by CTPA or V/Q if needed. If patients are likely to have nondiagnostic V/Q, they should undergo CT

    High (>50%): empirically start anticoagulation and obtain CTPA
  - If there is concern for recurrent PE, start with d-dimer if low PTP. If has +d-dimer or high PTP, CTPA should be obtained.

- *Imaging for diagnosis*
  - CTPA [3, 4]

    Advantages include filling defect definitively diagnoses PE, sensitivity and specificity of 80–90% and increased when combined with high PTP. It can also provide alternative diagnosis for clinical symptoms. In addition, CTPA can indicate clot burden and severity with RV/LV dimensions

    Disadvantages include the need for IV contrast (renal function, allergy), and can be suboptimal if patient has large body habitus, or with poor contrast bolus timing or artifact from metallic objects.
  - V/Q scan

    Main advantage is no need for contrast; disadvantage is that up to 30–40% can be read as indeterminate/intermediate probability
  - Other less common modalities

    Magnetic resonance pulmonary angiography, catheter-based pulmonary angiography
- *Clinical information and tests for risk stratification*
  - Vital signs
  - Cardiac echo

    Evidence of RV dysfunction may include RV hypokinesis, pulmonary hypertension, McConnell's sign
  - Biomarkers (troponin, BNP/proBNP, lactate)
- *Clinical severity definition help guide treatment* [5, 6]
  - *Massive PE* refers to patients with shock, defined as 15 minutes of sustained hypotension with systolic blood pressure < 90 mm Hg or 40 mm Hg lower than baseline or requiring inotropes
  - *Submassive PE* refers to patients without shock but has one or more of the following: RV dysfunction on echo (dilated or hypokinetic) or CT (RV/LV diameter > 0.9) or positive biomarkers suggestive of RV myocardial injury, with elevated troponin and BNP

    European Society of Cardiology (ESC) further divides submassive PE into intermediate-high (presence of positive biomarkers and RV dysfunction) and intermediate-low risks (presence of either/or) Elevated lactate has been associated with increased risk of PE-related complications (shock/hypotension, death) in patients with RV dysfunction and elevated biomarkers [7]

- *Low-risk PE* refers to patients who are normotensive, with normal biomarkers, and no RV dysfunction
- Studies have shown short-term mortality rates of up to 50% for massive vs 1% for low risk

• *Acute PE inpatient treatment*
  - *Interdisciplinary approach should be considered in patients with massive and submassive PE (Clinical Pearl)*
  - *In addition to systemic anticoagulation*, special considerations for massive and submassive PE are described below (See Table 19.1)
  - *Massive PE* [5, 6, 8]

    Systemic thrombolysis: agents approved are alteplase (tPA), streptokinase, and urokinase infused via peripheral intravenous catheter [5]

    • Alteplase (most commonly used): 100 mg IV over 2 hours
    • Streptokinase: 250,000 units IV over 30 minutes, then 100,000 units/hour for 24 hours
    • Urokinase: 4400 units/kg IV over 10 minutes, then 4400 units/kg/hour for 12 hours
    • UFH should be paused while giving systemic thrombolytics but can be resumed when activated partial thromboplastin time (aPTT) is less than twice upper limit of normal, or can resume heparin without bolus once thrombolytic infusion is completed
      - Contraindications to systemic thrombolysis [5]
      - Absolute

        Prior intracranial hemorrhage, structural intracranial cerebrovascular disease, ischemic stroke within 3 months, malignant

Table 19.1 Summarization of PE findings and treatment

	Findings	Treatment
Massive	Shock – 15 minutes of sustained hypotension with SBP <90 mm Hg or 40 mm Hg lower than baseline, or needing ionotropes	Systemic thrombolysis Catheter-directed thrombolysis Percutaneous mechanical thrombectomy Surgical embolectomy Hemodynamic support Systemic anticoagulation in all
Submassive	RV dysfunction on echo or CT (RV/LV diameter > 0.9) Positive biomarkers (troponin or BNP)	Half dose thrombolytics Catheter-directed thrombolysis Percutaneous mechanical thrombectomy Systemic anticoagulation in all
Low risk	Normotensive, normal biomarkers, no RV dysfunction	Systemic anticoagulation Sub-segmental and no proximal DVT can sometimes be managed with surveillance and no anticoagulation

intracranial mass, suspected aortic dissection, active bleeding, significant closed-head or facial injury, recent surgery near spinal cord or brain

– Relative

Current anticoagulation, pregnancy, prolonged CPR, recent internal bleeding, hypertension (systolic blood pressure > 180 or diastolic >110 mm Hg), major surgery within 3 weeks, ischemic stroke >3 months prior, minor head or facial trauma

- *Catheter-directed thrombolysis (CDT)*
  - Considered for relative contraindications to full dose thrombolytics
  - Currently the EKOS catheter is the only FDA-approved catheter-directed thrombolysis for PE with evidence of RV strain. It also uses ultrasound to break up clot fragments in addition to infusing a thrombolytic agent
- *Percutaneous mechanical thrombectomy (PMT)*
  - Techniques for mechanical thrombectomy include thrombus fragmentation, aspiration thrombectomy, rheolytic thrombectomy, and suction embolectomy
  - For use in patients with contraindication to any thrombolysis
  - Usually limited to main and lobar pulmonary artery branches
- *Surgical embolectomy on/off cardiopulmonary bypass*
  - It can be used when thrombolysis is contraindicated, or when there is paradoxical embolus, right atrial thrombus, or clot in transit that require excision. It is usually limited up to segmental arteries [5]
- Systemic thrombolysis is associated with reducing all-cause mortality and lower risk of recurrent PEs, but also associated with higher risk of major bleeding and intracranial hemorrhage; However, it is reasonable to use in massive PE (AHA Class IIa, ESC Class I)
- *If systemic thrombolysis fails or if there are contraindications to thrombolysis, patient can be considered for catheter-directed treatments or surgical embolectomy (AHA Class IIb, ESC Class IIa) (Clinical Pearl)*
- Hemodynamic support
  - Administration of IV fluids needs to be cautious because although initially may increase

preload and improve cardiac output, as the RV fails and becomes more distended, the septum will bow toward the left ventricle and decrease cardiac output

- Vasoactive support may be required with ionotropes to augment cardiac function
- Mechanical support with VA-ECMO may be needed as bridge to restore perfusion [9]

- *Submassive PE* [5, 6]

  Systemic thrombolysis can also be considered if has evidence of potential clinical decline or worse prognosis and low risk of bleeding (AHA Class IIb, ESC Class IIb)

  In patients with high-risk submassive PE, half dose thrombolytics, CDT, and catheter embolectomy can also be considered (Clinical Pearl)

  In patients with evidence of RV dysfunction on imaging/echo and positive troponin, fibrinolytic therapy (tenecteplase plus heparin) decreased death or hemodynamic decompensation compared with just heparin (2.6% vs. 5.6%) but associated with increased risk of major bleeding and stroke. 30-day mortality similar between the groups (PEITHO, NEJM 2014) [10]

  - Half dose tPA was associated with lower rate of pulmonary hypertension but not with death or recurrent PE. No bleeding was noted (MOPETT, ACC 2013) [11]

- *Low-risk PE*

  Main treatment is anticoagulation only

  Patients can be considered for early discharge and outpatient treatment [5, 12]

  In patients with low-risk PE, early discharge within 48 hours with rivaroxaban was not associated with increased risk of recurrent VTE or PE-related deaths within 3 months (HOT-PE, ESC 2019) [13]

- IVC filter considerations

  Indicated for acute PE/proximal DVT with contraindications to anticoagulation or having active bleed-

ing; however, anticoagulation should be resumed as soon as contraindication is resolved (AHA Class I)
Does not reduce PE recurrence in patients with acute PE and associated DVT versus anticoagulation alone (PREPIC2, JAMA 2015) [14] *(Clinical Pearl)*
  - Sub-segmental PE and no proximal DVT can be potentially managed with surveillance without anticoagulation [12]
  - Paradoxical embolization can occur in patients with patent foramen ovale (can be detected on echo with bubble study). It is an adverse predictor because of increased risk of death, stroke, and other arterial embolisms; hence, more aggressive treatment of PE should be considered [15]
- *Treatment at discharge*
  - Provoked vs. unprovoked [1]
    This is an important distinction because of prediction for risk of recurrence. Having risk factors is associated with half the risk of recurrence compared with not having risk factors
    Provoked VTE refers to both transient and persistent risk factors
    - Transient factors include surgery, leg injury with reduced mobility, pregnancy/estrogen use
    - Persistent factors include cancer and inflammatory bowel disease
  - Main stay is anticoagulation
    Options include unfractionated heparin (UFH), low molecular weight heparin (LMWH), vitamin K antagonists (VKA), and novel oral anticoagulants (NOAC) [12].
    - Approved NOACs include dabigatran, edoxaban, rivaroxaban, and apixaban. Of note, dabigatran and edoxaban require overlap with parenteral anticoagulation
    - In patients without cancer, NOACs are recommended over VKA and LMWH

- In cancer patients, LMWH is recommended over VKA and NOACs

Duration of treatment [12]

- For provoked VTE with transient risk factors, recommend anticoagulation for 3 months
- For provoked VTE with irreversible risk factor, recommend extended anticoagulation
- For unprovoked VTE, recommend extended anticoagulation if low risk of bleeding; if high risk of bleeding, recommend 3 months of anticoagulation
- For recurrent unprovoked VTE, if low or moderate risk of bleeding, recommend extended anticoagulation; if high risk of bleeding, recommend 3 months of anticoagulation

- *Post intervention care*
  - Patients who receive catheter-based intervention are at risk for access site bleeding
  - Follow-up echo should be obtained to evaluate for improvements in RV function
- *Pulmonary hypertension from pulmonary embolism*
  - With first episode of PE, chronic thromboembolic pulmonary hypertension (CTPH) occurs up to 4% at 2 years; systemic thrombolysis may decrease rate of pulmonary hypertension in submassive PE [11, 16]

Deep Vein Thrombosis

- *Anatomy*
  - Lower extremity DVT refers to thrombosis in veins that include anterior/posterior tibial, peroneal, popliteal, femoral, deep femoral, common femoral, external/internal iliac, common iliac, IVC, and pelvic veins

    Proximal DVT refers to popliteal, femoral, iliac veins, and above; whereas distal refers to no proximal component and below the knee. Proximal DVT has an increased risk of embolization

- Iliofemoral DVT (IFDVT)
  Defined as thrombosis of any part of iliac or common femoral vein; important distinction because it is associated with higher risk of recurrent DVT and severity of post-thrombotic syndrome [17, 18]
- Upper extremity DVT refers to thrombosis in veins that include ulnar, radial, interosseous, brachial, axillary, subclavian veins

• *Diagnosis* [2]
  - Low pretest probability (<10%): D-dimer to exclude
  - Intermediate probability (25 + 10%): lower extremity ultrasound. Can stop if whole leg US is negative, but if initial proximal ultrasound is negative, should be followed with repeat in 1 week if no alternative explanation
  - High probability (>50%): proximal or whole leg ultrasound followed by repeat ultrasound in 1 week if initial one was negative
  - Proximal duplex ultrasound has lower sensitivity for calf veins compared with whole leg ultrasound. Isolated pelvic vein DVT also may not be visualized (can consider venous CT or MRI)

• *Treatment Approach*
  - *Anticoagulation* is the main treatment with exception of contraindication [5, 6, 12]
    See duration above in PE
    For proximal lower extremity DVT, see anticoagulation duration in PE section
    Isolated distal DVT without severe symptoms can be managed with serial imaging in 2 weeks, and if no thrombus extension, can defer anticoagulation. If it has extension, then anticoagulation should be initiated
    Upper extremity DVT are usually associated with catheters. If catheter is to remain in, anticoagulation is recommended for the duration of catheter placement; otherwise, anticoagulate for 3 months
  - *Catheter-directed therapy (pharmacologic/mechanical)* [5]
    Should be considered in patients with phlegmasia cerulea dolens or with clot extension despite anticoagulation (AHA Class IIa). Systemic thrombolysis is

not routinely used in DVT management (AHA Class III) (Clinical Pearl)

CDT has not been shown to reduce post thrombotic syndrome (PTS) in acute DVT and is associated with more bleeding [19]

Should not be used routinely in chronic DVT symptoms

- *Percutaneous transluminal venous angioplasty and stent placement*

  It can be used in conjunction with CDT to treat obstructive lesions in iliac and common femoral veins (AHA Class IIa)

  If stent is placed, anticoagulation alone may be sufficient; however, if there is high risk of thrombosis (AHA Class IIa), additional antiplatelet agents may also be considered (AHA Class IIb)

- *IVC filter*

  If patient has contraindication to anticoagulation, IVC filter should be placed. Anticoagulation should be resumed when contraindication resolves (AHA class I)

- *Compression therapy*

  Elastic compression stockings may reduce rates of PTS and is recommended in IFDVT (AHA class I)

Key Learning Points

1. Massive PE is defined by hemodynamic instability and systemic thrombolytic is indicated unless contraindicated.
2. If systemic thrombolytics is contraindicated, other options include catheter-directed thrombolytics, and catheter or surgical embolectomy.
3. Advanced interventions such as half dose thrombolytics and catheter-directed therapies should be considered in high-risk submassive PE.
4. For low-risk PE, anticoagulation is the main treatment.
5. Catheter-directed therapy should also be considered in cases of extensive proximal DVT

References

1. Kearon C, Ageno W, Cannegieter SC, Cosmi B, Geersing G-J, Kyrle PA. Categorization of patients as having provoked or unprovoked venous thromboembolism: guidance from the SSC of ISTH. J Thromb Haemost. 2016;14(7):1480–3.
2. Lim W, Le Gal G, Bates S, Righini M, Haramati L, Lang E, et al. American Society of Hematology 2018 guidelines for management of venous thromboembolism: diagnosis of venous thromboembolism. Blood Adv. 2018;2(22):3226–56.
3. Perelas A, Dimou A, Saenz A, Rhee JH, Teerapuncharoen K, Rowden A, et al. Incidental findings on computed tomography angiography in patients evaluated for pulmonary embolism. Ann Am Thorac Soc. 2015;12(5):689–95.
4. Stein P, Fowler S, Goodman L, Gottschalk A, Hales C, Hull R, et al. Multidetector computed tomography for acute pulmonary embolism. N Engl J Med. 2006;354(22):2317–27.
5. Jaff M, McMurtry M, Archer S, Cushman M, Goldenberg N, Goldhaber S, et al. Management of massive and submassive pulmonary embolism, iliofemoral deep vein thrombosis, and chronic thromboembolic pulmonary hypertension. Circulation. 2011;123(16):1788–830.
6. Konstantinides S, Torbicki A, Agnelli G, Danchin N, Fitzmaurice D, Galiè N, et al. 2014 ESC guidelines on the diagnosis and management of acute pulmonary embolism. Eur Heart J. 2014;35(43):3033–80.
7. Vanni S, Jimenez D, Nazerian P, Morello F, Parisi M, Daghini E, et al. Short-term clinical outcome of normotensive patients with acute PE and high plasma lactate. Thorax. 2015;70(4):333–8.
8. Chatterjee S, Chakraborty A, Weinberg I, Kadakia M, Wilensky R, Sardar P, et al. Thrombolysis for pulmonary embolism and risk of all-cause mortality, major bleeding, and intracranial hemorrhage. JAMA. 2014;311(23):2414.
9. Corsi F, Lebreton G, Bréchot N, Hekimian G, Nieszkowska A, Trouillet J, et al. Life-threatening massive pulmonary embolism rescued by venoarterial-extracorporeal membrane oxygenation. Critical Care. 2017;21(1):76.
10. Meyer G, Vicaut E, Danays T, Agnelli G, Becattini C, Beyer-Westendorf J, et al. Fibrinolysis for patients with intermediate-risk pulmonary embolism. N Engl J Med. 2014;370(15):1402–11.

11. Sharifi M, Bay C, Skrocki L, Rahimi F, Mehdipour M. Moderate pulmonary embolism treated with thrombolysis (from the "MOPETT" trial). Am J Cardiol. 2013;111(2):273–7.
12. Kearon C, Akl E, Ornelas J, Blaivas A, Jimenez D, Bounameaux H, et al. Antithrombotic therapy for VTE disease. Chest. 2016;149(2):315–52.
13. Barco S, Schmidtmann I, Ageno W, Bauersachs RM, Becattini C, Bernardi E, et al. Early discharge and home treatment of patients with low-risk pulmonary embolism with the oral factor Xa inhibitor rivaroxaban: an international multicentre single-arm clinical trial. Eur Heart J. 2019;41:509.
14. Mismetti P, Laporte S, Pellerin O, Ennezat P, Couturaud F, Elias A, et al. Effect of a retrievable inferior vena cava filter plus anticoagulation vs anticoagulation alone on risk of recurrent pulmonary embolism. JAMA. 2015;313(16):1627.
15. Konstantinides S, Geibel A, Kasper W, Olschewski M, Blümel L, Just H. Patent foramen ovale is an important predictor of adverse outcome in patients with major pulmonary embolism. Circulation. 1998;97(19):1946–51.
16. Pengo V, Lensing A, Prins M, Marchiori A, Davidson B, Tiozzo F, et al. Incidence of chronic thromboembolic pulmonary hypertension after pulmonary embolism. N Engl J Med. 2004;350(22):2257–64.
17. Douketis J, Crowther M, Foster G, Ginsberg J. Does the location of thrombosis determine the risk of disease recurrence in patients with proximal deep vein thrombosis? Am J Med. 2001;110(7):515–9.
18. Kahn S. Determinants and time course of the postthrombotic syndrome after acute deep venous thrombosis. Ann Intern Med. 2008;149(10):698.
19. Vedantham S, Goldhaber S, Julian J, Kahn S, Jaff M, Cohen D, et al. Pharmacomechanical catheter-directed thrombolysis for deep-vein thrombosis. N Engl J Med. 2017;377(23):2240–52.

Chapter 20
Hypertension

Akanksha Agrawal and M. Carolina Gongora Nieto

Abbreviations

ABPM	Ambulatory blood pressure monitoring
ACE	Angiotensin converting enzyme
ARB	Angiotensin receptor blockers
ASCVD	Atherosclerotic cardiovascular disease
CAD	Coronary artery disease
CCB	Calcium channel blockers
CKD	Chronic kidney disease
DASH	Dietary approaches to stop hypertension
DBP	Diastolic blood pressure
HBPM	Home blood pressure monitoring
HELLP	Hemolysis, elevated liver enzymes, low platelet count
HFpEF	Heart failure with preserved ejection fraction
HFrEF	Heart failure with reduced ejection fraction
ICH	Intracranial hemorrhage
ICU	Intensive care unit
MRC	Medical Research Council
NHANES	National Health and Nutrition Examination Survey

A. Agrawal (✉) · M. C. G. Nieto
Department of Internal Medicine, Division of Cardiology, Emory University, Atlanta, GA, USA

B. J. Wells et al. (eds.), *Handbook of Inpatient Cardiology*, https://doi.org/10.1007/978-3-030-47868-1_20

PAD	Peripheral artery disease
SAH	Subarachnoid hemorrhage
SBP	Systolic blood pressure
SHEP	The systolic hypertension in the elderly program
SPRINT	Systolic pressure intervention trial
Syst-EUR	Systolic hypertension in Europe

Epidemiology of Hypertension

- Hypertension is an important public health challenge affecting almost 29% of the adult population in United States as per National Health and Nutrition Examination Survey (NHANES) data from 2015–2016 [1].
- Prevalence increases with age; age group 18–39 years, 7.5%; 40–59 years, 33.2%; and 60 and over, 63.1% [1].
- Prevalence of hypertension varies across different races; highest among non-Hispanic African American (40.3%), followed by non-Hispanic Caucasians (27.8%), Hispanic (27.8%), and non-Hispanic Asian (25%).
- Definition of hypertension used in NHANES 2015–16 classifies systolic blood pressure (SBP) ≥ 140 mm Hg or diastolic blood pressure (DBP) ≥ 90 mm Hg, or currently taking medication to lower BP. Among adults with hypertension, only 48.3% had controlled hypertension (SBP < 140 mm Hg and DBP < 90 mm Hg) [1].

Definition and Classification

The 2017 ACC/AHA guidelines define hypertension as SBP ≥ 130 mm Hg or DBP ≥ 80 mm Hg as hypertension [2]. Blood pressure is classified as normal, elevated, stage 1 or stage 2 hypertension (Table 20.1). The BP read is the average of ≥2 careful readings obtained on ≥2 separate occasions, measured with proper technique.

TABLE 20.1 Categories of BP in adults

BP category	Normal	Elevated	Hypertension Stage 1	Hypertension Stage 2
SBP	<120 mm Hg	120–129 mm Hg	130–139 mm Hg	≥140 mm Hg
	and	and	or	or
DBP	<80 mm Hg	<80 mm Hg	80–89 mm Hg	≥90 mm Hg

Primary Hypertension

- Formerly called essential hypertension, primary hypertension is diagnosed when there is not an identifiable anatomic or screening laboratory finding that identifies a cause of hypertension. It corresponds to approximately 90% of patients with hypertension.

Secondary Hypertension

- In approximately 10% of patients with hypertension, a specific, reversible cause of hypertension can be identified. Table 20.2 enlists the common causes of secondary hypertension along with their screening and diagnostic tests.
- *Who to screen for secondary causes of hypertension?*

  (i) Difficult to control hypertension in adults (≥3 drugs)
  (ii) New onset or abrupt onset
  (iii) Age < 30 years
  (iv) Target organ damage such as cerebral vascular disease, retinopathy, left ventricular hypertrophy, heart failure with preserved ejection fraction (HFpEF), coronary artery disease (CAD), chronic kidney disease (CKD), peripheral artery disease (PAD), and albuminuria
  (v) Onset of diastolic hypertension in older adults
  (vi) Unprovoked or excessive hypokalemia

TABLE 20.2 Causes of secondary hypertension and their diagnostic screening tests and additional/confirmatory tests

Cause	Screening tests	Additional/ confirmatory tests
Renal parenchymal disease	Renal ultrasound	Evaluate etiology renal disease
Renovascular disease	Renal duplex Doppler ultrasound, MRA, abdominal CT	Bilateral selective renal intra-arterial angiography
Primary aldosteronism	Plasma aldosterone/ renin ratio under standardized conditions	Oral sodium loading test (with 24-hour urine aldosterone) or IV saline infusion test with plasma aldosterone at 4 hours of infusion. Adrenal CT scan, adrenal vein sampling
Obstructive sleep apnea	Berlin Questionnaire, Epworth Sleepiness Score, overnight oiximetry	Polysomnography
Drug or alcohol induced	Urinary drug screen	Response to withdrawal of suspected agent
Pheochromocytoma/ paraganglioma	24-hour urinary fractionated metanephrines or plasma metanephrines under standard conditions	CT or MRI scan of abdomen/pelvis
Cushing's syndrome	Overnight 1 mg dexamethasone suppression test	24-hour urinary free cortisol excretion (preferably multiple); midnight salivary cortisol

TABLE 20.2 (continued)

Cause	Screening tests	Additional/ confirmatory tests
Hypothyroidism	Thyroid-stimulating hormone; free thyroxine	TPO antibodies
Hyperthyroidism	Thyroid-stimulating hormone; free thyroxine	Radioactive iodine uptake and scan
Aortic coarctation (undiagnosed or repaired)	Echocardiogram	Thoracic and abdominal CT angiogram or MRA
Primary hyperparathyroidism	Serum calcium	Serum parathyroid hormone
Congenital adrenal hyperplasia	Hypertension and hypokalemia with low or normal aldosterone and renin	11-beta-OH; elevated deoxycorticosterone (DOC), 11-deoxycortisol, and androgens 17-alpha-OH; decreased androgens and estrogen; elevated deoxycorticosterone and corticosterone
Mineralocorticoid excess syndromes other than primary aldosteronism	Low aldosterone and renin	Urinary cortisol metabolites; genetic testing
Acromegaly	Serum growth hormone ≥1 ng/mL during oral glucose load	Elevated age and sex matched IGF-1 level; MRI scan of the pituitary

White Coat Hypertension/Isolated Clinic Hypertension/Office Hypertension

- Defined as average BP readings in the office of ≥130/80 mm Hg and out of office readings <130/80 mm Hg determined by home measurements or ambulatory blood pressure monitoring (ABPM).
- Adults with untreated systolic BP between 130 and 160 mm Hg or diastolic between 80 and 100 mm Hg should be screened for the presence of white coat hypertension using either daytime ABPM or home blood pressure monitoring (HBPM).

Masked Hypertension

- In contrast to white coat hypertension, masked hypertension is characterized by normal BP office readings but consistently elevated out-of-office or ABPM readings. Adults with elevated office BP (120–129/<80 mm Hg) but not meeting criteria for hypertension screening for masked hypertension with daytime ABPM or HBPM is reasonable.

Resistant Hypertension

- Resistant hypertension = uncontrolled blood pressure while being on ≥3 different classes of antihypertensive agents, one of them being a diuretic OR blood pressure controlled with ≥3 medications.
- The term "refractory hypertension" has been defined as failure to control BP despite use of at least five antihypertensive agents of different classes, including a long-acting thiazide-type diuretic, such as chlorthalidone, and a mineralocorticoid receptor antagonist, such as spironolactone.

Clinical Pearl
Uncontrolled blood pressure while being on ≥3 different classes of antihypertensive agents (one of them being a diuretic), OR blood pressure controlled with ≥3 medications is termed as resistant hypertension.

Management

Who to Treat?

- Non-pharmacological interventions are recommended for all patients with hypertension.
- Threshold to start pharmacologic therapy is defined by the calculated atherosclerotic cardiovascular disease (ASCVD) risk level.
- Target blood pressure of <130/80 mm Hg is recommended. Use of BP-lowering medications are recommended in following scenarios:
  - (i) Adults with established cardiovascular disease and SBP ≥ 130 mm Hg or DBP ≥ 80 mm Hg
  - (ii) Adults with SBP ≥ 130 mm Hg or DBP ≥ 80 mm Hg and estimated 10-year ASCVD risk of ≥10%
  - (iii) Adults with SBP ≥ 140 mm Hg or DBP ≥ 90 mm Hg and with estimated 10-year ASCVD risk <10%

Non-pharmacological Management

- All patients with BP > 120/80 mm Hg should receive lifestyle modification counseling.
- Non-pharmacological interventions include weight loss, DASH (dietary approaches to stop hypertension) diet, sodium reduction, potassium supplementation, increased physical activity, smoking cessation, and reduction in alcohol consumption.

- Lifestyle changes can reduce SBP by 4–5 mm Hg and DBP by 2–4 mg; low sodium and saturated fat diet and increased fruits, vegetables, and grains consumption may decrease SBP by approximately 11 mm Hg.

Pharmacological Management

- First-line antihypertensive agents include thiazide diuretics, calcium channel blockers (CCBs), angiotensin converting enzyme (ACE) inhibitors, or angiotensin receptor blockers (ARBs). The choice of one over the other is guided by patients' comorbidities such as chronic kidney disease, diabetes, heart failure (HF), albuminuria, and race.
- As the initial agent, the thiazide-type diuretic chlorthalidone was superior to the CCB amlodipine and ACE inhibitor lisinopril in a large head-to-head comparison study [3]. For African American patients, ACE inhibitors showed less effectiveness in preventing HF and strokes when compared to CCBs [4, 5]. Additionally, nondihydropyridine CCBs are not recommended for treating hypertension in patients with HFrEF. In adults with CKD Stage 3 or higher or Stage 1 and 2 with albuminuria (≥300 mg/d, or ≥ 300 mg/g albumin-to-creatinine ratio), ACE inhibitor slowed kidney disease progression. When ACE inhibitor is not tolerated, ARB should be used [6].
- In African American adults with hypertension, but without HF or CKD, first-line antihypertensive agent should include a thiazide-type diuretic or CCB, rather than ACE inhibitor.
- Choosing two first-line agents of different classes, either as separate agents or in a fixed dose combination, is recommended for adults with stage 2 hypertension and average BP more than 20/10 mm Hg above their BP target.

Clinical Pearl

Combination of non-pharmacological and pharmacological interventions is used to achieve a target blood pressure of <130/80 mm Hg.

Special Populations

- *Elderly*
  - Multiple randomized clinical trials including SHEP, Syst-EUR, and MRC have shown clear benefit in treating hypertension in older adults including those over 80 years of age [7–9]. The aim of therapy in these trials was to either reduce SBP by 20 mm Hg or below 160 mm Hg.
  - In the Systolic Pressure Intervention Trial (SPRINT), at 3.1 years, rates of both the primary cardiovascular endpoint and all-cause mortality were significantly lower among those assigned more intensive group (goal of <120 mm Hg; mean achieved systolic blood pressure 123 mm Hg) versus less intensive group (goal of <140 mm Hg; mean achieved systolic blood pressure 135 mm Hg) systolic blood pressure lowering (2.6% versus 3.8% and 1.8% versus 2.6%, respectively) [10].
  - As per the most updated 2017 ACC/AHA guidelines, in noninstitutionalized ambulatory community-dwelling adults (≥65 years of age), a goal of <130 mm Hg is recommended.
- *Women and Pregnancy*
  - As per a large meta-analysis including 31 randomized controlled trials (RCTs), no significant differences in cardiovascular disease outcomes were observed between men and women with hypertension [11].

- Women with hypertension who become pregnant or are planning pregnancy should be transitioned to nifedipine and/or labetalol during pregnancy. Agents like Hydralazine and Methyldopa can be also used.
- In patients with concomitant HF, CAD, or other indication for beta blockers, these agents can be continued. Atenolol is the beta blocker that carries more concerns about association with low birth weight and should be avoided.
- ACE inhibitors, ARBs, and direct renin inhibitors should not be used as antihypertensive agents during pregnancy (Class III – Harm).

- *Post Kidney Transplantation*
  - Patients with kidney transplant have high incidence of hypertension due to the preexisting kidney disease, immunosuppressive medication (calcineurin inhibitors), and presence of allograft pathology.
  - Post-transplant, treatment of hypertension with CCB is recommended based on improved GFR and kidney survival [12].
- *Cerebrovascular Disease*
  - Management of BP in patients with stroke is complex and challenging due to its heterogenous causes and hemodynamic consequences. The stroke type, acuity, and therapeutic objectives guide the management of BP in a patient with stroke.
  - *Acute Intracerebral Hemorrhage*: In patients with ICH and SBP >220 mm Hg, continuous intravenous antihypertensive should be used to lower in patients presenting within 6 hours of symptom onset (Class IIa). Reducing BP to <140 mm Hg has shown to be harmful (Class III).
  - *Acute Ischemic Stroke (within 72 hours of symptom onset)*: Management depends on whether patient qualifies for intravenous (IV) thrombolysis therapy.

Qualifies for thrombolysis: The SBP should be lowered to <185 mm Hg and DBP <110 mm Hg before initiation of IV thrombolysis (Class I), and maintained at <180/105 mm Hg after thrombolysis for the first 24 hours (Class I).
Does not qualify for thrombolysis: If BP is >220/110, it should be lowered by 15% during the first 24 hours (Class IIb). However, if BP ≤ 220/110 mm Hg, initiating or reinitiating treatment for hypertension is ineffective in preventing death (Class III – no benefit).
BP management after 72 hours in a patient with stroke: In patients with previously diagnosed or treated hypertension, the BP goal remains <130/80 mm Hg. In patients with no previous history of hypertension, with established SBP ≥ 140 mm Hg or DBP ≥ 90 mm Hg, antihypertensive treatment should be initiated aiming for a BP goal of <130/80 mm Hg. If SBP < 140 mm Hg and DBP < 90 mm Hg, the usefulness of starting antihypertensive treatment remains not well established (Class IIb).

Hypertensive Crisis and Management

- Hypertensive crises are sudden, severe elevation in blood pressure with or without associated target-organ dysfunction.
- Hypertensive emergencies are characterized by BP >180/110 mm Hg with presence or impendence of target organ dysfunction. Hypertensive urgencies on the other hand have similar elevation in BP but without associated target organ dysfunction [13].

- Examples of target organ dysfunction include cardiovascular (acute pulmonary edema, acute coronary syndrome), neurologic (cerebral infarction, hypertensive encephalopathy, intracranial hemorrhage (ICH), or subarachnoid hemorrhage (SAH)), renal (acute kidney injury), hepatic (liver enzyme elevation, hemolysis, low platelet count during pregnancy (HELLP syndrome)), ocular (retinal hemorrhage or exudate), and vascular (aortic dissection, eclampsia).
- Management of patients with hypertensive emergency requires admission to intensive care unit (ICU) with continuous blood pressure monitoring and parenteral administration of antihypertensive agents.
- Guidelines recommend reduction of SBP by no more than 25% within the first hour; then, if stable, to 160/100 mm Hg within the next 2–6 hours; and then cautiously to normal during the following 24–48 hours.
- Special circumstances such as severe preeclampsia or eclampsia or pheochromocytoma require reduction of SBP to <140 mm Hg during the first hour and to <120 mm Hg in the case of aortic dissection (Table 20.3).

TABLE 20.3 Management of hypertensive emergency

Acute aortic dissection	**Eclampsia or pheochromocytoma**	**All other hypertensive emergency (non-stroke)**
Reduce SBP to <120 mm Hg in first hour	Reduce SBP to <140 mm Hg in first hour	Reduce SBP by 25% max in first hour Reduce BP to 160/110 over next 2–6 hours Reduce to normal NP over next 24–48 hours

- In patients without target organ damage (hypertensive urgency), the oral antihypertensive regimen should be reinstituted or intensified to achieve BP control. The preferred antihypertensive agent during hypertensive emergency in selected circumstances has been enlisted in Table 20.4.

Clinical Pearl
Hypertensive crises are sudden, severe elevation in blood pressure with or without associated target-organ dysfunction. Management of patients with hypertensive emergency requires admission to intensive care unit with continuous blood pressure monitoring and parenteral administration of antihypertensive agent.

Key Learning Points

- Normal BP is defined as <120/<80 mm Hg; elevated BP 120–129/<80 mm Hg; hypertension stage 1 is 130–139 systolic or 80–89 mm Hg diastolic; and hypertension stage 2 is ≥140 systolic or ≥90 mm Hg diastolic.
- First-line antihypertensive agents include thiazide diuretics, calcium channel blockers (CCBs), angiotensin converting enzyme (ACE) inhibitors, or angiotensin receptor blockers (ARBs). The choice of one over the other is guided by patients' comorbidities such as chronic kidney disease, diabetes, heart failure (HF), albuminuria, and race.
- Management of BP in a patient with stroke is complex. The stroke type, acuity, and therapeutic objectives guide the management of BP in a patient with stroke.

Table 20.4 Preferred intravenous antihypertensive drug in patients with hypertensive emergency with specific comorbidities

Comorbidity	Preferred drug	Dosing	Comments
Acute aortic dissection	Esmolol, labetalol	Esmolol: Loading dose 500–1000 mcg/kg/min over 1 min followed by 50 mcg/kg/min infusion. For additional dosing, the bolus dose is repeated and the infusion increased in 50 mcg/kg/min increments as needed to a maximum of 200 mcg/kg/min Labetalol: Initial 0.3–1.0 mg/kg dose (maximum 20 mg) slow IV injection every 10 min or 0.4–1.0 mg/kg/hour IV infusion up to 3 mg/kg/hour. Adjust rate up to total cumulative dose of 300 mg. This dose can be repeated every 4–6 hours	Beta blockade should precede vasodilator (e.g., nicardipine or nitroprusside) administration to prevent reflex tachycardia or inotropic effect

Acute pulmonary edema	Clevidipine, nitoglycerine, nitroprusside	Clevidipine: Initial 1–2 mg/hour, doubling every 90 seconds until BP approaches target, then increasing by less than double every 5–10 min; maximum dose 32 mg/hour; maximum duration 72 hours Nitroglycerin: Initial 5 mcg/min; increase in increments of 5 mcg/min every 3–5 min to a maximum of 20 mcg/min Nitroprusside: Initial 0.3–0.5 mcg/kg/min; increase in increments of 0.5 mcg/kg/min to achieve BP target; maximum dose 10 mcg/kg/min; duration of treatment as short as possible	Beta blockers are contraindicated

(continued)

TABLE 20.4 (continued)

Comorbidity	Preferred drug	Dosing	Comments
Acute coronary syndrome	Esmolol, Nitroglycerine [a]Alternative: labetalol, nicardipine	Nicardipine: Initial 5 mg/hour, increasing every 5 min by 2.5 mg/hour to maximum 15 mg/hour	Contraindications to beta blockers include moderate-to-severe LV failure with pulmonary edema, bradycardia (<60 bpm), hypotension (SBP <100 mm Hg), poor peripheral perfusion, second- or third-degree heart block, and reactive airways disease
Acute renal failure	Clevidipine, [a]fenoldopam, nicardipine	Fenoldopam: Initial 0.1–0.3 mcg/kg/min; may be increased in increments of 0.05–0.1 mcg/kg/min every 15 min until target BP is reached. Maximum infusion rate 1.6 mcg/kg/min	–

Eclampsia or preeclampsia	Hydralazine, [a]labetalol, nicardipine	–	ACE inhibitors, ARBs, renin inhibitors, and nitroprusside contraindicated
Acute sympathetic discharge or catecholamine excess states (e.g., pheochromocytoma, post-carotid endarterectomy status)	Phentolamine, clevidipine, [a]nicardipine	Phentolamine: IV bolus dose 5 mg. Additional bolus doses every 10 min as needed to lower BP to target	–

[a]Dosing is not repeated in the table if the name of medication gets repeated

References

1. Fryar CD, Ostchega Y, Hales CM, Zhang G, Kruszon-Moran D. Hypertension prevalence and control among adults: United States, 2015–2016. NCHS Data Brief No. 289, October 2017. https://www.cdc.gov/nchs/products/databriefs/db289.htm.
2. Whelton PK, Carey RM, Aronow WS, Casey DE, Collins KJ, Himmelfarb CD, DePalma SM, Gidding S, Jamerson KA, Jones DW, MacLaughlin EJ, Muntner P, Ovbiagele B, Smith SC, Spencer CC, Stafford RS, Taler SJ, Thomas RJ, Williams KA, Williamson JD, Wright JT. 2017 ACC/AHA/AAPA/ABC/ACPM/AGS/APhA/ASH/ASPC/NMA/PCNA guideline for the prevention, detection, evaluation, and management of high blood pressure in adults. J Am Coll Cardiol. 2018;71(19):e127–248. https://doi.org/10.1016/j.jacc.2017.11.006.
3. ALLHAT Officers and Coordinators for the ALLHAT Collaborative Research Group. Major outcomes in high-risk hypertensive patients randomized to angiotensin-converting enzyme inhibitor or calcium channel blocker vs diuretic: the antihypertensive and lipid-lowering treatment to prevent heart attack trial (ALLHAT). JAMA. 2002;288:2981–97.
4. Ogedegbe G, Shah NR, Phillips C, et al. Comparative effectiveness of angiotensin-converting enzyme inhibitor-based treatment on cardiovascular outcomes in hypertensive blacks versus whites. J Am Coll Cardiol. 2015;66:1224–33.
5. Leenen FHH, Nwachuku CE, Black HR, et al. Clinical events in high-risk hypertensive patients randomly assigned to calcium channel blocker versus angiotensin-converting enzyme inhibitor in the antihypertensive and lipid-lowering treatment to prevent heart attack trial. Hypertension. 2006;48:374–84.
6. Contreras G, Greene T, Agodoa LY, et al. Blood pressure control, drug therapy, and kidney disease. Hypertension. 2005;46:44–50.
7. Probstfield JL, Applegate WB, Borhani NO, David Curb J, Cutler JA, Davis BR, Furberg CD, Morton Hawkins C, Lakatos E, Page LB, Mitchell Perry H, Schron E, McFate Smith W. The systolic hypertension in the elderly program (SHEP): an intervention trial on isolated systolic hypertension. Clin Exp Hypertens A. 1989;11(5–6):973–89.

8. Staessen JA, Fagard R, Thijs L, Celis H, Arabidze GG, Birkenhager WH, Bulpitt CJ, deLeeuw PW, Dollery CT, Fletcher AE, Forette F, Leonetti G, Nachev C, ETO B, Rosenfeld J, Rodicio JL, Tuomilehto J, Zanchetti A, Systolic Hypertension in Europe (Syst-Eur) Trial Investigators. Randomized double- blind comparison of placebo and active treatment for older patients with isolated systolic hypertension. Lancet. 1997;350(9080):757–64.
9. MRC Working Party. Medical Research Council trial of treatment of hypertension in older adults: principal results. BMJ. 1992;304(6824):405–12.
10. The SPRINT Research Group. A randomized trial of intensive versus standard blood- pressure control. N Engl J Med. 2015;373:2103–16.
11. Turnbull F, Woodward M, Neal B, et al. Do men and women respond differently to blood pressure-lowering treatment? Results of prospectively designed overviews of randomized trials. Eur Heart J. 2008;29:2669–80.
12. Cross NB, Webster AC, Masson P, et al. Antihypertensive treatment for kidney transplant recipients. Cochrane Database Syst Rev. 2009;(3):CD003598.
13. Benken ST. Hypertensive emergencies. CCSAP 2018 Book 1, Medical Issues in the ICU.

Chapter 21
Commonly Encountered Congenital Heart Disease

Logan Eberly and Maan Jokhadar

Abbreviations

ASD	Atrial Septal Defect
CHD	Congenital Heart Disease
ECG	Electrocardiogram
IVC	Inferior Vena Cava
PFO	Patent Foramen Ovale
PVR	Pulmonary Vascular Resistance
Qp:Qs	Ratio of pulmonary to systemic flow
SVC	Superior Vena Cava
TEE	Transesophageal Echocardiogram
TOF	Tetralogy of Fallot
TTE	Transthoracic Echocardiogram
VSD	Ventricular Septal Defect

L. Eberly (✉) · M. Jokhadar
Department of Medicine, Division of Cardiology, Emory University, Atlanta, GA, USA
e-mail: logan.mark.eberly@emory.edu; maan.jokhadar@emory.edu

B. J. Wells et al. (eds.), *Handbook of Inpatient Cardiology*,
https://doi.org/10.1007/978-3-030-47868-1_21

Atrial Septal Defect (ASD)

Introduction

- 10% of CHD
- Typically results in a left-to-right shunt.
- 4 different sub-types (Fig. 21.1). We will discuss ostium secundum and sinus venosus ASDs (isolated ostium primum ASDs and coronary sinus defects are rare and beyond the scope of this text).

Ostium Secundum ASD

- Definition/Presentation:
  - Defects of the fossa ovalis—60% of ASDs
  - May be asymptomatic for years—often first present in adulthood (depending on size)

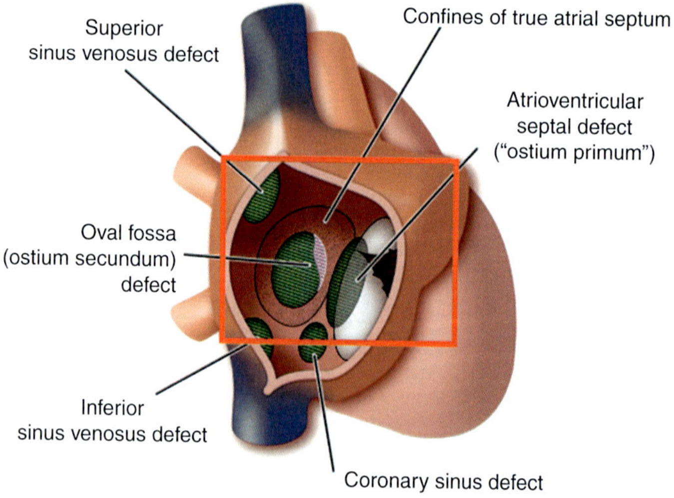

FIGURE 21.1 Schematic diagram outlines the different types of interatrial shunting that can be encountered (with permissions from Zipes et al. [2])

- May be asymptomatic at diagnosis (diagnosed by physical exam, see below); if symptomatic, most common presentation is progressive exertional dyspnea and/or palpitations

Clinical Pearl
Consider ASD in your differential diagnosis of an adult patient with otherwise unexplained exertional dyspnea and/or palpitations.

- Complications—atrial fibrillation/flutter, right heart failure, pulmonary hypertension, and paradoxical embolism
- Any condition that increases left atrial pressure (i.e. left ventricular dysfunction or mitral valve disease) increases the left-to-right shunt and worsens symptoms.

- Physical Exam
  - Loud S1, a widely split and fixed S2, pulmonary systolic ejection murmur loudest at the left upper sternal border, and a tricuspid mid-diastolic murmur loudest at the left lower sternal border (due to increased flow across the tricuspid valve)
  - If right-sided heart failure/pulmonary hypertension is present, exam may show signs of elevated jugular venous pressure and right ventricular heave
- Investigations
  - Electrocardiogram (ECG)—Look for sinus node dysfunction, prolonged PR interval, right axis deviation, rSR' pattern in V1, and large P waves.
  - Transthoracic echocardiogram (TTE)—Evaluate for color flow across the inter-atrial septum (as well as positive bubble study), and/or a dilated right ventricle. Perform a Doppler estimate of pulmonary artery pressure and an assessment for associated defects.

- Transesophageal echocardiogram (TEE)—often best characterizes the ASD (precise size, margins, etc.) and identifies the pulmonary veins (to assess for associated partial anomalous pulmonary venous return).
- Cardiac catheterization—performed to calculate pulmonary vascular resistance and determine the ratio of pulmonary to systemic flow (Qp:Qs); also often performed to evaluate for concomitant coronary artery disease prior to ASD repair.

- ASD Closure
  - Indications for ASD closure—evidence of right heart volume overload, left-to-right shunt ratio greater than or equal to 1.5:1, size greater than 10 mm, or prevention of recurrent paradoxical embolism
  - Contradictions to ASD closure—significant pulmonary vascular disease, severe left ventricular dysfunction, and significant mitral valve disease
  - Often can be closed percutaneously or surgically

Sinus Venosus ASD

- Caused by defects of the infolding of the atrial wall at the site of the superior vena cava (SVC) or inferior vena cava (IVC)—superior is more common than inferior
- Superior sinus venosus ASD—the defect in the atrial wall leads to the SVC communicating with both atria—invariably associated with anomalous right-sided pulmonary venous return whereby the right-sided pulmonary veins drain into the SVC near its junction with the right atrium.
- 2–3% of ASDs
- Similar presentation to ostium secundum ASDs
- TEE—performed both to evaluate the defect and to identify anomalous pulmonary venous drainage; MRI or CT may be required if the pulmonary venous return is not clearly seen on TEE

- Same indications for closure as ostium secundum ASDs; however, sinus venosus ASDs are not suitable for percutaneous closure because of the lack of rim around the defect as well as the associated anomalous pulmonary venous return.

Patent Foramen Ovale (PFO)

- PFO is common—found in up to 25% of the population—it is usually clinically silent
- Results from failure of fusion of the valve of the foramen ovale with the inter-atrial septum after birth when the left atrial pressure exceeds that of the right atrium; unlike ASDs—there is no defect in atrial septal tissue
- Most are found incidentally; however, paradoxical embolism can be a cause of cryptogenic stroke in young adults
- Detected on contrast echocardiogram—agitated saline is injected intravenously while an echocardiogram is obtained (can be TTE or TEE). A PFO is likely if, with Valsalva, bubbles appear within the left atrium within 5 heartbeats
- Patients with PFO who have had prior embolic stroke and have risk factors for venous thrombosis appear to benefit from PFO closure (which can be done percutaneously similar to ostium secundum ASD closure). However, a thorough evaluation of risk factors for alternative etiology of stroke should be performed prior to PFO closure.

Clinical Pearl
PFO's are commonly diagnosed on echocardiogram during the inpatient workup for stroke. However, one must complete a comprehensive evaluation to identify possible alternative etiologies for stroke before referral for PFO closure. If an alternative etiology is found, the patient is unlikely to benefit from PFO closure.

Ventricular Septal Defect (VSD)

- *Definition/Prevalence*
  - Interventricular septum is composed of 4 parts: inlet septum, outlet septum, muscular (also known as trabecular) septum, and membranous septum. VSDs can arise from defects in any of these components (Fig. 21.2).
  - Most common congenital heart defect—membranous VSDs are the most common type

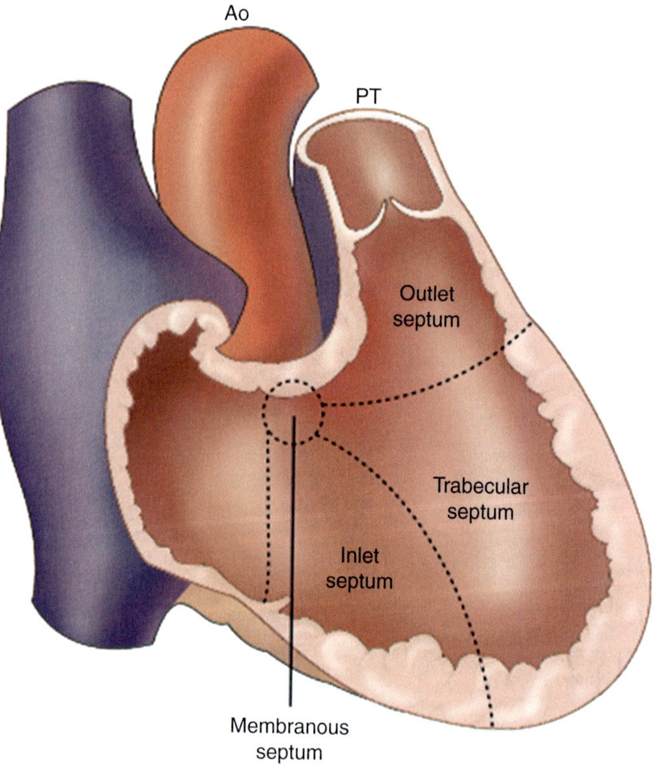

FIGURE 21.2 Four components of the ventricular septum are shown here from the right ventricular aspect. *Ao*, aorta; *PT*, pulmonary trunk (With permissions from Zipes et al. [2])

  - Can occur in isolation, in association with other lesions, or as part of a more complex condition (such as tetralogy of Fallot)
- *Presentation*
  - Depends upon the size and hemodynamic effects of the defect
  - Restrictive VSDs describe small defects with a high pressure gradient between the left and right ventricles and a small shunt of no hemodynamic significance.
  - Larger defects are hemodynamically significant and cause left ventricular volume overload and progressive increase in pulmonary vascular resistance (PVR).
  - In adults, un-operated restrictive VSDs are often asymptomatic but cause a loud murmur. Survivors of large un-operated VSDs are likely to have developed significant pulmonary hypertension and possibly Eisenmenger syndrome.
- *Physical Exam*
  - Small restrictive VSDs cause a high-frequency pansystolic murmur loudest at the left sternal border, with palpable thrill.
  - Moderate-to-large nonrestrictive VSDs cause a displaced cardiac apex and a pansystolic murmur, as well as an apical diastolic murmur and S3 (from increased flow through the mitral valve).

Clinical Pearl
The intensity of the systolic murmur due to a VSD is inversely proportional to the size of the VSD because of the increased turbulence and flow velocity produced by a smaller defect.

- *Investigations*
  - ECG—large VSDs cause right axis deviation and biventricular hypertrophy; ECG often unremarkable in small defects

  - TTE—characterizes the size, location, and hemodynamic consequences of the VSD and identifies associated lesions; moderate-sized VSDs cause left atrial and left ventricular volume overload, which leads to dilation of these chambers. Large VSDs that have already resulted in increased PVR cause right ventricular pressure overload, which leads to right ventricular hypertrophy.
  - Cardiac catheterization—performed to calculate the size of the shunt as well as PVR.
- *VSD Closure*
  - Indications for closure—symptoms and Qp:Qs greater than 1.5:1, ventricular dysfunction with right ventricular pressure or left ventricular volume overload, or a previous episode of endocarditis.
  - Selected membranous and muscular VSDs are suitable for percutaneous closure; however, surgical repair is usually necessary when indicated.
  - Damage to the conduction system is relatively common during VSD closure (either percutaneous or surgical), especially for membranous VSDs. Right bundle branch block is common post-procedure and complete heart block can occur, and if it is persistent, a pacemaker is required.

Tetralogy of Fallot (TOF)

Introduction

- The underlying abnormality in TOF is the antero-cephalad deviation of the outlet ventricular septum. This leads to the four features (Fig. 21.3):
  - VSD
  - Sub-pulmonary stenosis
  - Aorta that overrides the inter-ventricular septum
  - Secondary right ventricular hypertrophy
- TOF—most common cyanotic congenital heart defect

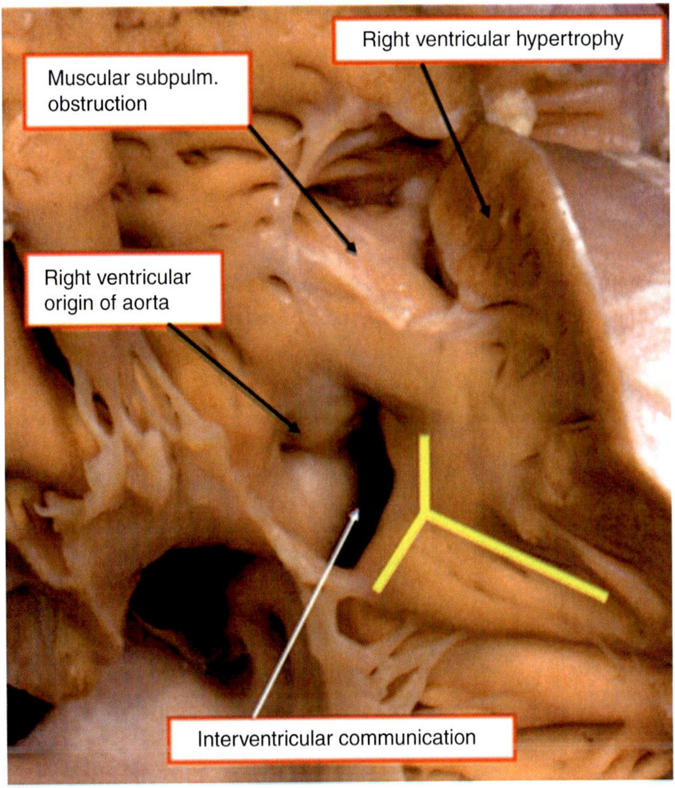

FIGURE 21.3 The photograph, taken from the apex of the right ventricle looking towards the base, shows the features of tetralogy of Fallot. The infundibulum is inserted to the antero-cephalad limb of the septomarginal trabeculation (*yellow* Y). (With permissions from Anderson [3])

Natural History (Un-Operated)

- Survival past 40 years of age is rare.
- Survival into adulthood without repair is dependent upon mild right ventricular outflow tract obstruction in childhood. Patients with severe obstruction have cyanosis early in life and don't survive to adulthood without repair.

- Complications
  - Cyanosis
  - Arrhythmia (atrial or ventricular)
  - Ascending aortic dilation and aortic regurgitation
  - Endocarditis
- Physical exam
  - Cyanosis and clubbing
  - Right ventricular heave
  - Palpable thrill and loud systolic ejection murmur (from the right ventricular outflow tract obstruction)
  - Soft P2
- Investigations
  - ECG—right axis deviation and right ventricular hypertrophy
  - Chest x-ray—look for boot-shaped heart and decreased pulmonary vascularity.
  - Echocardiography makes the diagnosis.

TOF Repair

- Surgical repair involves:
  - Patch closure of the VSD
  - Resection of the infundibular stenosis
  - Transannular patch to enlarge the pulmonary valve annulus in most patients
- Most adults with TOF have undergone repair and have a good prognosis. However, lifetime follow-up is required due increased risk of complications, particularly relating to the pulmonary valve and the need for pulmonary valve replacement.
- Possible sequelae of repair
  - Right bundle branch block

    Occurs in almost all patients because the right bundle runs in the floor of the VSD and is damaged during surgery
  - Pulmonary regurgitation (more on this below)
  - Late complete heart block

- Residual right ventricular outflow tract obstruction
- Aortic dilation and aortic regurgitation
- Endocarditis
- Arrhythmia and arrhythmogenic sudden death

Pulmonary Regurgitation After TOF Repair

- Most patients with TOF repair have severe pulmonary regurgitation that results from the relief of pulmonary stenosis and RVOT obstruction at the time of repair (transannular patch). Severe pulmonary regurgitation is usually well tolerated for several years or decades but most will eventually require pulmonary valve replacement. Pulmonary valve replacement is not a usual part of initial TOF repair.
- Signs of severe pulmonary regurgitation
  - Loss of sinus rhythm
  - Signs of right heart failure (elevated jugular venous pressure, hepatomegaly, peripheral edema, etc.)
  - Right ventricular heave
  - Soft or absent P2 (single S2)
  - To and fro systolic and diastolic murmur of pulmonary regurgitation (the diastolic murmur is often missed when it is short with rapid decrescendo)
- Investigations
  - With few exceptions, ECG shows RBBB with QRS widening. Varying degrees of atrioventricular block can also be present. Longer QRS duration is associated with more severe RV dilation and arrhythmia risk.
  - In addition to demonstrating the severe pulmonary regurgitation, echocardiography is important to evaluate for other abnormalities, including ventricular dysfunction, paradoxical inter-ventricular septal motion, residual VSD, aortic root dilation, aortic regurgitation, and residual right ventricular outflow tract obstruction.

- Indications for pulmonary valve replacement
  - Severe pulmonary regurgitation and any of the following:
    - Increasing symptoms
    - Impaired exercise tolerance on cardio-pulmonary exercise testing
    - Arrhythmias
    - Progressive right ventricular dilation or dysfunction

> **Clinical Pearl**
> Severe pulmonary regurgitation after TOF repair can be asymptomatic for years. Indications for referral for pulmonary valve replacement include worsening symptoms, objective evidence of exercise intolerance, or right ventricular dilation or dysfunction.

Cyanotic Heart Disease—The Basics

Introduction

- There are many specific defects that cause cyanosis other than TOF. Detailed discussion of each specific condition is beyond the scope of this text. Nevertheless, there are some general principles that apply to the care of the hospitalized cyanotic patient with which adult providers should be familiar. These patients are typically followed at tertiary referral centers; however, they often live far away from these centers and when acutely ill may present and be admitted locally initially for stabilization. This underlies the need for the adult inpatient provider to have a basic understanding of cyanotic heart disease.

- Cyanosis is present when there is a right-to-left shunt. The shunt can occur at any level—intra-cardiac, between the great vessels, or intrapulmonary.
- Cyanosis is typically clinically detectable when oxygen saturations are less than 85%.

General Principles for Inpatients with Cyanotic Heart Disease

- Supplemental oxygen should be used primarily for symptom relief and/or to maintain baseline oxygen saturations; oxygen is a pulmonary vasodilator and depending on the patient's anatomy, excessive oxygen may cause pulmonary edema.
- Use 0.22 micron air filters on all intravenous lines and use infusion pumps with a bubble detector to prevent paradoxical bubble emboli
- Maintain adequate hemoglobin concentration to optimize oxygen-carrying capacity
- Only perform phlebotomy if there are signs and symptoms of hyperviscosity (headache, confusion, etc.) due to very high hemoglobin concentration; phlebotomy can cause a relative iron deficiency anemia, which can increase thromboembolic risk
- Vasodilators can worsen hypoxia and should only be used with caution and under the supervision of an adult congenital cardiologist.

Clinical Pearl
One must be aware of the common pitfalls in caring for cyanotic patients—avoid the following: 1) excessive supplemental oxygen, 2) vasodilators, and 3) excessive phlebotomy.

Common Inpatient Emergencies in Cyanotic Heart Disease

- Tachyarrhythmias
  - Atrial arrhythmias are often atypical.
  - Tachyarrhythmias are generally not well tolerated.
  - Electrical cardioversion is often safer and more effective than anti-arrhythmic therapy.
- Hemoptysis
  - Can be life-threatening and warrants inpatient admission
  - One of the leading causes of death in cyanotic patients, especially in those with pulmonary hypertension.
  - Chest CT should be obtained.
  - Systemic blood pressure may need to be lowered.
    - In patients with Eisenmenger syndrome, the systemic blood pressure is essentially equal to the pulmonary arterial pressure, and it is important to lower the pressure in a bleeding pulmonary vessel.
    - IV beta blockers are typically the most appropriate pharmacologic agent; as noted above, vasodilators generally should be avoided.
  - Emergency management for severe hemoptysis is complicated and requires emergent adult congenital cardiology consultation. In general, bronchoscopy, intubation, and mechanical ventilation should be avoided if at all possible. Urgent transfer to a tertiary center is usually required.
  - Possible sources of hemoptysis—pulmonary artery thrombus, bleeding from a pulmonary arteriovenous malformation, bleeding collateral vessels, or chest infection

Key Learning Points

1. There are currently more adults than children living with CHD in the United States; therefore, adult inpatient providers need to be familiar with commonly encountered congenital heart defects.
2. ASDs comprise about 10% of CHD, and the diagnosis should be considered in patients with otherwise unexplained exertional dyspnea.
3. VSD is the most common congenital heart defect, and auscultation of the systolic murmur can lead to the diagnosis in asymptomatic patients.
4. Severe pulmonary regurgitation is common after TOF repair, and pulmonary valve replacement will eventually be needed in most patients, once indications arise, which include signs or symptoms of RV dilation and dysfunction.
5. For patients with cyanotic CHD, excessive oxygen supplementation, unnecessary phlebotomy, and vasodilators should be avoided, and 0.22 micron air filters should be used on all IVs. Arrhythmias should be treated aggressively, and hemoptysis can be life-threatening and warrants transfer to an adult congenital heart disease center.

References

1. Moons P, Bovijn L, Budts W, Belmans A, Gewillig M. Temporal trends in survival to adulthood among patients born with congenital heart disease from 1970 to 1992 in Belgium. Circulation. 2010;122(22):2264–72. https://doi.org/10.1161/circulationaha.110.946343.
2. Zipes DP, Libby P, Bonow RO, Mann DL, Tomaselli GF, Braunwald E. Braunwalds heart disease a textbook of cardiovascular medicine. Philadelphia: Elsevier; 2019.
3. Anderson RH. Paediatric cardiology. Philadelphia: Churchill Livingstone/Elsevier; 2010.
4. Thorne S, Bowater S. Adult congenital heart disease. Oxford: Oxford University Press; 2017.

Chapter 22
Pregnancy and Heart Disease

An Young, Mariana Garcia, and Gina Lundberg

Abbreviations

ACOG	American College of Obstetricians and Gynecologists
ACS	Acute coronary syndrome
BP	Blood pressure
CABG	Coronary artery bypass graft
CHF	Congestive heart failure
CT	Computed tomography
ECG	Electrocardiogram
HCM	Hypertrophic cardiomyopathy
MI	Myocardial infarction
PMHx	Past medical history
PPCM	Peripartum cardiomyopathy
SCAD	Spontaneous coronary artery dissection
TTE	Transthoracic echocardiogram
US	Ultrasound

A. Young (✉) · M. Garcia · G. Lundberg
Division of Cardiovascular Disease,
Emory University School of Medicine, Atlanta, GA, USA
e-mail: an.young@emory.edu; mariana.garcia@emory.edu; gina.lundberg@emory.edu

B. J. Wells et al. (eds.), *Handbook of Inpatient Cardiology*,
https://doi.org/10.1007/978-3-030-47868-1_22

Epidemiology

- Cardiovascular disease is one of the leading causes of morbidity and mortality in pregnant women in the United States, [1, 2] complicating between 1% and 4% of pregnancies and accounting for 26.5% of maternal mortality [3–5].

Physiologic Changes During Pregnancy

- Many hemodynamic changes (Table 22.1) occur during the first 5–8 weeks of pregnancy, peaking toward the end of the second trimester, and do not normalize until 3–6 months postpartum [6–8].

Evaluation and Diagnosis of Cardiac Disease in Pregnancy

- Physiologic changes in pregnancy make it difficult to differentiate between normal pregnancy and heart disease. A list of the various signs and symptoms of normal versus abnormal pregnancy as adapted from the American College of Obstetricians and Gynecologists (ACOG) 2019 Guideline is included in Table 22.2 [9]. Those with abnor-

Table 22.1 Hemodynamic changes during pregnancy

Parameter	Percentage of change	
Intravascular volume	40–50%	Increase
Heart rate	15–25%	Increase
Stroke volume	30%	Increase
Cardiac output	30–50%	Increase
Systemic vascular resistance	20%	Decrease
Diastolic blood pressure	20%	Decrease

TABLE 22.2 Signs and symptoms of normal versus abnormal pregnancy

Normal	Abnormal
Dyspnea, fatigue, exercise intolerance, peripheral edema	S4 and diastolic murmurs
Right ventricle dilation	Sustained tachycardia with heart rate ≥120
Increased splitting of S2 due to increased volume on the right side of heart	Ventricular tachycardias
Systolic ejection murmur, S3, or venous hum	Bradyarrhythmias
Mild left axis deviation on EKG	Elevated jugular venous pressure
Limited ectopy: atrial or ventricular premature beats, supraventricular tachycardias	Gallop
	Marked edema
	Exertional or unprovoked syncope
	Systolic blood pressure ≥160

Adapted from the 2019 American College of Obstetricians and Gynecologists Practice Bulletin

mal symptoms require prompt evaluation with electrocardiogram (ECG), echocardiography, and cardiology consult.

Clinical Pearls

When evaluating a pregnant patient or assessing risk of maternal complications, it is important to check the following: [10]

- Family history: sudden death, myocardial infarction (MI), maternal heart disease, hypertrophic cardiomyopathy (HCM), congestive heart failure (CHF), long QT syndrome, arrhythmogenic right ventricular dysplasia
- Past medical history (PMHx): prior cardiac events, arrhythmia, syncope, aortopathy, vascular or connective tissue disorder, complications in pregnancy, preeclampsia

- Rule out thyroid disease (Hashimoto's thyroiditis/Grave's disease can flare up during pregnancy or postpartum) or anemia [11–13]
- ECG for any palpitations as well as those with a family history of sudden death/arrhythmias
- Transthoracic echocardiogram (TTE) for those with a family history or PMHx of HCM, CHF, or maternal heart disease
- Computed tomography (CT) scan or magnetic resonance imaging (MRI) for those with FH or PMHx of aortopathy

Acquired Cardiac Disorders During Pregnancy

Peripartum Cardiomyopathy (PPCM)

- PPCM presents with heart failure secondary to left ventricular systolic dysfunction, with most of the cases diagnosed postpartum and left ventricular ejection fraction usually <45%. Specific time frames along with echocardiographic cut-offs are arbitrary and may lead to underdiagnosis of PPCM, which is why simplified definitions have been proposed [14].
- Predisposing factors include multiparity, preeclampsia, advanced age, teenage pregnancy, African-American ethnicity, smoking, diabetes, and malnutrition [15].

Clinical Presentation and Diagnosis

- PPCM is a diagnosis of exclusion and should be considered whenever a patient, without a prior history of CHF, presents with paroxysmal nocturnal dyspnea, new regurgitant murmurs, pulmonary edema, elevated jugular venous pressure, and hepatomegaly during the peripartum period.

Clinical Pearls

- Consider PPCM in a pregnant female without known history of structural or cardiac disease who presents with ventricular tachycardia or ventricular fibrillation.
- Echocardiography is the imaging modality of choice.

Management

- In advanced CHF with hemodynamic instability, urgent delivery, irrespective of gestation, should be considered [16].
- After delivery, the principles of managing CHF due to PPCM are similar to CHF secondary to other etiologies [14, 17]. The essential therapies for patients with acute PPCM have been summarized as the BOARD regimen: Bromocriptine, Oral heart failure therapies, Anticoagulants, vasoRelaxing agents, and Diuretics [18].
- Addition of bromocriptine to standard HF therapy may improve LV recovery and clinical outcome in women with acute severe PPCM.
- Long-acting metoprolol is safe during both pregnancy and lactation. Newborns can be sensitive to angiotensin-converting enzyme inhibitors, and these agents should not be used during the first few weeks postpartum if breast-feeding. Angiotensin receptor blockers have not been studied during lactation and should be avoided. Loop diuretics can be used during pregnancy, but they have not been well studied during lactation; thiazide diuretics appear to be safe in both.
- Inotropes can be used in patients with severely reduced cardiac output; anticoagulation may be indicated if ejection fraction falls below 35%.

Acute Coronary Syndrome (ACS)

- ACS complicating pregnancy is rare but accounts for >20% of all maternal cardiac deaths [10] and the risk is especially increased during pregnancy compared to age-matched non-pregnant women [5, 19–21].

- The etiology of coronary artery disease in pregnancy has a non-atherosclerotic mechanism in its majority, including spontaneous coronary artery dissection (43%), angiographically normal coronary arteries (18%), and coronary thrombosis (17%) [22, 23].

Management

- ACS management in pregnancy is similar to that in the general population. Percutaneous coronary intervention (PCI) can be performed safely in pregnancy due to low fetal radiation dose (<0.1 Gy) [24].
- In the event of maternal cardiac arrest, resuscitation and delivery should be performed per existing guidelines [25].
- Low-dose aspirin appears to be safe; clopidogrel should be used only when strictly needed (after stenting), and glycoprotein IIb/IIIa inhibitors and statins should be avoided [23]. The benefits of short-term heparinization during PCI outweigh the risk of bleeding complications.
- Clopidogrel does not increase the risk of fetal bleeding; however, it can cause bleeding if administered within 7 days of surgery. Some experts recommend discontinuation 1 week before delivery [26]. The risk of stent thrombosis from early cessation of dual antiplatelet therapy should be weighed against the risk of bleeding at delivery.
- In pregnancy, coronary artery bypass grafting (CABG) is generally avoided due to elevated fetal mortality associated with cardiopulmonary bypass [27, 28]. However, bypass grafting is sometimes necessary in cases of hemodynamic instability, obstructed coronary blood flow, or PCI failure. Bypass grafting without cardiopulmonary bypass or delivery before CABG can be considered during pregnancy [29].

Spontaneous Coronary Artery Dissection (SCAD)

- SCAD is a sudden separation between the layers of a coronary artery wall, creating an intimal flap and intramural hematoma, obstructing intraluminal blood flow distally and resulting in acute MI [22].
- MI complicates approximately 1 in 16,000 pregnancies in the United States [19] and SCAD is the most common cause of pregnancy-associated MI (43%) [30].
- The majority of pregnancy-associated SCAD events occur in the third trimester or early postpartum period, although it has been reported as early as 5 weeks of gestation and up to several months to a year postpartum, particularly in lactating women and is associated with fibromuscular dysplasia.

Clinical Presentation and Diagnosis

- Presentation of SCAD in pregnancy can vary, from asymptomatic to cardiogenic shock or sudden death. Most (91%) report chest pain, diaphoresis, nausea, and dyspnea; some with ventricular arrhythmias [22, 31].
- Diagnosis requires a high degree of suspicion with coronary or CT angiography. Accurate differentiation of ACS due to SCAD from ACS due to atherosclerosis is crucial, because approaches to both acute and long-term management are different [32].
- Acute SCAD patients undergoing PCI have markedly reduced technical success rates compared to atherosclerotic ACS (62% versus 92%) [22].

Management

- The substantial rate of spontaneous vascular healing suggests a role for conservative management in stable SCAD patients with preserved distal coronary flow, with generally favorable outcomes [22, 34]. However, careful inpatient monitoring (4–5 days) is needed because of a small early threat of dissection progression.

- Revascularization procedures are limited to patients with obstructed coronary blood flow or hemodynamic instability [35].
- After PCI, dual antiplatelet therapy with low-dose aspirin and clopidogrel is generally recommended for at least 12 months. Low-dose aspirin (100 mg daily or less) is not associated with adverse maternal or fetal outcomes, can be given throughout pregnancy, and does not require discontinuation before delivery [36].

Hypertension (HTN)

- There are four hypertensive disorders that occur in pregnancy: [9]
  - Chronic HTN: occurs before 20 weeks of gestation or persists >12 weeks postpartum.
  - Preeclampsia-eclampsia: syndrome of new onset HTN and proteinuria or end-organ dysfunction with or without proteinuria, most often after 20 weeks of gestation in a previously normotensive woman. Eclampsia includes seizures.
  - Preeclampsia-eclampsia superimposed on chronic HTN: those with chronic HTN who develops worsening HTN with proteinuria or other features of preeclampsia.
  - Gestational HTN: elevated BP after 20 weeks of gestation without proteinuria or other features of preeclampsia.

Management

- *Chronic hypertension*
  - Women with chronic HTN who are normotensive or mildly hypertensive on medications can continue, taper, or stop during pregnancy, with close monitoring of the maternal BP response [9, 10].
  - ACOG recommends withholding antihypertensive therapy unless BP is severely elevated (systolic ≥160 mmHg and/or diastolic ≥110 mmHg), or patient has significant comorbidities/impaired renal function [9].

- Severe HTN in pregnancy (defined as systolic ≥160 and/or diastolic ≥110 mmHg) should be treated to protect the mother from serious complications, such as stroke, heart failure, pulmonary edema, hypertensive encephalopathy, or renal failure.
- Antihypertensive therapy with labetalol, nifedipine, or methyldopa is preferred [10].

Clinical Pearls: Preeclampsia and Gestational Hypertension

- Delivery is the definitive treatment for preeclampsia.
- Avoid antihypertensive for mild HTN associated with preeclampsia.
- Start antihypertensives for systolic BP ≥150 mmHg and diastolic BP ≥100 mmHg.
- For acute therapy, intravenous labetalol or hydralazine are first-line agents.
- Nitroglycerin can be used for the treatment of HTN with pulmonary edema.

Aortic Dissection

- Aortic dissection, although rare in pregnancy, typically occurs in the third trimester or postpartum [37–39].
- Hemodynamic changes during pregnancy lead to increased shear stress and estrogen can weaken the aortic wall structure [40–42].
- Those with connective tissue disorder, i.e., Ehlers-Danlos and Marfan syndromes, aortic valve abnormalities, dilated aortic root, coarctation, and HTN have elevated risk [38, 39].

Clinical Presentation and Diagnosis

- Symptoms typically include sudden-onset ripping chest or intrascapular pain, syncope, nausea, vomiting, and diaphoresis [43, 44].

- CT angiography or MRI can be used when clinical suspicion is high [10, 33, 45]. Iodinated contrast is not teratogenic but can cross the placenta leading to transient suppression of fetal thyroid [33]. Very little (≤1% of iodinated contrast) is excreted in breast milk, so it is also safe to use during lactation [33].

Management

- Treatment strategy is dependent on the type of dissection similar to the general population.

Clinical Pearls

- Type A dissections (ascending aorta) require emergent surgical intervention.
- Type B (descending aorta) can be managed medically if there is no rupture or visceral ischemia.
- Strict BP control; beta-blocker can be used to lower heart rate [10].
- Patients with aortopathy should be monitored with echocardiography at regular intervals during pregnancy and 6 months postpartum [10].

Valvular Heart Disease

- Patients with unrepaired mitral stenosis (usually rheumatic heart disease) or bicuspid aortic valve can present in the first or third trimester with heart failure symptoms due to increased cardiac output [46–48].
- Women with mitral and aortic stenosis and moderate to severe symptoms (NYHA>II, valve area <1 cm, or pulmonary artery pressure >50 mmHg) require valvular repair prior to pregnancy [10, 46, 49]. Ideally, the valve type should be chosen prior to conception dependent on the woman's desire for childbearing.
- Bioprosthetic valves are recommended for those who desire pregnancy due to lower complication rates, but has less durability [50, 51].

Management

- *Unrepaired mitral or aortic stenosis:* Medical management includes beta-1-selective blockers (metoprolol or bisoprolol) and low-dose diuretics for significant heart failure symptoms [3, 10]. Those with significant symptoms and stenosis can undergo balloon valvuloplasty during pregnancy, preferably after 20 weeks [50]. C-section is recommended for those with severe mitral stenosis [10, 50].
- *Mechanical valve:* The third trimester is peak time for complications due to increased hypercoagulability near term [10, 50, 52]. The European Society of Cardiology (ESC) guidelines recommend the following anticoagulation management: [10, 50]

Clinical Pearls

- Low-dose warfarin ($\leq$5 mg per day), is associated with a low risk of warfarin embryopathy and a low risk of fetal complications and can be continued throughout pregnancy and switched to unfractionated heparin (UFH) at 36 weeks in preparation for delivery.
- Warfarin doses $\geq$5 mg per day warrant change to low molecular weight heparin (LMWH) with weekly monitoring of anti-Xa level in the first trimester, and can then be switched back to warfarin during the second trimester, with consideration for C-section due to increased risk of fetal intracranial hemorrhage with vaginal delivery [53, 54]. If anti-Xa levels cannot be monitored regularly, UFH can be used instead of LMWH.

Arrhythmias

- Common arrhythmias in pregnancy include premature atrial and ventricular complexes; ventricular tachycardia or fibrillation is extremely rare [55].
- ECG should be performed on all patients with palpitations or syncopal symptoms with exclusion for thyroid disease [10, 56].

Management

- Table 22.3 provides a summary of key management strategies based on ESC guidelines [10].

Table 22.3 Management of arrhythmias in pregnancy

Arrhythmia	Initial management	Secondary management
Limited PAC or PVC without underlying cardiac disease	Reassure	Beta-blocker only if symptomatic
SVT	Vagal stimulation if stable Beta-blockers and digoxin if recurrent	Adenosine and cardioversion if unstable Flecainide, propafenone Rule out structural heart disease
SVT or atrial fibrillation with WPW	Cardioversion in acute situations	Flecainide, propafenone for long-term control
Atrial fibrillation Atrial flutter	Beta-1 selective blocker Anticoagulants	Cardioversion Rule out thyroid disease
Ventricular tachycardia Ventricular fibrillation	Cardioversion	EKG to rule out long QT Echocardiogram for postpartum cardiomyopathy Beta-blocker, anti-arrhythmic Implantable cardioverter defibrillator

Table 22.3 (continued)

Arrhythmia	Initial management	Secondary management
High-degree AV block	Temporary pacing in acute situation	Check for structural heart disease or myocarditis Pacemaker if persistent

Adapted from the European society of cardiology 2018 Guidelines for management of Cardiovascular disease in pregnancy

Abbreviations: *PAC* premature atrial tachycardia, *PVC* premature ventricular tachycardia, *SVT* supraventricular tachycardia, *WPW* Wolff-Parkinson-White, *AV* atrioventricular

Clinical Pearls

- Adenosine and direct cardioversion are safe during pregnancy [57]. Pregnant women who require cardioversion in the third trimester should be intubated prior to the procedure to decrease risk of aspiration [10, 56].
- Rate control of atrial fibrillation and flutter are similar to supraventricular tachycardia. Anticoagulate based on stroke risk with LMWH or UFH in the event of urgent delivery or surgery. Avoid direct oral anticoagulants [58–60].
- Women with long QT syndrome are at increased risk of VT and require treatment with beta-blocker throughout pregnancy and at least 40 weeks postpartum [61].
- Amiodarone should be avoided due to risk of fetal thyroid suppression [58].

Venous Thromboembolism

- Pregnancy is a hypercoagulable state, with elevated risk for venous thromboembolism (VTE) peripartum [62, 63].
- Risk factors for VTE in pregnancy are similar to nonpregnant patients, which include a history of prior VTE, FH of VTE, thrombophilia, age >35, obesity, and smoking [64, 65].

- Pregnant women with multi-gestation, preeclampsia, prolonged labor, hemorrhage, immobility, infection, or C-section have increased risk [64].
- If high risk (>3 risk factors such as prior unprovoked VTE or estrogen-related VTE, antiphospholipid antibodies, and thrombophilia), prevention is recommended with LHWH and compression stockings [65, 66].

Clinical Presentation and Diagnosis

- Risk prediction tools such as Wells and Geneva scores have not been validated in pregnant females and D-dimer testing is inaccurate as levels increase throughout pregnancy [67, 68].
- In a pregnant female with acute chest pain and shortness of breath, think pulmonary embolism. Low-dose CTA of chest is the gold standard. Ventilation/perfusion scan can also be used, although it can potentially expose the fetus to higher radiation dose but well below the threshold of teratogenicity [69–71].

Management

- In pregnant and postpartum patients, use LMWH or UFH in the event of urgent delivery, surgery, or poor renal function [72].
- In postpartum women with recent pulmonary embolism, heparin treatment should be restarted 6 hours after vaginal delivery and 12 hours after C-section [10]. If no significant bleeding has occurred, warfarin can be overlapped with LMWH for at least 5 days and continued for 3–6 months [10].

Cardiovascular Medications During Pregnancy

- When initiating cardiovascular medications during pregnancy and lactation, keep in mind the necessity, urgency, timing during gestation, and effects on the fetus or infant [58]. Start at the lowest dose. See Fig. 22.1.

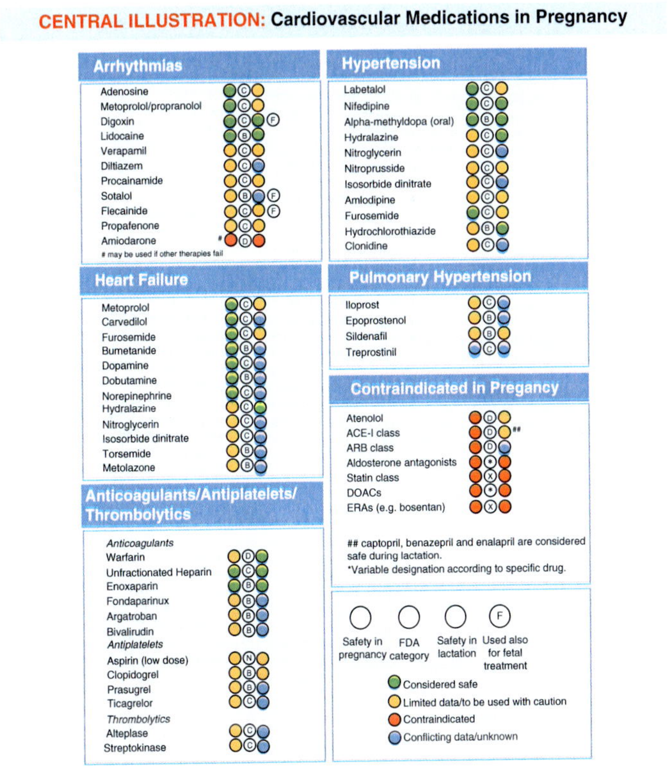

Halpern, D.G. et al. J Am Coll Cardiol. 2019;73(4):457-76.

FIGURE 22.1 Cardiovascular Medications in Pregnancy summarizes some of the more common CVD medications used during pregnancy, potential adverse events, former FDA category, and the compatibility of the drug with breastfeeding. Former Food and Drug Administration ABCDX categories: A) no demonstrated risk to the fetus based on well-controlled human studies; B) no demonstrated risk to the fetus based on animal studies; C) animal studies have demonstrated fetal adverse effects, no human studies, potential benefits may warrant use of the drug; D) demonstrated human fetal risk, potential benefits may warrant use of the drug; and X) demonstrated high risk for human fetal abnormalities outweighing potential benefit; N) nonclassified; F) Used also for fetal treatment

Key Learning Points

- Physiologic changes in pregnancy can predispose women to cardiac complications.
- Pregnancy is a hypercoagulable state, especially during the peripartum period, which increases the risk for thromboembolism and other cardiac conditions.
- Overall, treatment of major acquired heart disease including aortic dissection, ACS, PPCM, arrhythmia, and VTE is similar to the general population.
- In emergent situations, life-saving drugs not typically recommended in pregnancy should not be withheld. Fetal survival is optimized with maternal survival.

References

1. Benjamin EJ, et al. Heart disease and stroke statistics-2019 update: a report from the American Heart Association. Circulation. 2019;139(10):e56–e528.
2. McAloon CJ, et al. The changing face of cardiovascular disease 2000-2012: an analysis of the world health organisation global health estimates data. Int J Cardiol. 2016;224:256–64.
3. Elkayam U, et al. High-risk cardiac disease in pregnancy: part I. J Am Coll Cardiol. 2016;68(4):396–410.
4. Hameed AB, et al. Pregnancy-related cardiovascular deaths in California: beyond peripartum cardiomyopathy. Am J Obstet Gynecol. 2015;213(3):379 e1–10.
5. Creanga AA, et al. Pregnancy-related mortality in the United States, 2011-2013. Obstet Gynecol. 2017;130(2):366–73.
6. Sanghavi M, Rutherford JD. Cardiovascular physiology of pregnancy. Circulation. 2014;130(12):1003–8.
7. Kampman MA, et al. Cardiac adaption during pregnancy in women with congenital heart disease and healthy women. Heart. 2016;102(16):1302–8.
8. Chapman AB, et al. Temporal relationships between hormonal and hemodynamic changes in early human pregnancy. Kidney Int. 1998;54(6):2056–63.
9. ACOG Practice Bulletin No. 212: pregnancy and heart disease. Obstet Gynecol. 2019;133(5):e320–56.

10. Regitz-Zagrosek V, et al. 2018 ESC Guidelines for the management of cardiovascular diseases during pregnancy. Kardiologia Polska (Polish Heart Journal). 2019;77(3):245–326.
11. Lazarus JH. Thyroid disorders associated with pregnancy. Treat Endocrinol. 2005;4(1):31–41.
12. Wilson KL, et al. Subclinical thyroid disease and the incidence of hypertension in pregnancy. Obstet Gynecol. 2012;119(2):315–20.
13. Kaaja RJ, Greer IA. Manifestations of chronic disease during pregnancy. JAMA. 2005;294(21):2751–7.
14. Sliwa K, et al. Current state of knowledge on aetiology, diagnosis, management, and therapy of peripartum cardiomyopathy: a position statement from the Heart Failure Association of the European Society of Cardiology Working Group on peripartum cardiomyopathy. Eur J Heart Fail. 2010;12(8):767–78.
15. Elkayam U. Clinical characteristics of peripartum cardiomyopathy in the United States: diagnosis, prognosis, and management. J Am Coll Cardiol. 2011;58(7):659–70.
16. McNamara DM, et al. Clinical outcomes for peripartum cardiomyopathy in North America: results of the IPAC Study (Investigations of Pregnancy-Associated Cardiomyopathy). J Am Coll Cardiol. 2015;66(8):905–14.
17. Bauersachs J, et al. Pathophysiology, diagnosis and management of peripartum cardiomyopathy: a position statement from the Heart Failure Association of the European Society of Cardiology Study Group on peripartum cardiomyopathy. Eur J Heart Fail. 2019;21:827.
18. Arrigo M, et al. Bromocriptine for the treatment of peripartum cardiomyopathy: welcome on BOARD. Eur Heart J. 2017;38(35):2680–2.
19. James AH, et al. Acute myocardial infarction in pregnancy. Circulation. 2006;113(12).1564–71.
20. Petitti DB, et al. Incidence of stroke and myocardial infarction in women of reproductive age. Stroke. 1997;28(2):280–3.
21. Petersen EE, et al. Vital signs: pregnancy-related deaths, United States, 2011–2015, and strategies for prevention, 13 states, 2013–2017. Morb Mortal Wkly Rep. 2019;68(18):423.
22. Tweet MS, et al. Clinical features, management, and prognosis of spontaneous coronary artery dissection. Circulation. 2012;126(5):579–88.
23. Elkayam U, et al. Pregnancy-associated acute myocardial infarction: a review of contemporary experience in 150 cases between 2006 and 2011. Circulation. 2014;129(16):1695–702.

24. Colletti PM, Lee KH, Elkayam U. Cardiovascular imaging of the pregnant patient. Am J Roentgenol. 2013;200(3):515–21.
25. Jeejeebhoy FM, et al. Cardiac arrest in pregnancy: a scientific statement from the American Heart Association. Circulation. 2015;132(18):1747–73.
26. Chernoguz A, et al. Cessation of clopidogrel before major abdominal procedures. Arch Surg. 2011;146(3):334–9.
27. Pomini F, et al. Cardiopulmonary bypass in pregnancy. Ann Thorac Surg. 1996;61(1):259–68.
28. Bernal JM, Miralles PJ. Cardiac surgery with cardiopulmonary bypass during pregnancy. Obstet Gynecol Surv. 1986;41(1):1–6.
29. Sundaram V, et al. Emergent cesarean section in the catheterization laboratory for spontaneous coronary artery dissection. Am J Cardiol. 2015;115(12):1777–8.
30. Hayes SN, et al. Spontaneous coronary artery dissection: current state of the science: a scientific statement from the American Heart Association. Circulation. 2018;137(19):e523–57.
31. Vijayaraghavan R, et al. Pregnancy-related spontaneous coronary artery dissection. Circulation. 2014;130(21):1915–20.
32. Tweet MS, Gulati R, Hayes SN. What clinicians should know αbout spontaneous coronary artery dissection. In: Mayo Clinic Proceedings: Elsevier; 2015.
33. Obstetricians, A.C.o. and Gynecologists. Guidelines for diagnostic imaging during pregnancy and lactation: committee opinion no. 723. Obstet Gynecol. 2017;130:e210–6.
34. Alfonso F, et al. Spontaneous coronary artery dissection: long-term follow-up of a large series of patients prospectively managed with a "conservative" therapeutic strategy. J Am Coll Cardiol Intv. 2012;5(10):1062–70.
35. Tweet MS, et al. Spontaneous coronary artery dissection: revascularization versus conservative therapy. Circ Cardiovasc Interv. 2014;7(6):777–86.
36. CLASP Collaborative Group CLASP Coordinating Centre, R.I., Oxford. Low dose aspirin in pregnancy and early childhood development: follow up of the collaborative low dose aspirin study in pregnancy. Br J Obstet Gynaecol. 1995;102(11):861–8.
37. Fabricius A, et al. Acute aortic dissection during pregnancy. Thorac Cardiovasc Surg. 2001;49(01):56–7.
38. Immer FF, et al. Aortic dissection in pregnancy: analysis of risk factors and outcome. Ann Thorac Surg. 2003;76(1):309–14.
39. Zhu J-M, et al. Aortic dissection in pregnancy: management strategy and outcomes. Ann Thorac Surg. 2017;103(4):1199–206.

40. Anderson R, Fineron P. Aortic dissection in pregnancy: importance of pregnancy-induced changes in the vessel wall and bicuspid aortic valve in pathogenesis. BJOG Int J Obstet Gynaecol. 1994;101(12):1085–8.
41. Manalo-Estrella P, Barker AE. Histopathologic findings in human aortic media associated with pregnancy. Arch Pathol. 1967;83(4):336.
42. Kamel H, et al. Pregnancy and the risk of aortic dissection or rupture: a cohort-crossover analysis. Circulation. 2016;134(7):527–33.
43. Thalmann M, et al. Acute type A aortic dissection and pregnancy: a population-based study. Eur J Cardiothorac Surg. 2011;39(6):e159–63.
44. McGregor AJ, Barron R, Rosene-Montella K. The pregnant heart: cardiac emergencies during pregnancy. Am J Emerg Med. 2015;33(4):573–9.
45. De Wilde J, Rivers A, Price D. A review of the current use of magnetic resonance imaging in pregnancy and safety implications for the fetus. Prog Biophys Mol Biol. 2005;87(2–3):335–53.
46. Hameed A, et al. The effect of valvular heart disease on maternal and fetal outcome of pregnancy. J Am Coll Cardiol. 2001;37(3):893–9.
47. Samiei N, et al. Echocardiographic evaluation of hemodynamic changes in left-sided heart valves in pregnant women with valvular heart disease. Am J Cardiol. 2016;118(7):1046–52.
48. Drenthen W, et al. Predictors of pregnancy complications in women with congenital heart disease. Eur Heart J. 2010;31(17):2124–32.
49. Silversides CK, et al. Cardiac risk in pregnant women with rheumatic mitral stenosis. Am J Cardiol. 2003;91(11):1382.
50. Baumgartner H, et al. 2017 ESC/EACTS guidelines for the management of valvular heart disease. Eur Heart J. 2017;38(36):2739–91.
51. Lawley CM, et al. Prosthetic heart valves in pregnancy, outcomes for women and their babies: a systematic review and meta-analysis. BJOG Int J Obstet Gynaecol. 2015;122(11):1446–55.
52. Vause S, et al. Pregnancy outcomes in women with mechanical prosthetic heart valves: a prospective descriptive population based study using the United Kingdom Obstetric Surveillance System (UKOSS) data collection system. BJOG Int J Obstet Gynaecol. 2017;124(9):1411–9.

53. Van Driel D, et al. Teratogen update: fetal effects after in utero exposure to coumarins overview of cases, follow-up findings, and pathogenesis. Teratology. 2002;66(3):127–40.
54. Schaefer C, et al. Vitamin K antagonists and pregnancy outcome. Thromb Haemost. 2006;95(06):949–57.
55. Vaidya VR, et al. Burden of arrhythmia in pregnancy. Circulation. 2017;135(6):619–21.
56. Enriquez AD, Economy KE, Tedrow UB. Contemporary management of arrhythmias during pregnancy. Circ Arrhythm Electrophysiol. 2014;7(5):961–7.
57. Wang YC, et al. The impact of maternal cardioversion on fetal haemodynamics. Eur J Obstet Gynecol Reprod Biol. 2006;126(2):268–9.
58. Halpern DG, et al. Use of medication for cardiovascular disease during pregnancy: JACC state-of-the-art review. J Am Coll Cardiol. 2019;73(4):457–76.
59. Lau E, Yeh DD. Management of high risk cardiac conditions in pregnancy: anticoagulation, severe stenotic valvular disease and cardiomyopathy. Trends Cardiovasc Med. 2019;29(3):155–61.
60. Agewall S, Camm J. New ESC/EACTS guidelines for the management of atrial fibrillation. Eur Heart J Cardiovasc Pharmacother. 2017;3(2):71.
61. Rashba EJ, et al. Influence of pregnancy on the risk for cardiac events in patients with hereditary long QT syndrome. Circulation. 1998;97(5):451–6.
62. James A. Practice bulletin no. 123: thromboembolism in pregnancy. Obstet Gynecol. 2011;118(3):718–29.
63. Sultan AA, et al. Risk of first venous thromboembolism in and around pregnancy: a population-based cohort study. Br J Haematol. 2012;156(3):366–73.
64. Sultan AA, et al. Risk factors for first venous thromboembolism around pregnancy: a population-based cohort study from the United Kingdom. Blood. 2013;121(19):3953–61.
65. Obstetricians, R.C.o. and Gynaecologists. Reducing the risk of thrombosis and embolism during pregnancy and the puerperium. Green-top Guideline. 2009(37).
66. Bauersachs RM, et al. Risk stratification and heparin prophylaxis to prevent venous thromboembolism in pregnant women. Thromb Haemost. 2007;98(12):1237–45.
67. Rodger MA, et al. Clinical decision rules and D-Dimer in venous thromboembolism: current controversies and future research priorities. Thromb Res. 2014;134(4):763–8.

68. Van der Pol L, et al. Use of clinical prediction rules and D-dimer tests in the diagnostic management of pregnant patients with suspected acute pulmonary embolism. Blood Rev. 2017;31(2):31–6.
69. Shahir K, et al. Pulmonary embolism in pregnancy: CT pulmonary angiography versus perfusion scanning. Am J Roentgenol. 2010;195(3):W214–20.
70. Greer IA. Pregnancy complicated by venous thrombosis. N Engl J Med. 2015;373(6):540–7.
71. Matthews S. Imaging pulmonary embolism in pregnancy: what is the most appropriate imaging protocol? Br J Radiol. 2006;79(941):441–4.
72. Bates SM, et al. Guidance for the treatment and prevention of obstetric-associated venous thromboembolism. J Thromb Thrombolysis. 2016;41(1):92–128.

Chapter 23
Cardio-oncology

Devinder S. Dhindsa and Anant Mandawat

Introduction

- As cancer survivorship continues to improve due to advancements in treatment and screening, a large number of cancer survivors are entering the population [1]. Many of these individuals are subject to cardiovascular (CV) complications, which are critical for the hospitalist to be aware of both at the time of, and years after, therapy [2].

D. S. Dhindsa (✉)
Emory Clinical Cardiovascular Research Institute, Division of Cardiology, Department of Medicine, Emory University School of Medicine, Atlanta, GA, USA
e-mail: devinder.singh.dhindsa@emory.edu

A. Mandawat
Emory Clinical Cardiovascular Research Institute, Division of Cardiology, Department of Medicine, Emory University School of Medicine, Atlanta, GA, USA

Winship Cancer Institute, Department of Hematology and Medical Oncology, Emory University School of Medicine, Atlanta, GA, USA
e-mail: anant.mandawat@emory.edu

B. J. Wells et al. (eds.), *Handbook of Inpatient Cardiology*,
https://doi.org/10.1007/978-3-030-47868-1_23

Screening and Prevention

- Obtain complete history and physical exam detail, including baseline clinical assessment based on established risk factors and anticipated cancer treatment [3].
- Cardiac risk factor optimization for all patients [4].
- Consider baseline assessment of left ventricular ejection fraction (LVEF) based on risk factors and anticipated cancer treatments [5].
- If there is baseline left ventricular dysfunction, engage cardiology and oncology providers regarding selection of chemotherapy options with lower risk of cardiotoxicity or additional cardioprotective drugs (e.g., beta blocker or angiotensin-converting enzyme inhibitors (ACE-i)) [4, 6].

Cardiac Toxicities of Cancer Therapies

Heart Failure

- Myocardial dysfunction can present early after exposure or after several years due to myocardial injury that occurred at the time of oncological therapy [7–9].
- Cardiotoxicity is defined as > 10% point decrease of LVEF to a value below the lower limit of normal (usually LVEF <50%) by echocardiography or nuclear cardiac imaging (MUGA). A > 15% relative percentage reduction from baseline of global longitudinal strain (GLS) can also suggest cardiotoxicity.

Clinical Pearl
Global longitudinal strain measured by echo may help detect more subtle myocardial dysfunction than monitoring for changes with LVEF.

- Chemotherapies associated with myocardial dysfunction, as well as incidence of LV dysfunction associated with each agent, are presented in Table 23.1 [3].
- Screening for detection of cardiotoxicity includes cardiac imaging through echocardiography, nuclear imaging, cardiac magnetic resonance imaging, or through biomarkers (i.e., brain natriuretic peptide, troponin) [7, 10–12].
- Timing and frequency of monitoring depend on specific treatment, cumulative dose of chemotherapy, duration of therapy, and patient's baseline CV risk [3].
- Of note, LV dysfunction with immunotherapies, such as the anti-*HER2* monoclonal antibody trastuzumab, is usually reversible with interruption of chemotherapy and treatment with heart failure therapies; rechallenge is often well tolerated. This is *in contrast* to the cardiotoxicity associated with anthracyclines, which often leads to an irreversible dilated cardiomyopathy.

Table 23.1 Chemotherapies associated with myocardial dysfunction

Agents associated with myocardial dysfunction (incidence % of LV dysfunction)
Anthracyclines – dose-dependent effect [e.g., doxorubicin (3–48%), idarubicin (5–18%), epirubicin (0.9–11.4%), mitoxantrone (2.6%)]
Alkylating agents [e.g., cyclophosphamide (7–28%), ifosfamide (0.5–17%)]
Antimetabolites [e.g., clofarabine (27%)]
Antimicrotubule agents [e.g., docetaxel (2.3–13%), paclitaxel (<1%)]
Monoclonal antibodies [e.g., *anti-HER2*: trastuzumab (1.7–20.1%), pertuzumab (0.7–1.2%); *anti-VEGF:* bevacizumab (1.6–4%)]
Small molecule tyrosine kinase inhibitors [e.g., sunitinib (2.7–19%), sorafenib (4–8%), dasatinib (2–4%), imatinib (0.2–2.7%)]
Proteosome inhibitors [e.g., carfilzomib (11–25%), bortezomib (2–5%)]
Immune checkpoint inhibitors – associated with myocarditis in 1.1%

- Immune checkpoint inhibitors (pembrolizumab, nivolumab, ipilimumab, tremelimumab, atezolizumab, avelumab, durvalumab) have an uncommon but severe association with myocarditis presenting within 3 months of starting therapy [13]. Patients presenting with this require cessation of the agent, high-dose steroids, and urgent cardiology/cardio-oncology consultation.

Clinical Pearl
Immune checkpoint inhibitor myocarditis is associated with a poor prognosis. Keep a high index of suspicion and treat early.

- If LV dysfunction or heart failure occurs during therapy, patients are likely to benefit from traditional heart failure management like ACE-i/ARB and beta-blocker therapy [6]. Recommend risk-benefit discussion with cardiology and oncology provider regarding interruption of cancer therapy or adjustment of chemotherapeutic strategy [5].
- In addition to managing overall cardiovascular risk, specific strategies to reduce chemotherapy-induced cardiotoxicity can vary by agent.
  - For anthracyclines and analogs, limiting cumulative dose, altering delivery system (e.g., liposomal doxorubicin) and continuous infusions, use of dexrazoxane with anthracyclines to reduce anthracycline toxicity in appropriate patients, cardioprotective medications (ACE-i/ARBs, beta-blockers, statins), and aerobic exercise can reduce the risk of cardiotoxicity.
  - For trastuzumab, cardioprotective medications (ACE-i/ARBs) are an important consideration [3].

Coronary Artery Disease/Therapy-Related Ischemia

- Myocardial ischemia can occur through a number of mechanisms from cancer therapies, including vasospasm, endothelial injury, acute arterial thrombosis, or through premature atherosclerosis [14–16].
- Therapies associated with myocardial ischemia are listed in Table 23.2 [14, 15, 17–20].
- Baseline screening for preexisting CVD is important as preexisting CVD increases the risk of developing treatment-related CVD [16].
- For patients who develop signs or symptoms of ischemia on cancer therapy, in particular pyrimidine analogs (e.g., 5-FU, capecitabine), consider withholding treatment and referral to cardiology for evaluation and discussion with oncology regarding the risk benefit of continued use given the high rates of symptom recurrence [3, 14, 21].
- Additionally, patients treated with radiation therapy can develop premature atherosclerotic disease. Consensus documents suggest regular screening beginning 5–10 years after receiving radiation therapy [22].
- Management with antiplatelets and anticoagulants is particularly challenging in this population, given the prevalence of treatment-related thrombocytopenia [23]. An individualized risk-benefit discussion is recommended.

TABLE 23.2 Therapies associated with myocardial ischemia

Therapy	Mechanism of ischemia
Fluoropyrimidines (e.g., 5-FU, capecetabine, gemcitabine)	Endothelial injury, vasospasm
Cisplatin	Procoagulant, direct endothelial toxicity
VEGF inhibitors (bevacizumab, sorafenib, sunitinib)	Endothelial injury, arterial thrombosis, vasospasm
Radiotherapy	Endothelial injury, plaque rupture, thrombosis

Clinical Pearl

- When possible, avoid premature/unnecessary cessation as this may affect cancer curability. In addition to optimizing preexisting cardiovascular disease/risk factors for patients receiving fluoropyrimidines, screening treadmill may not be sufficient, and coronary CT angiogram or left heart catheterization should be considered. Coronary spasm due to fluoropyrimidines is usually reversible but usually recurrent upon reexposure if not treated with nitrates-/calcium-channel blockers

Valvular Disease

- Radiation therapy can be associated with fibrosis and calcification of the aortic root or cardiac valves [16, 20, 24].
- Echocardiography is the imaging test of choice for assessing for valvular disease, though cardiac MRI or computed tomography (CT) may also be used [25, 26].
- If valve repair is required, surgery is often challenging due to fibrosis and impaired wound healing. Transcatheter options may be a suitable alternative [27].

Arrhythmia

- Patients treated with chemotherapy can experience a number of arrhythmias during their treatment course, including tachyarrhythmias or bradyarrhythmias and conduction disturbances [28].
- QT prolongation has been associated with arsenic trioxide and tyrosine kinase inhibitors, in particular vandetanib [29–31]. Management consists of correction of any electrolyte abnormalities (hypocalcemia, hypokalemia, hypomagnesemia) and avoidance or withdrawal of any QT-prolonging medication.

- Conduction disturbances, including complete heart block, have been noted with paclitaxel and thalidomide [32].
- Atrial fibrillation/flutter (AF/AFL) can occur due to comorbidities and malignancy, as well as ibrutinib [33]. Management of this rhythm generally requires anti-coagulation, though this can be challenging in this population due to thrombocytopenia.

Arterial Hypertension

- Arterial hypertension can be associated with VEGF inhibitors [34]. Early and aggressive management is warranted with ACE-i/ARB, beta-blocker, or dihydropyridine calcium channel blocker to avoid CV complications, such as heart failure [35].
- If blood pressure remains uncontrolled, the VEGF inhibitor should be held or reduced until blood pressure is adequately controlled (<140/90 mmHg or lower in case of overt proteinuria), at which point the VEGF inhibitor can be restarted [31, 35].

Thromboembolic Disease

- Malignancy contributes to a pro-thrombotic state, placing cancer patients at risk for both arterial and venous thrombosis [36].
- Low molecular weight heparin is preferred currently due to lower rates of recurrent venous thrombosis in those patients who are able to be anticoagulated (CLOT, 2003) [37]. Direct oral anticoagulants are being studied within this population [38]. If recurrence of thrombosis occurs despite therapy, the provider can consider adjusting anti-coagulation strategy or consider placement of an inferior vena cava filter [39].

Peripheral Vascular Disease and Stroke

- Severe atherosclerotic and non-atherosclerotic peripheral arterial disease can occur with nilotinib, ponatinib, or *BCR-ABL* tyrosine kinase inhibitors [40].
- Ischemic stroke has also been associated with head and neck radiotherapy [41, 42].
- Risk factor control is critical. In cases of severe PAD, the decision for revascularization should be individualized with multidisciplinary input from cardio-oncology, vascular surgery, and hematology/oncology [43].
- Patients irradiated for head and neck cancer are at higher risk for developed cerebrovascular disease following radiation therapy [44].

Pulmonary Hypertension

- Pulmonary hypertension can occur following dasatinib therapy, stem cell bone marrow transplantation, or alkylating agent therapy (due to veno-occlusive disease) [45, 46].
- Baseline echocardiogram should be considered prior to dasatinib therapy [47].
- Signs of elevated pulmonary artery pressure may require cardiology or a pulmonary hypertension team assessment, as etiology of pulmonary hypertension may affect therapy

Key Learning Points

- The CV effects of cancer and cancer-related therapies are a challenging reality of the treatment of these conditions.
- There should be a particular emphasis on screening and optimization of cardiac risk factors prior to receiving potentially cardiotoxic treatments.
- It is important to recognize that the CV effects can occur early or years after oncological treatment.

References

1. Shapiro CL. Cancer survivorship. N Engl J Med. 2018;379(25):2438–50.
2. de Azambuja E, Ameye L, Diaz M, Vandenbossche S, Aftimos P, Bejarano Hernandez S, et al. Cardiac assessment of early breast cancer patients 18 years after treatment with cyclophosphamide-, methotrexate-, fluorouracil- or epirubicin-based chemotherapy. Eur J Cancer (Oxford, England: 1990). 2015;51(17):2517–24.
3. Zamorano JL, Lancellotti P, Rodriguez Muñoz D, Aboyans V, Asteggiano R, Galderisi M, et al. 2016 ESC position paper on cancer treatments and cardiovascular toxicity developed under the auspices of the ESC Committee for Practice Guidelines: the task force for cancer treatments and cardiovascular toxicity of the European Society of Cardiology (ESC). Eur Heart J. 2016;37(36):2768–801.
4. Barac A, Murtagh G, Carver JR, Chen MH, Freeman AM, Herrmann J, et al. Cardiovascular health of patients with cancer and cancer survivors: a roadmap to the next level. J Am Coll Cardiol. 2015;65(25):2739–46.
5. Cardinale D, Colombo A, Lamantia G, Colombo N, Civelli M, De Giacomi G, et al. Anthracycline-induced cardiomyopathy: clinical relevance and response to pharmacologic therapy. J Am Coll Cardiol. 2010;55(3):213–20.
6. Cardinale D, Colombo A, Bacchiani G, Tedeschi I, Meroni CA, Veglia F, et al. Early detection of anthracycline cardiotoxicity and improvement with heart failure therapy. Circulation. 2015;131(22):1981–8.
7. Armstrong GT, Plana JC, Zhang N, Srivastava D, Green DM, Ness KK, et al. Screening adult survivors of childhood cancer for cardiomyopathy: comparison of echocardiography and cardiac magnetic resonance imaging. J Clin Oncol. 2012;30(23):2876–84.
8. Hequet O, Le QH, Moullet I, Pauli E, Salles G, Espinouse D, et al. Subclinical late cardiomyopathy after doxorubicin therapy for lymphoma in adults. J Clin Oncol. 2004;22(10):1864–71.
9. Steinherz LJ, Steinherz PG, Tan CT, Heller G, Murphy ML. Cardiac toxicity 4 to 20 years after completing anthracycline therapy. JAMA. 1991;266(12):1672–7.
10. Cardinale D, Sandri MT. Role of biomarkers in chemotherapy-induced cardiotoxicity. Prog Cardiovasc Dis. 2010;53(2):121–9.

11. Ledwidge M, Gallagher J, Conlon C, Tallon E, O'Connell E, Dawkins I, et al. Natriuretic peptide-based screening and collaborative care for heart failure: the STOP-HF randomized trial. JAMA. 2013;310(1):66–74.
12. Mitani I, Jain D, Joska TM, Burtness B, Zaret BL. Doxorubicin cardiotoxicity: prevention of congestive heart failure with serial cardiac function monitoring with equilibrium radionuclide angiocardiography in the current era. J Nucl Cardiol. 2003;10(2):132–9.
13. Mahmood SS, Fradley MG, Cohen JV, Nohria A, Reynolds KL, Heinzerling LM, et al. Myocarditis in patients treated with immune checkpoint inhibitors. J Am Coll Cardiol. 2018;71(16):1755–64.
14. Frickhofen N, Beck FJ, Jung B, Fuhr HG, Andrasch H, Sigmund M. Capecitabine can induce acute coronary syndrome similar to 5-fluorouracil. Ann Oncol. 2002;13(5):797–801.
15. Choueiri TK, Schutz FA, Je Y, Rosenberg JE, Bellmunt J. Risk of arterial thromboembolic events with sunitinib and sorafenib: a systematic review and meta-analysis of clinical trials. J Clin Oncol. 2010;28(13):2280–5.
16. Hull MC, Morris CG, Pepine CJ, Mendenhall NP. Valvular dysfunction and carotid, subclavian, and coronary artery disease in survivors of hodgkin lymphoma treated with radiation therapy. JAMA. 2003;290(21):2831–7.
17. Moore RA, Adel N, Riedel E, Bhutani M, Feldman DR, Tabbara NE, et al. High incidence of thromboembolic events in patients treated with cisplatin-based chemotherapy: a large retrospective analysis. J Clin Oncol. 2011;29(25):3466–73.
18. McEniery PT, Dorosti K, Schiavone WA, Pedrick TJ, Sheldon WC. Clinical and angiographic features of coronary artery disease after chest irradiation. Am J Cardiol. 1987;60(13):1020–4.
19. Virmani R, Farb A, Carter AJ, Jones RM. Comparative pathology: radiation-induced coronary artery disease in man and animals. Semin Interv Cardiol. 1998;3(3–4):163–72.
20. McGale P, Darby SC, Hall P, Adolfsson J, Bengtsson NO, Bennet AM, et al. Incidence of heart disease in 35,000 women treated with radiotherapy for breast cancer in Denmark and Sweden. Radiother Oncol. 2011;100(2):167–75.
21. Kosmas C, Kallistratos MS, Kopterides P, Syrios J, Skopelitis H, Mylonakis N, et al. Cardiotoxicity of fluoropyrimidines in different schedules of administration: a prospective study. J Cancer Res Clin Oncol. 2008;134(1):75–82.

22. Lancellotti P, Nkomo VT, Badano LP, Bergler J, Bogaert J, Davin L, et al. Expert consensus for multi-modality imaging evaluation of cardiovascular complications of radiotherapy in adults: a report from the European Association of Cardiovascular Imaging and the American Society of Echocardiography. J Am Soc Echocardiogr. 2013;26(9):1013–32.
23. Xu XR, Yousef GM, Ni H. Cancer and platelet crosstalk: opportunities and challenges for aspirin and other antiplatelet agents. Blood. 2018;131(16):1777–89.
24. Hering D, Faber L, Horstkotte D. Echocardiographic features of radiation-associated valvular disease. Am J Cardiol. 2003;92(2):226–30.
25. Plana JC, Galderisi M, Barac A, Ewer MS, Ky B, Scherrer-Crosbie M, et al. Expert consensus for multimodality imaging evaluation of adult patients during and after cancer therapy: a report from the American Society of Echocardiography and the European Association of Cardiovascular Imaging. Eur Heart J Cardiovasc Imaging. 2014;15(10):1063–93.
26. Groarke JD, Nguyen PL, Nohria A, Ferrari R, Cheng S, Moslehi J. Cardiovascular complications of radiation therapy for thoracic malignancies: the role for non-invasive imaging for detection of cardiovascular disease. Eur Heart J. 2014;35(10):612–23.
27. Nishimura RA, Otto CM, Bonow RO, Carabello BA, Erwin JP, Fleisher LA, et al. 2017 AHA/ACC focused update of the 2014 AHA/ACC guideline for the management of patients with valvular heart disease. A report of the American College of Cardiology/American Heart Association Task Force on Clinical Practice Guidelines. J Am Coll Cardiol. 2017;70(2):252–89.
28. Tamargo J, Caballero R, Delpon E. Cancer chemotherapy and cardiac arrhythmias: a review. Drug Saf. 2015;38(2):129–52.
29. Soignet SL, Frankel SR, Douer D, Tallman MS, Kantarjian H, Calleja E, et al. United States multicenter study of arsenic trioxide in relapsed acute promyelocytic leukemia. J Clin Oncol. 2001;19(18):3852–60.
30. Shah RR, Morganroth J, Shah DR. Cardiovascular safety of tyrosine kinase inhibitors: with a special focus on cardiac repolarisation (QT interval). Drug Saf. 2013;36(5):295–316.
31. Chandrasekhar S, Fradley MG. QT interval prolongation associated with cytotoxic and targeted cancer therapeutics. Curr Treat Options Oncol. 2019;20(7):55.

32. Lenihan DJ, Kowey PR. Overview and management of cardiac adverse events associated with tyrosine kinase inhibitors. Oncologist. 2013;18(8):900–8.
33. Farmakis D, Parissis J, Filippatos G. Insights into onco-cardiology: atrial fibrillation in cancer. J Am Coll Cardiol. 2014;63(10):945–53.
34. Izzedine H, Ederhy S, Goldwasser F, Soria JC, Milano G, Cohen A, et al. Management of hypertension in angiogenesis inhibitor-treated patients. Ann Oncol. 2009;20(5):807–15.
35. Maitland ML, Bakris GL, Black HR, Chen HX, Durand JB, Elliott WJ, et al. Initial assessment, surveillance, and management of blood pressure in patients receiving vascular endothelial growth factor signaling pathway inhibitors. J Natl Cancer Inst. 2010;102(9):596–604.
36. Rickles FR. Mechanisms of cancer-induced thrombosis in cancer. Pathophysiol Haemost Thromb. 2006;35(1–2):103–10.
37. Lee AYY, Levine MN, Baker RI, Bowden C, Kakkar AK, Prins M, et al. Low-molecular-weight heparin versus a coumarin for the prevention of recurrent venous thromboembolism in patients with cancer. N Engl J Med. 2003;349(2):146–53.
38. Gerotziafas GT, Mahe I, Elalamy I. New orally active anticoagulant agents for the prevention and treatment of venous thromboembolism in cancer patients. Ther Clin Risk Manag. 2014;10:423–36.
39. Barginear MF, Gralla RJ, Bradley TP, Ali SS, Shapira I, Greben C, et al. Investigating the benefit of adding a vena cava filter to anticoagulation with fondaparinux sodium in patients with cancer and venous thromboembolism in a prospective randomized clinical trial. Support Care Cancer. 2012;20(11):2865–72.
40. Valent P, Hadzijusufovic E, Schernthaner GH, Wolf D, Rea D, le Coutre P. Vascular safety issues in CML patients treated with BCR/ABL1 kinase inhibitors. Blood. 2015;125(6):901–6.
41. De Bruin ML, Dorresteijn LD, van't Veer MB, Krol AD, van der Pal HJ, Kappelle AC, et al. Increased risk of stroke and transient ischemic attack in 5-year survivors of Hodgkin lymphoma. J Natl Cancer Inst. 2009;101(13):928–37.
42. Plummer C, Henderson RD, O'Sullivan JD, Read SJ. Ischemic stroke and transient ischemic attack after head and neck radiotherapy: a review. Stroke. 2011;42(9):2410–8.
43. Fokkema M, den Hartog AG, Bots ML, van der Tweel I, Moll FL, de Borst GJ. Stenting versus surgery in patients with carotid

stenosis after previous cervical radiation therapy: systematic review and meta-analysis. Stroke. 2012;43(3):793–801.

44. Gujral DM, Shah BN, Chahal NS, Senior R, Harrington KJ, Nutting CM. Clinical features of radiation-induced carotid atherosclerosis. Clinical Oncol (Royal College of Radiologists (Great Britain)). 2014;26(2):94–102.
45. Limsuwan A, Pakakasama S, Rochanawutanon M, Hong-eng S. Pulmonary arterial hypertension after childhood cancer therapy and bone marrow transplantation. Cardiology. 2006;105(3):188–94.
46. Montani D, Bergot E, Gunther S, Savale L, Bergeron A, Bourdin A, et al. Pulmonary arterial hypertension in patients treated by dasatinib. Circulation. 2012;125(17):2128–37.
47. Montani D, Bergot E, Günther S, Savale L, Bergeron A, Bourdin A, et al. Pulmonary arterial hypertension in patients treated by dasatinib. Circulation. 2012;125(17):2128–37.

Part II
Clinical Approach to the Patient Chief Complaint

Chapter 24
Chest Pain

Serge Korjian and C. Michael Gibson

Abbreviations

ACS	Acute coronary syndrome
CAD	Coronary artery disease
CTA	Computed tomography angiogram
CXR	Chest X-ray
ECG	Electrocardiogram
MI	Myocardial infarction
NSTEMI	Non-ST-elevation myocardial infarction
NTG	Nitroglycerin
PE	Pulmonary embolism
PTX	Pneumothorax
STEMI	ST-elevation myocardial infarction
TTE	Transthoracic echocardiogram

Introduction

- Given the broad differential diagnosis of chest discomfort, the initial evaluation of chest pain can be challenging.

S. Korjian (✉) · C. M. Gibson
Cardiovascular Division, Department of Medicine, Beth Israel Deaconess Medical Center, Harvard Medical School, Boston, MA, USA
e-mail: skorjian@bidmc.harvard.edu

B. J. Wells et al. (eds.), *Handbook of Inpatient Cardiology*,
https://doi.org/10.1007/978-3-030-47868-1_24

- The internist must to be able to identify life-threatening conditions promptly in order to prevent major morbidity and mortality.
- A thorough history and physical examination can often limit unnecessary testing, particularly in patients who are at a low risk for serious cardiovascular disease.

Initial Evaluation

- The initial evaluation of any patient with chest pain should promptly identify evidence of hemodynamic or respiratory instability and rule out conditions that require immediate intervention (Fig. 24.1).
- In a stable patient, take the time to obtain a focused history, which may limit your diagnostic testing in certain situations where life-threatening etiologies are highly unlikely such as esophageal disorders, musculoskeletal disease, or pleural and pericardial inflammatory conditions.
- A focused physical examination should include the following:
  - Vital signs with blood pressure measurement in both arms
  - Peripheral oxygen saturation
  - Cardiac and pulmonary auscultation
  - Abdominal examination
  - Evaluation of signs of peripheral perfusion (pulses, temperature of extremities, and capillary refill)
- Further testing should invariably include an electrocardiogram (ECG) to identify patients with ischemic heart disease, particularly those with ST-elevation myocardial infarctions that require immediate intervention.
- A chest X-ray should be obtained for patients with shortness of breath, new or worsening oxygen requirement, and concomitant signs or symptoms of congestive heart failure or active lung disease.
- Cardiac biomarkers may also be obtained among patients with concern for acute coronary syndromes (ACS) or patients without an evident non-cardiac etiology of chest pain in order to rule out ACS.

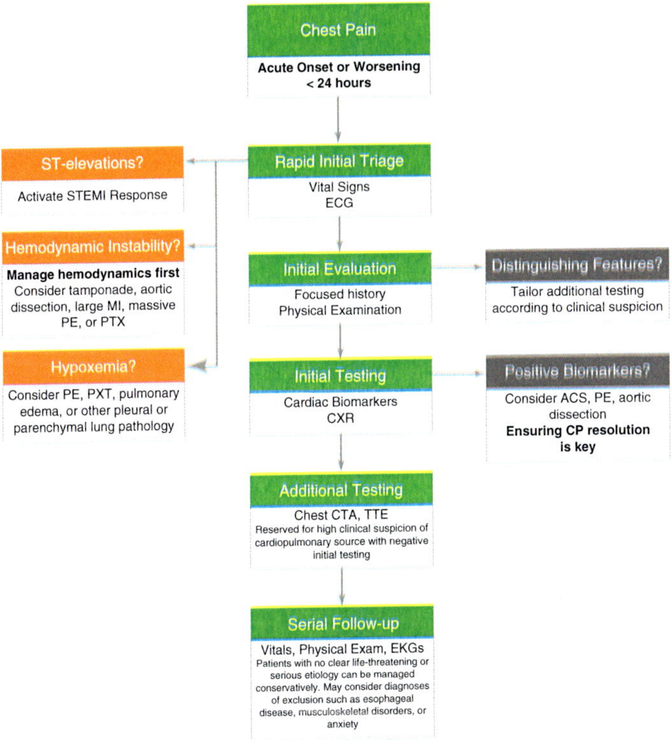

FIGURE 24.1 Approach to patient with acute chest pain. *Abbreviations:* ACS acute coronary syndrome, CTA computed tomography angiogram, CXR chest X-ray, ECG electrocardiogram, NTG nitroglycerin, PE pulmonary embolism, PTX pneumothorax, TTE transthoracic echocardiogram

   - Cardiac troponins are highly sensitive and specific for myocardial tissue injury but may be elevated in conditions other than ACS including acute decompensated heart failure, myocarditis, renal failure (due to reduced clearance), septic shock, and acute strokes [1].
- Further diagnostic testing should be guided by the clinical impression.

Etiologies of Chest Pain

Angina and Acute Coronary Syndromes

- Anginal chest pain is often substernal and does not localize to a small area of the chest.
- It is described as a pressure, heaviness, tightness, or a squeezing sensation; it is less commonly described as a sharp pain.
- The pain may radiate to any area between the maxilla and the umbilicus, but more commonly involves the epigastrium, arms, shoulders, neck, or jaw.
- Associated symptoms may include shortness of breath, diaphoresis, and palpitations.
- Chest pain can be classified into three distinct categories: typical angina, atypical angina, and non-cardiac chest pain.
  - *Typical angina* is defined as a characteristic substernal chest discomfort provoked by exertion or emotion, and relieved by rest or nitroglycerin. This combination of characteristics is highly suggestive of cardiac chest pain.
  - *Atypical angina* is defined as any chest discomfort that meets two of the three cardinal features of typical angina.
  - *Non-cardiac chest pain* has one or none of these features [1–3].
  - While typical angina is the most common presentation of ischemic heart disease, atypical angina is more common in certain patient populations such as the elderly, women, and patients with diabetes mellitus [4–6].
  - Features suggesting non-cardiac chest pain include sharp discomfort localized to a very small area of the chest, fleeting pain that lasts only a few seconds, and pain that is reliably recreated with palpation.
- Ischemic chest pain can clinically present as either stable angina or ACS, i.e., unstable angina, non-ST-elevation myocardial infarction (NSTEMI), or ST-elevation myocardial infarction (STEMI).

- Pain that is acute in onset, increasing in severity, occurring at rest, and lasting longer than 20 minutes is suggestive of ACS [7].
- Stable angina is chronic, stable in severity, occurs relatively reliably with a similar level of exertion, and resolves within a few minutes with rest or nitroglycerin.
- ST-segment deviations and T-wave inversions present at rest are more suggestive of ACS particularly in the setting of active chest pain. Cardiac biomarkers (particularly troponin T & I) may also help identify a myocardial infarction.

Clinical Pearl
Among patients with anginal chest pain and positive biomarkers, it is crucial to ensure resolution of chest pain given that it is often a sign of ongoing myocardial injury.

- History may identify traditional risk factors for CAD such as advanced age, hypertension, hyperlipidemia, diabetes mellitus, obesity, smoking history, family history of premature CAD, and post-menopausal female gender.
- The physical examination of patients with stable angina may have a normal exam or findings suggestive of atherosclerotic disease in other vascular beds such as vascular bruits or diminished peripheral pulses.
- Patients with ACS may have tachycardia or bradycardia, hypotension, crackles (suggestive of pulmonary edema), a new systolic murmur (suggestive of mitral regurgitation), S3/S4 gallop, as well as signs of decreased peripheral perfusion.
- Once ACS is ruled out, additional diagnostic studies in the form of cardiac stress testing may help distinguish ischemic disease from other causes of chest pain.

Pericarditis and Myopericarditis

- Chest pain associated with pericarditis is often substernal, sharp in character and pleuritic.
- Radiation to the trapezius ridge is more specific for pericarditis, given the joint phrenic-nerve innervation.

Clinical Pearl
Radiation to the trapezius ridge may suggest pericarditis, given the joint phrenic-nerve innervation.

- The pain is often worse in the supine position and alleviated when sitting up and leaning forward.
- A pericardial friction rub may be notable on physical examination and is heard best at the end expiration with the patient leaning forward.
- If a significant pericardial effusion is present, the patient may complain of concomitant shortness of breath and the exam may reveal signs of cardiac tamponade (Beck's triad, hypotension, muffled heart sounds, and distended neck veins).
- In cases of myopericarditis, the exam may show signs of congestive heart failure.
- The pathognomonic ECG finding in pericarditis is diffuse upward concave ST-segment elevations due to subepicardial inflammation as well as PR-segment depressions. Conduction abnormalities may suggest myopericarditis.
- Cardiac biomarkers are negative in cases of pericarditis. When biomarkers are elevated, this is termed myopericarditis [8].

Aortic Dissection

- Aortic dissection has high in-hospital mortality, particularly when not identified promptly.
- The pain associated with aortic dissection has classically been described as a ripping or tearing sensation, although majority of patients report sharp chest pain.
- In cases of *type A dissection* (involving the ascending aorta), the pain is usually anterior and substernal similar to angina.
- Pain associated with *type B dissection* (involving only the descending aorta) is usually more localized to the back or abdomen, although half of patients still report anterior chest pain.
- Approximately 90% of patients presenting for aortic dissection report an abrupt onset of pain described as severe or the worst they have experienced.
- Three out of four patients with aortic dissection are hypertensive at the time of presentation. Hypotension is a poor prognostic sign and may suggest the presence of cardiac tamponade.
- A variation of greater than 20 mmHg in the systolic blood pressure may be noted between arms due to decreased blood flow from an obstructive intimal flap.
- Patients with *type A dissection* may have an early diastolic murmur suggestive of aortic regurgitation, a pulse deficit between distal vascular beds, signs of congestive heart failure, and focal neurological deficits.
- The ECG may show ST-segment and T-wave abnormalities, although only 10–15% are associated with cardiac ischemia.
- A chest X-ray may show a widened mediastinum, an abnormal aortic contour, or new pleural effusions [9].
- A computed tomography angiogram of the aorta is the gold standard for the diagnosis of aortic dissection when suspected.
- Although very non-specific, a D-dimer may help rule out aortic dissection due to sensitivity of approximately 95% [10].

Pulmonary Embolism

- Chest pain has been associated with increased mortality among patients with PE.
- The pain is often sharp in character, does not radiate, and is pleuritic.
- Associated symptoms may include hemoptysis or syncope. Patients may report lower extremity swelling, redness, or pain in cases of concomitant deep vein thrombosis.
- Tachypnea and hypoxemia are present in approximately 75% of patient, while tachycardia is present in 50% of cases. Hypotension is a marker of massive pulmonary embolization observed in approximately 10% of patients.
- The physical examination may also demonstrate elevated jugular venous pressure due to increased pulmonary and right ventricular pressures and a right-sided S3 gallop.
- Evidence of deep vein thrombosis on physical examination also increases the likelihood of PE [11].
- The most common ECG finding among patients with PE is sinus tachycardia, observed in 60–70% of patients. Other findings include new right bundle branch block, right axis deviation, atrial fibrillation, anterior and inferior T-wave inversions, and ST-segment depressions, which indicate right ventricular strain.
- S1-Q3-T3 pattern (large S-wave in lead I, deep Q-wave and inverted T-wave in lead III) is neither sensitive nor specific for acute PE [12, 13].
- Dedicated lung perfusion imaging such as a computed tomography angiogram (CTA) of the chest or a ventilation-perfusion (V/Q) lung scan is essential in diagnosing PE.
- In select patients among whom the risk of PE is low to intermediate, a D-dimer may be sufficient in ruling out a PE due to its high diagnostic sensitivity [14, 15].

Other Lung Diseases

- Conditions such as tension pneumothorax, pneumonia, and pleuritis may be associated with significant chest discomfort.
- The pain is more commonly ipsilateral to the lung involved due to the anatomic separation of the lungs and is often pleuritic in nature.
- A very abrupt onset of sharp pain may suggest a spontaneous pneumothorax, although the pain often progresses to a dull ache.
- The presence of fever, chills, cough, and sputum production suggests pneumonia.
- The physical exam may be notable for tachypnea, tachycardia, low peripheral oxygen saturation, increased work of breathing, as well as diminished breath sounds, rales, or a pleural rub upon auscultation.
- The chest X-ray is essential in identifying lung opacities, pleural effusions, or loss of lung markings due to a pneumothorax.

Gastrointestinal Diseases

- Gastrointestinal diseases, particularly esophageal conditions, are the most common causes of non-cardiac chest pain due to similar visceral innervation to the heart via the vagus nerve and the thoracic sympathetic trunk [16].
- Patients may report a substernal burning sensation, acidic or unpleasant taste in the mouth, and hoarseness. Symptoms are often exacerbated by food intake.
- Intense substernal chest pain triggered by food intake may suggest diffuse esophageal spasm.
  - Patients may sometimes report radiation of the pain to the throat or jaw.
  - Esophageal spasm pain may be relieved by anti-anginal medications such as nitrates and calcium channel blockers.

- Severe chest pain triggered by vomiting may be suggestive of esophageal rupture known as Boerhaave's syndrome [17–20].
- Non-esophageal causes of gastrointestinal chest pain include peptic ulcer disease, biliary colic, and pancreatitis. Similar to esophageal disease, close correlation of the pain to food intake increases clinical suspicion for these conditions.

Miscellaneous Causes

- Non-visceral causes of chest pain are common and include musculoskeletal disease, herpes zoster, and postherpetic neuralgia, and anxiety.
  - Costochondritis and intercostal muscle spasms are often underdiagnosed and lead to excessive and unnecessary testing for chest pain. The pain is often sharp and lasts for only a few seconds and is exacerbated by certain positions and by direct palpation. Some patient may also report a chronic, dull ache. The pain is usually localized to a small area in the chest and is very rarely diffuse in nature [16].
  - Herpes zoster often presents with a visible rash in a dermatomal distribution, which makes the diagnosis less challenging. In a small number of cases, patient may experience significant chest discomfort prior to the appearance of the pathognomonic vesicular rash. The pain is usually unilateral and localized to a single dermatome. It is described as very intense and constant, and burning, sharp, or pin-like in character.
  - Anxiety and panic disorders may cause chest tightness and shortness of breath, which is often difficult to differentiate from true visceral pain. Anxiety should always be a diagnosis of exclusion but should be considered in young patients with no significant risk factors for cardiovascular disease, patients with history of psychiatric disease, and patients with a history of extensive negative diagnostic testing.
- Common causes and features of chest pain are summarized in Table 24.1.

Table 24.1 Common causes of chest pain

Diagnosis	Characteristics of pain	Provoking factors	Alleviating factors	Associated symptoms	Findings
Stable angina	Substernal Diffuse Heaviness/tightness May radiate anywhere from maxilla to umbilicus Crescendo onset	Exertion Emotional stress	Rest Nitroglycerin (NTG)	Diaphoresis Shortness of breath Palpitations	ECG may be normal Positive stress testing
Acute coronary syndrome (ACS)	Substernal Diffuse Lasts >20 minutes Heaviness/tightness Radiates anywhere from maxilla to umbilicus Variable onset but often acute	Exertion Emotional stress	Rest NTG Symptoms may persist despite rest and NTG	Diaphoresis Shortness of breath Palpitations Nausea/ vomiting	Ischemic changes on ECG Positive cardiac biomarkers

(continued)

Table 24.1 (continued)

Diagnosis	Characteristics of pain	Provoking factors	Alleviating factors	Associated symptoms	Findings
Pericarditis	Anterior chest Sharp Radiates to trapezius ridge Variable onset	Lying down Inspiration (pleuritic pain)	Sitting up and leaning forward	Viral prodrome	Diffuse ST elevations and PR depressions Friction rub Pericardial effusion on TTE
Aortic dissection	Anterior or posterior chest Sharp, ripping Radiates to back or abdomen Severe Abrupt onset	None	None	Syncope Focal weakness Palpitations	Hypertension Tamponade ACS Stroke CTA confirms dissection
Pulmonary embolism (PE)	Localized or diffuse Sharp Variable onset	Inspiration (pleuritic pain)	None	Dyspnea Syncope Palpitations	Tachycardia, tachypnea, hypoxia Heart failure Right heart strain on ECG, Echo CTA confirms PE

Pneumothorax (PTX)	Localized Sharp initially, then dull ache Acute onset	Inspiration (pleuritic pain)	Shallow breathing	Dyspnea	Hemodynamic collapse if tension PTX Tachypnea CXR showing PTX
Pneumonia	Localized Dull ache Subacute onset	Inspiration (pleuritic pain)	Shallow breathing	Dyspnea Cough Fever	Infiltrate on CXR
Esophageal disorders	Substernal Tightness or burning May radiate to jaw or throat Variable onset	Triggered by food intake	Water intake Nitroglycerin Calcium channel blockers	Acid reflux Vomiting Abdominal pain	Normal exam Thrush in the case of *Candida* spp. esophagitis
Musculoskeletal disease	Localized to focal area Dull at rest, sharp with movement	Movement and positioning Direct palpation	Rest Analgesics Stretching	Arthritis	Pain reproducible with palpation

Abbreviations: ACS acute coronary syndrome, *CTA* computed tomography angiogram, *CXR* chest X-ray, *ECG* electrocardiogram, *NTG* nitroglycerin, *PE* pulmonary embolism, *PTX* pneumothorax, *TTE* transthoracic echocardiogram

Key Learning Points

1. A focused history and exam, ECG, and basic testing including a CXR and cardiac biomarkers can help adequately triage the majority of patients complaining of chest pain.
2. Life-threatening conditions such as acute myocardial infarction, aortic dissection, pulmonary embolism, and tension pneumothorax need to be recognized promptly in order to prevent major morbidity and mortality.
3. When in doubt, serial testing with frequent vitals, ECGs at 30 to 60 minute intervals, and cardiac biomarker monitoring may identify the etiology of the chest pain.

References

1. Fihn SD, Gardin JM, Abrams J, Berra K, Blankenship JC, Dallas AP, et al. ACCF/AHA/ACP/AATS/PCNA/SCAI/STS guideline for the diagnosis and management of patients with stable ischemic heart disease: executive summary: a report of the American College of Cardiology Foundation/American Heart Association task force on practice guidelines, and the American College of Physicians, American Association for Thoracic Surgery, Preventive Cardiovascular Nurses Association, Society for Cardiovascular Angiography and Interventions, and Society of Thoracic Surgeons. Circulation. 2012;126(25):3097–137.
2. Prinzmetal M, Kennamer R, Merliss R, Wada T, Bor N. Angina pectoris. I. A variant form of angina pectoris; preliminary report. Am J Med. 1959;27:375–88.
3. Braunwald E, Jones RH, Mark DB, Brown J, Brown L, Cheitlin MD, et al. Diagnosing and managing unstable angina. Agency for Health Care Policy and Research. Circulation. 1994;90(1):613–22.
4. McSweeney JC, Cody M, O'Sullivan P, Elberson K, Moser DK, Garvin BJ. Women's early warning symptoms of acute myocardial infarction. Circulation. 2003;108(21):2619–23.

5. Culic V, Eterovic D, Miric D, Silic N. Symptom presentation of acute myocardial infarction: influence of sex, age, and risk factors. Am Heart J. 2002;144(6):1012–7.
6. Canto JG, Shlipak MG, Rogers WJ, Malmgren JA, Frederick PD, Lambrew CT, et al. Prevalence, clinical characteristics, and mortality among patients with myocardial infarction presenting without chest pain. JAMA. 2000;283(24):3223–9.
7. Thygesen K, Alpert JS, Jaffe AS, Simoons ML, Chaitman BR, White HD, et al. Third universal definition of myocardial infarction. Glob Heart. 2012;7(4):275–95.
8. Troughton RW, Asher CR, Klein AL. Pericarditis. Lancet. 2004;363(9410):717–27.
9. Hagan PG, Nienaber CA, Isselbacher EM, Bruckman D, Karavite DJ, Russman PL, et al. The International Registry of Acute Aortic Dissection (IRAD): new insights into an old disease. JAMA. 2000;283(7):897–903.
10. Weber T, Hogler S, Auer J, Berent R, Lassnig E, Kvas E, et al. D-dimer in acute aortic dissection. Chest. 2003;123(5):1375–8.
11. Anderson FA Jr, Wheeler HB, Goldberg RJ, Hosmer DW, Patwardhan NA, Jovanovic B, et al. A population-based perspective of the hospital incidence and case-fatality rates of deep vein thrombosis and pulmonary embolism. The Worcester DVT Study. Arch Intern Med. 1991;151(5):933–8.
12. Stein PD, Terrin ML, Hales CA, Palevsky HI, Saltzman HA, Thompson BT, et al. Clinical, laboratory, roentgenographic, and electrocardiographic findings in patients with acute pulmonary embolism and no pre-existing cardiac or pulmonary disease. Chest. 1991;100(3):598–603.
13. Chan TC, Vilke GM, Pollack M, Brady WJ. Electrocardiographic manifestations: pulmonary embolism. J Emerg Med. 2001;21(3):263–70.
14. Szucs MM Jr, Brooks HL, Grossman W, Banas JS Jr, Meister G, Dexter L, et al. Diagnostic senstivity of laboratory findings in acute pulmonary embolism. Ann Intern Med. 1971;74(2):161–6.
15. Wells PS, Anderson DR, Rodger M, Stiell I, Dreyer JF, Barnes D, et al. Excluding pulmonary embolism at the bedside without diagnostic imaging: management of patients with suspected pulmonary embolism presenting to the emergency department by using a simple clinical model and d-dimer. Ann Intern Med. 2001;135(2):98–107.

16. Fruergaard P, Launbjerg J, Hesse B, Jorgensen F, Petri A, Eiken P, et al. The diagnoses of patients admitted with acute chest pain but without myocardial infarction. Eur Heart J. 1996;17(7):1028–34.
17. Traube M, Albibi R, McCallum RW. High-amplitude peristaltic esophageal contractions associated with chest pain. JAMA. 1983;250(19):2655–9.
18. Ho KY, Ng WL, Kang JY, Yeoh KG. Gastroesophageal reflux disease is a common cause of noncardiac chest pain in a country with a low prevalence of reflux esophagitis. Dig Dis Sci. 1998;43(9):1991–7.
19. McDonald GB, Sharma P, Hackman RC, Meyers JD, Thomas ED. Esophageal infections in immunosuppressed patients after marrow transplantation. Gastroenterology. 1985;88(5):1111–7.
20. Kikendall JW. Pill esophagitis. J Clin Gastroenterol. 1999;28(4):298–305.

Chapter 25
Palpitations

Dustin Staloch and Mikhael El Chami

Abbreviations

AV	Atrioventricular
ECG	Electrocardiogram
EPS	Electrophysiologic study
ILR	Implanted loop recorder
LV	Left ventricle
PAC	Premature atrial contraction
PVC	Premature ventricular contraction
TTE	Transthoracic echocardiography

Background

- An awareness of the heart beat often described as an uncomfortable sensation of pulsation or chest movement.

D. Staloch (✉)
Department of Medicine, Division of Cardiology, Emory University Hospital, Atlanta, GA, USA
e-mail: dustin.allen.staloch@emory.edu

M. El Chami
Medicine, Division of Cardiology, Emory University Hospital-Midtown, Atlanta, GA, USA

B. J. Wells et al. (eds.), *Handbook of Inpatient Cardiology*,
https://doi.org/10.1007/978-3-030-47868-1_25

- It is estimated that palpitations are the primary reason for emergency department visits for 5.8 per 1000 patients [1].
- Most evaluation of palpitations occurs in the outpatient setting. The need for hospitalization is rare but might be required when high-risk features exist such as syncope, low ejection fraction, and abnormal ECG are present.
- In up to 15% of cases, no etiology of palpitations is identified despite recommended evaluation.

Etiologies

Electrical Cardiac Disease

- Symptoms such as “heart fluttering,” “heart stopping,” or “irregular heartbeat” correlate with higher likelihood of an arrhythmic source of palpitations. Presentation with dizziness, lightheadedness, or presyncope/syncope with episodes also raises concern [2].
- Palpitations often arise from abnormal heart rhythms (Table 25.1), but may arise from simple awareness of sinus rhythm. Though frequently due to primary electrical cardiac abnormalities, deviations from normal sinus rhythm may arise due to structural heart disease or non-cardiac causes (Table 25.2).
- Paroxysmal SVT is often sensed in the side of the neck or upper sternum, with a classic sudden onset and sudden termination description.
- With extrasystole (i.e., PVCs), some may sense the extra beat itself (often more powerful). Supraventricular beats are more often sensed than ventricular beats. Fullness in the neck is a common sensation with PVCs due to ventricular contraction when cardiac valves are closed.
- Bradyarrhythmias are a rare cause of palpitations but palpitation could be reported due to irregularities in pulse (i.e., Wenckebach or post PAC or PVC pause). In the setting of complete heart block, neck pulsation is accentuated due to AV dissociation and ventricular contraction against closed AV valves.

TABLE 25.1 Cardiac rhythms commonly identified with palpitations

Primary causes of palpitations
Premature atrial or ventricular beats
Atrial fibrillation/flutter
Inappropriate sinus tachycardia
Awareness of normal sinus rhythm
Supraventricular or ventricular tachycardias
Pacemaker-mediated tachycardia (PMT)
Bradyarrhythmias

TABLE 25.2 Common causes of palpitations and identified arrhythmias

Underlying conditions associated with palpitations
Structural heart disease
Electrical cardiac disease
Systemic disorders
Psychosomatic disorders
Induced by drugs (prescription or illicit)

Clinical Pearl
PVCs and PACs make up the largest burden of arrhythmia-related causes of palpitations, accounting for an estimated 40.8% of patients.

Structural Heart Disease

- Structural heart disease (including varied valvular pathologies, congenital heart disease, and cardiomyopathies) are infrequent causes of palpitations but are of high prognostic and therapeutic importance.

- Valvular disorders often associated with palpitations include mitral valve prolapse, severe mitral regurgitation, and aortic regurgitation.
- Congenital heart disease such as undiagnosed atrial or ventricular septal defects and undiagnosed tetralogy of Fallot should be considered.
- Cardiomyopathies such as hypertrophic cardiomyopathy, arrythmogenic right ventricular dysplasia, and varied sources of heart failure with reduced ejection fraction should also be considered as predisposing to arrhythmias or as a source of palpitations by themselves.

Systemic Conditions

- Systemic disease may manifest palpitations via sinus tachycardia or increased contractility. In the correct context, the below listed causes (not an exhaustive list) should be considered [3]:
  - Hypoglycemia
  - Hyperthyroidism
  - Postmenopausal syndrome
  - Fever
  - Anemia
  - Hypovolemia
  - Orthostatic syndromes (orthostatic hypotension or syncope, postural orthostatic tachycardia syndrome)
  - Pheochromocytoma
  - Arteriovenous fistula

Psychosomatic Disorders

- Psychosomatic disorders are common in patients evaluated for palpitations, with an estimated prevalence of 15–30%.
- Predominating causes are anxiety and panic attacks, though depression or somatization can share palpitations as a symptom. Palpitations may be sensed either from induced sinus tachycardia or from increased perception of otherwise normal heartbeats [3].

Clinical Pearl
The presence of psychiatric disease does not exclude alternative causes; arrhythmias and psychiatric disorders often coexist. Thorough investigation should be conducted to exclude other causes, as many patients with arrhythmias are wrongly diagnosed as suffering panic attacks.

Drug-Induced

- Many drugs, prescription or illicit, may lead to palpitations at initiation, titration, or discontinuation. The temporal relationship between symptoms and drug ingestion or medication changes should be established.
- Sinus tachycardia and palpitations may be induced by anticholinergic agents, hydralazine, sympathomimetics, and vasodilators. With discontinuation of beta-blockers, rebound increased sympathetic tone and sinus tachycardia may result; alternatively, their uptitration may cause a perceivable increase in stroke volume and/or extrasystole.
- Hyperadrenergic states may also be induced through legal or illicit recreational drugs, such as stimulants including caffeine, nicotine, marijuana, LSD, or heroin.
- Medication reconciliation should be conducted of potential sources for drug-induced QT prolongation [3].

Evaluation

- Initial evaluation of all patients with palpitations includes history, physical exam, and standard 12-lead ECG. This is usually appropriately conducted in the outpatient setting. Indications for specialist evaluation and hospital admission include known or suspected severe structural heart disease, known or suspected inherited cardiomyopathies or arrhythmia syndromes, or family history of sudden cardiac death. Hospital admission is also indicated for patients with device malfunction, identified arrhythmias requiring pacemaker/ICD implantation or catheter ablation, heart failure symptomatology, hemodynamic compromise (including syncope or chest pain), or severe systemic causes [3]. Further evaluation is predicated on initial findings and aims to efficiently diagnose and risk stratify patients (Fig. 25.1).

- Physical exam outside of the symptomatic period is most often unrevealing, though attention should be paid to identifying structural heart disease (murmurs, vascular disease, heart failure findings) or evidence of systemic causes. When examination occurs during a symptomatic

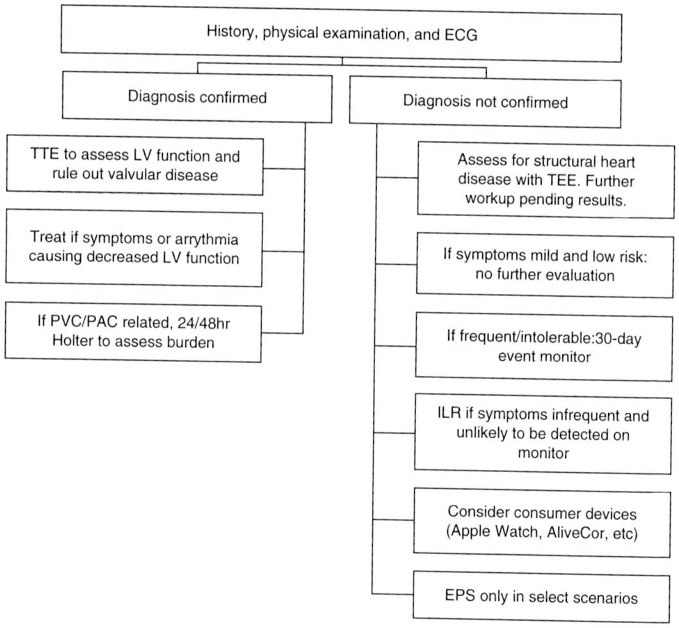

Figure 25.1 A proposed algorithm for evaluation of palpitations. ECG electrocardiogram (12-lead), TTE transthoracic echocardiography, LV left ventricle, PVC premature ventricular contraction, PAC premature atrial contraction, ILR implanted loop recorder, EPS electrophysiologic study

period, use of vagal maneuvers may elucidate culprit arrhythmias due to termination in arrhythmias involving the atrioventricular node or simple rate reduction with atrial tachycardia, fibrillation, or flutter [4].

- The gold standard for diagnosis is 12-lead ECG conducted during palpitations. Attention should be paid to the morphology and relationships between P waves and the QRS segments, as well as the QT interval. Correct QT interval >0.46 s is suggestive of long QT syndrome, while <0.32 is suggestive of short QT syndrome. Findings of high voltage in the precordium as well as Q waves and ST changes lend suspicion to hypertrophic cardiomyopathy. Brugada syndrome should be suspected when a right bundle branch morphology is accompanied by coved- or saddle-type ST segment elevations in the V1-V3. Arrythmogenic right ventricular cardiomyopathy should be suspected in those with ventricular ectopy of left bundle morphology and right axis deviation, as well as with the presence of epsilon waves or T-wave inversions with QRS duration >110 ms in V1–V3.
- If palpitations are unexplained after history, exam, and ECG, no further evaluation is required if symptoms are tolerably rare and the patient is with low likelihood of electrical or structural heart.
- If initial evaluation is unrevealing and concern for heart disease remains, or if the initial 12-lead ECG is abnormal, advanced testing may be indicated. In such patients, a transthoracic echocardiogram is advised. Exertional symptomology should raise concern for ischemic heart or structural heart disease. In this setting as well as in athletes, stress testing is indicated in addition to echocardiography. More advance cardiac imaging such as cardiac magnetic resonance imaging should be considered based on suspected diagnoses and in conjunction with expert consultation [3].
- External ambulatory ECG monitoring typically follows the above evaluation when palpitations are unexplained, severe, and frequent. Options include telemetry (for those warranting hospitalization otherwise), Holter monitor, or

event recorders with selection based on frequency of symptoms. Electrophysiologic study should usually follow ambulatory ECG monitoring at the end of evaluation. Exceptions include patients at high risk for adverse outcome (those presenting with or with substantial structural heart disease) owing to expedited diagnosis and therapeutic intervention. If the above evaluation remains non-diagnostic, implanted loop recorders may be considered [5].

Clinical Pearl
In 50% of patient, an initial evaluation of history, exam, and ECG leads to probable diagnosis or excludes diagnoses of important prognostic implication.

Management

- Management of palpitations is dictated by identified etiology, culprit arrhythmia, severity of symptoms, and the presence of structural heart disease.
- In most cases, management of palpitations follows the management of the identified arrhythmia, psychosomatic disorder, structural heart disease, or systemic condition.
- 24 or 48 hour Holter is important when symptoms are related to PVCs as it will help determine the burden of PVCs (>20% is considered high burden).

Clinical Pearl
For PVC- or PAC-mediated palpitations, elimination of lifestyle triggers such as caffeine or tobacco is often effective. Consideration is given to treatment with beta-blockers, calcium channel blockers, antiarrhythmic drugs, or catheter ablation if symptoms are unresponsive to lifestyle changes and remain severe, extrasystole burden exceeds 20%, or PVC-mediated cardiomyopathy is identified.

Key Learning Points

1. Most patients with palpitations can safely be evaluated outpatient. Inpatient workup seeks to identify or treat electrical and structural diseases in high-risk populations.
2. History, physical examination, and standard 12-lead ECG identify the source of palpitations or exclude diagnoses of prognostic importance in most patients.
3. Further evaluation should follow an algorithmic approach based on risk of adverse outcome or salient features.
4. Management is based on and flows from accurate diagnosis of the underlying etiology of palpitations.

References

1. Robst MA, Mower WR, Kanzaria HK, Hoffman JR, Buch EF, Sun BC. Analysis of emergency department visits for palpitations (from the National Hospital Ambulatory Medical Care Survey). Am J Cardiol. 2014;113(10):1685–90.
2. Barsky AJ, Clear PD, Barnett MS, Christiansen CL, Ruskin JN. The accuracy of symptom reporting by patients complaining of palpitations. Am J Med. 1994;97(3):214–21.
3. Raviele A, Giada F, Bergfeld L, Blanc JJ, Blomstrom-Lundqvist C, Mont L, et al. Management of patients with palpitations: a position paper from the European Heart Rhythm Association. Europace. 2011;13(7):920–34.
4. Page RL, Joglar JA, Caldwell MA, Calkins H, Conti JB, Deal BJ, et al. 2015 ACC/AHA/HRS guideline for the management of adult patients with supraventricular tachycardia: a report of the American College of Cardiology/American Heart Association task force on clinical practice guidelines and the Heart Rhythm Society. Circulation. 2016;133(14):e506–74.
5. Kadish AH, Buxton AE, Kennedy HL, Knight BP, Mason JW, Schuger CD, et al. ACC/AHA clinical competence statement on electrocardiography and ambulatory electrocardiography:

a report of the ACC/AHA/ACP-ASIM task force on clinical competence (ACC/AHA Committee to develop a clinical competence statement on electrocardiography and ambulatory electrocardiography) endorsed by the International Society for Holter and noninvasive electrocardiology. Circulation. 2001;104(25):3169–78.

Chapter 26
Syncope

Shu Yang and Peter Zimetbaum

Abbreviations

AS	Aortic stenosis
BP	Blood pressure
CSP	Carotid sinus pressure
CSS	Carotid sinus syndrome
CT	Computed tomography
CVA	Cerebrovascular accident
ECG	Electrocardiogram
ED	Emergency department
ELR	External loop recorder
ESC	European Society of Cardiology
HCM	Hypertrophic cardiomyopathy
ILR	Implantable loop recorder
LVOT	Left ventricular outflow tract

S. Yang (✉) · P. Zimetbaum
Department of Medicine, Beth Israel Deaconess Medical Center, Boston, MA, USA
e-mail: syang2@bidmc.harvard.edu

B. J. Wells et al. (eds.), *Handbook of Inpatient Cardiology*,
https://doi.org/10.1007/978-3-030-47868-1_26

MCOT	Mobile cardiac outpatient telemetry
MI	Myocardial infarction
MRI	Magnetic resonance imaging
MS	Mitral stenosis
PCI	Percutaneous coronary intervention
PE	Pulmonary embolus
proBNP	Pro-brain natriuretic peptide
SSRI	Selective serotonin reuptake inhibitor
TdP	Torsades de pointes
TIA	Transient ischemic attack
TLOC	Transient loss of consciousness

Introduction to Syncope

Definition

- Syncope is a transient, abrupt, and self-limited loss of consciousness.
- Resolves without any intervention and can be associated with loss of postural tone.
- The sentence refers to the fact that Syncope is a specific form of transient loss of consciousness and should be distinguished from other types of transient loss of conciousness (TLOC) (Table 26.1).
- Syncope should also be recognized as distinct from presyncope, which can be caused by similar underlying pathologies, but does not involve loss of consciousness.

Epidemiology

- Syncope comprises 1-2% of hospital admissions from the emergency department (ED). Annual cost of syncope-related hospitalizations estimated as nearly 2.5 billion dollars, rivaling that of asthma, HIV, and COPD, individually [1].

TABLE 26.1 Causes of syncope

Other causes of TLOC

- Neurologic
  - General tonic-clonic seizure
  - Stroke/transient ischemic attack
- Intoxications
- Metabolic
  - Hypoxia/hypercarbia
  - Infection
  - Uremia
  - Hypoglycemia
- Traumatic
  - Concussion
- Psychiatric
  - Psychogenic non-epileptic Seizure
  - Cataplexy

Orthostatic syncope

- Hypovolemia-mediated
- Medication-induced
  - Angiotensin converting enzyme inhibitors (ACEis)
  - Angiotensin receptor blockers (ARBs)
  - Alpha-1 antagonists
  - Dihydropyridine calcium channel blockers (CCBs)
- Autonomic predispositions
  - Diabetic neuropathy
  - Parkinsonism
  - Multi-system atrophy
  - Amyloidosis

Reflex syncope

- Situational syncope
  - Micturition syncope
  - Swallowing-associated
- Post-exertional
- Emotion-mediated
  - Pain
  - Fear
  - Anxiety
- Carotid sinus syndrome
- Other stimuli-driven

Cardiogenic syncope

Arrhythmogenic

- Bradyarrhythmia and heart block
  - Sinus node dysfunction
  - Tachy-brady syndrome
  - Beta blocker toxicity
- Tachyarrhythmias in the setting of:
  - Channelopathies (LQTS)
  - CPVT
  - Infiltrative disease (sarcoidosis)
  - Cardiomyopathies (ARVC) Pacemaker malfunction

Mechanical / obstructive

- Severe systolic/diastolic cardiomyopathies
- Severe valvular disease
  - Aortic or mitral stenosis
- Hypertrophic cardiomyopathy with LVOT obstruction
- Pericardia effusion/tamponade
- Sub/massive pulmonary embolism
- Aortic dissection

Ischemic

- Rarely manifests as syncope
- Acute ischemic systolic/diastolic dysfunction
- Malignant ventricular tachyarrhythmia
- Heart block/bradyarrhythmia
  - Due to transient rise in vagal tone (inferior ischemia) or necrosis of local conduction system (anterior infarction)

TLOC Transient Loss Of Consciousness, *LQTS* Long QT Syndrome, *CPVT* Catecholaminergic Polymorphic Ventricular Tachycardia, *ARVC* Arrhythmogenic Right Ventricular Cardiomyopathy, *LVOT* Left Ventricular Outflow Tract

Mechanisms and Causes of Syncope

- Syncope can be caused by a long list of specific conditions (Table 26.1), although ~40% have no identifiable cause [2, 3].
- Primary mechanism of syncope is cerebral hypoperfusion
  - Can result from inadequate cardiac output and/or inappropriately low peripheral vascular resistance.
  - Can be further subdivided by physiologic categories, outlined below and in Fig. 26.1.
- Orthostatic syncope:
  - Can occur immediately following trigger (i.e., change in position from supine to standing) or in delayed fashion (i.e., following a period of prolonged standing).

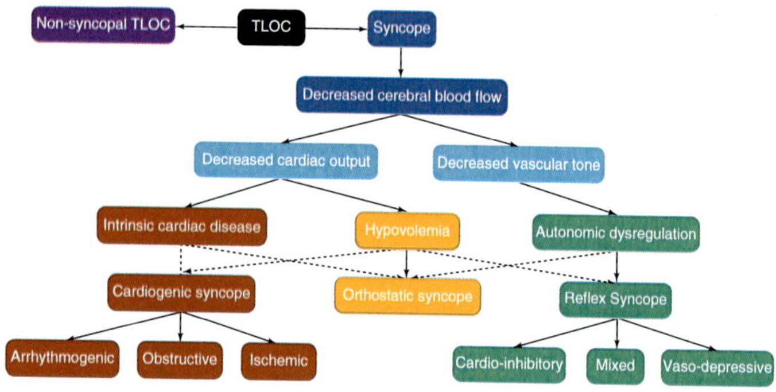

FIGURE 26.1 Mechanism of syncope. Syncope is a specific form of transient loss of consciousness (TLOC) resulting from a decrease in cerebral blood flow. This can be due to impaired cardiac output, which primarily results from hypovolemia and intrinsic cardiac disease, if present. Reduction in cerebral perfusion can also arise from decreased vascular tone, typically a function of autonomic dysregulation. Cardiogenic, orthostatic, and reflex syncope are predominantly caused by underlying intrinsic cardiac disease, hypovolemia, and dysautonomia, respectively (*solid arrows*). However, there is significant overlap in contributing pathophysiology underlying each of these conditions (*dashed lines*). Cardiogenic and reflex causes of syncope can further be sub-classified by mechanism

  - Hypovolemia and autonomic insufficiency predispose to orthostatic syncope. Commonly exacerbated by use of diuretic and vasoplegic agents.

- Reflex (formerly vasovagal or neutrally mediated) syncope:
  - Most common form of syncope [4].
  - Occurs in response to certain stimuli and characterized by exaggerated shifts in autonomic balance toward predominance of vagal tone.
  - Can be subdivided into three major categories:
    - Cardio-inhibitory: Characterized by a profound, negative chronotropic response leading to severe bradycardia and potentially asystole.

- Vaso-depressive: Dysregulated vasodilatory mechanisms lead to low vascular resistance and inadequate cerebral blood flow, despite effective augmentation of cardiac output.
  - Proposed mechanisms: Rapid withdrawal of sympathetic tone and abnormal baroreceptor sensitivity [5, 6].
- Mixed: Cardio-inhibition and vaso-depression both present. Upregulation of endogenous adenosine may play a pathophysiologic role [7].

– Reflex syncope occurs in response to an extensive list of triggers, detailed in Table 26.2.

- Cardiogenic syncope:
  - Arrhythmogenic:
    - Most common cause of cardiogenic syncope, accounting for 26% of all syncope [3].

TABLE 26.2 High- and low-risk features in history and exam

	Low-risk features (favoring benign etiology)	High-risk features (favoring cardiogenic syncope)

Clinical presentation	• Prodome typical of reflex syncope (nausea, vomiting, lightheadedness, diaphoresis, flushing)
	• Syncope in response to discrete trigger
	  • Abrupt change in position (orthostatic)
	  • Prolonged standing (orthostatic or reflex)
	  • Strong emotion, unpleasant odor or sight or pain (reflex)
	  • Head rotation or pressure on carotid sinuses (reflex)
	  • Micturition, defecation, vomiting (reflex)
	  • Syncope after exercise/during recovery (reflex)
	• Prolonged period of fatigue during recovery period (reflex)
		• Severe associated physical injuries, particularly with associated facial trauma
		• Short or absent prodrome
		• No clear triggger
		• Concurrent symptoms suggestive of:
		  • Pulmonary embolus, gastrointestinal bleeding, myocardial infarction, aortic dissection, pulmonary embolus
		• Sudden/rapid recovery following event
		• New onset syncope
		• Syncope from a supine position
		• Syncope during exercise
		• History of cardiac disease

Prior history	• No known cardiac risk factors
	• History recurrent syncope over long period of time (reflex)
		• History of known cardiac disease
		  • Severe valvular disease
		  • Hypertrophic cardiomyopathy
		  • Coronary artery disease
		  • Cardiomyopathy
		• Family history of sudden cardiac death

Exam	• Orthostatic vital signs
	• Presence of carotid hypersensitivity
		• Persistenly abnormal vital signs
		  • Systolic BP <90 mmHg
		  • Heart rate <40 bpm
		• New systolic murmur

ADAPTED FROM BRIGNOLE ET AL. [16]

    - Arrhythmias result from wide range of pathologies. Presence of structural cardiac abnormalities should raise suspicions (Table 26.1).

- Mechanical/obstructive:
    - Reduction in cardiac output due to:
        - Primary systolic and diastolic failure.
        - Physical obstruction of blood flow from heart into systemic circulation.
            - Structural cardiac pathologies: Severe aortic stenosis (AS) and mitral stenosis (MS), and hypertrophic cardiomyopathy (HCM) with left ventricular outflow tract (LVOT) obstruction.
            - Extrinsic conditions: Pericardial effusion/tamponade and sub/massive pulmonary embolism (PE).
            - Aortic dissection.
                - Potentially via complications of cardiac tamponade or massive stroke (proximal dissection extending into carotid arteries) [8].
- Ischemic:
    - Acute coronary ischemia is rare in patients presenting with syncope (~7%) [9].
    - Potential mechanisms:
        - Acute mechanical dysfunction
        - Malignant ventricular arrhythmias
        - Heart block (more likely increased vagal tone with inferior ischemia and myocardial necrosis with anterior MIs) [10, 11].

Clinical Pearl
Acute stroke and transient ischemic attack (TIA) infrequently cause syncope. Given that cerebral blood supply is deliberately redundant, with ample collateral circulation, syncope due to cerebrovascular accidents (CVA) occurs only in the presence of severe, chronic multi-vessel occlusions. Vertebro-basilar insufficiency can manifest as "drop attacks," which mimic the loss of postural tone and physical collapse often associated with syncope, but do not involve any loss of consciousness.

Diagnosis of Syncope

Initial Evaluation

- Initial diagnostic evaluation (Fig. 26.2) should include thorough *history, physical exam, and electrocardiogram (ECG).*
- Primary goals:
  - Differentiate between cardiogenic and non-cardiogenic etiologies
  - Risk stratify patients by identifying high- and low-risk features (Table 26.2)

History

- Obtaining a clear and accurate history is critical in work-up of syncope. Seek out collateral information from bystanders and witnesses
  - Confirm the presence of true syncope:
    - Distinguish syncope from other causes of TLOC, given significant management implications

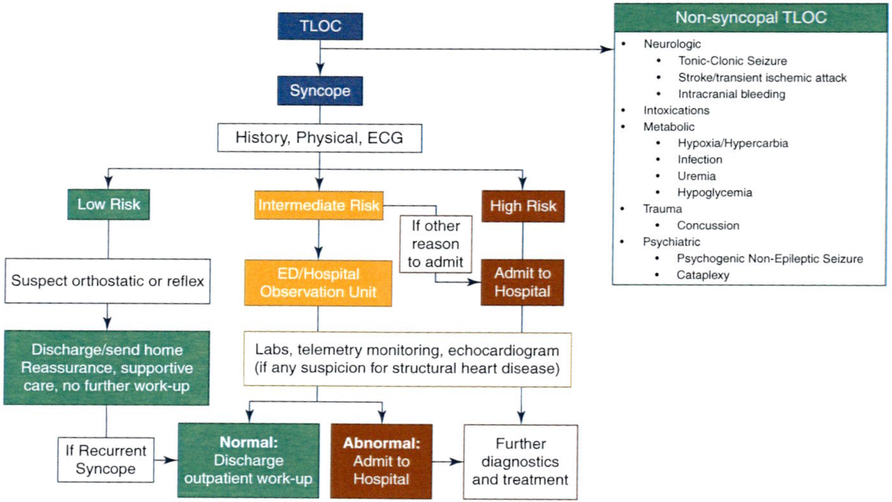

FIGURE 26.2 Diagnostic and management approach to syncope. Management of syncope begins with confirming diagnosis of true syncope versus non-syncopal transient loss of consciousness (TLOC). All patients should receive history, physical, and electrocardiography (ECG). If any high-risk features are present, patients should be admitted to the hospital for further evaluation. If only low-risk features present, he/she can be sent home with supportive care and reassurance, unless symptoms recur. If neither high- nor low-risk features (intermediate risk) and there is no other reason to warrant admission, patient should be sent to an observation unit for $\geq$24 hours of close monitoring prior to final triage decision

- Elicit potential triggers:
  - Provoking events can shed light into mechanism of syncope and underlying condition (Table 26.2).
- Assess for prodrome (and post-drome):
  - Absence or brief duration increases concern for significant injury and sudden death. Potential explanations:
    - Sudden onset of lethal arrhythmias
    - Inability to recognize and protect against impending loss of consciousness and subsequent fall
      - Characteristic prodromes (nausea, vomiting, diaphoresis, flushing) carry considerable diagnostic value for more benign causes

> **Clinical Pearl**
> Reflex syncope is the most common form of syncope and can be distinguished from other forms of syncope by the presence of an often prolonged period of fatigue and feeling "washed out," which is in direct contrast to the brisk recovery seen typically in arrhythmogenic syncope [12].

- Obtain full past medical, social, family, medication, and allergy histories to identify important predisposing factors
  - History of autonomic insufficiency (i.e., diabetic neuropathy or Parkinsonism) increases odds of orthostatic/reflex syncope.
  - Recurrent syncopal episodes over many years suggests against malignant cause [13].
  - High-risk features supporting cardiogenic syncope:
    - Significant personal cardiac history [14]
    - Family history of sudden or unexplained death, particularly at a young age

- Elucidate other "red-flags" (Table 26.2):
  - Presence of significant physical injury (i.e., facial trauma or motor vehicle accident)
    - Suggests insufficient time and/or awareness to protect oneself
  - Syncope from supine position suggestive of arrhythmogenic cause
  - Concomitant chest pain, dyspnea, or limb weakness consistent with other medical conditions warranting urgent assessment

> **Clinical Pearl**
> Syncope while driving is particularly concerning given risk for severe/fatal injury. This can be due to increased pressure on carotid baroreceptors with head turning against seatbelts or underlying arrhythmia. However, falling asleep while driving should be an important consideration. This can be supported by descriptions of skid marks on the road (often gathered as collateral information) as drivers who fall asleep often have sufficient time to recover and engage the brakes, in contrast to those who suffer true syncope [15].

Physical Exam

- In addition to complete set of vital signs and standard physical evaluation, particular attention should be paid to the following.
  - Abnormal vital signs:
    - Persistent bradycardia (heart rate <40 beats/minute) may reflect underlying conduction disease/heart block [16]

- Systolic blood pressure (BP) <90 mmHg is an independent predictor of adverse outcomes [17, 18]

- Orthostatic challenge:
  - Definition: Fall in systolic BP ≥20 mmHg or diastolic BP ≥10 mmHg, measured ≥2 minutes after position change [19].
    - 2018 European Society of Cardiology (ESC) guidelines added systolic BP ≤90 mmHg to criteria.
      - Reproduction of pre-/syncope during challenge enhances post-test probability of orthostatic syncope [16].
      - Presence of orthostatic hypotension does not preclude simultaneous cardiogenic or other cause of syncope. Red-flag features still must be assessed.
        - In one study, 10-25% of patients in the ED diagnosed with cardiogenic syncope also met criteria for orthostatic hypotension [20].
    - New cardiac murmur:
      - Should evaluate for structural cardiac pathology
    - Carotid sinus pressure (CSP):
      - Indicated in patients >40 years old to evaluate for carotid sinus syndrome (CSS) [16, 21].
      - Diagnosing CSS requires (Fig. 26.3):
        - Ventricular pause lasting >3 seconds and/or decrease in systolic BP >50 mmHg following CSP
        - Reproduction of pre-/syncopal symptoms (typically requires pauses of >6 seconds) [22].

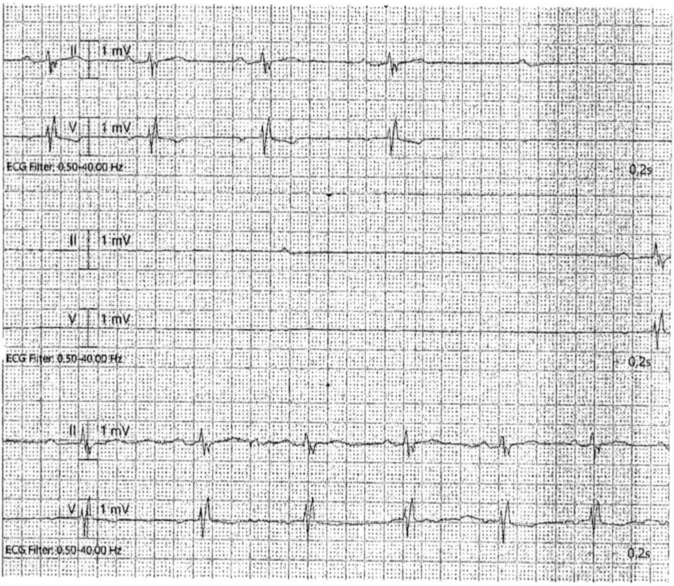

FIGURE 26.3 Carotid sinus syndrome. A 70 year-old man with a history of recurrent syncope of unclear etiology and unrevealing prior work-up including cardiovascular imaging, ischemic evaluation, and multiple rounds of ambulatory ECG monitoring. He had one prior episode of syncope while driving, following which he was not permitted to drive by state law. Upon reinstatement of his license, he had a second episode of syncope while driving (resulting in motor vehicle accident the week prior to planned implantable loop recorder placement). This telemetry strip was obtained during application of carotid sinus pressure, which promptly resulted in an 8.8 second pause and reproduction of syncope, making the diagnosis of carotid sinus syndrome. He was subsequently treated with implantation of a dual chamber pacemaker

- Contraindications to CSP [16]:
  - Significant carotid bruit/carotid stenosis
  - Recent MI
  - Prior ventricular arrhythmia

Electrocardiogram

- Resting 12-lead ECG should be obtained in *all patients presenting with syncope.*
- Evaluate for presence/absence of:
  - Acute cardiac ischemia, arrhythmia, or conduction disease
  - Evidence of chronic structural heart disease, cardiomyopathies, or channelopathies [16, 21].
  - Detailed list of high-risk electrocardiographic features outlined in Table 26.3.

Table 26.3 High-risk features on ECG

Concerning electrocardiographic (ECG) findings
• Heart rates <40 bpm
• Sinus rhythm or otherwise
• Changes consistent with acute ischemia
• Evidence of prior infarction-asociated ECG changes
• Evidence of infranodal conduction disease
• Bundle branch blocks, intraventricular conduction delays
• ECG evidence of structural heart disease
• Left/right ventricular hypertrophy, hypertrophic cardiomyopathy, infiltrative disease
• Atrioventricular block
• Mobitz type II, high gradem and complete heart block
Ventricular arrhythmias
• Sustained and non-sustained ventricular tachycardia (VT)
• Risk factors for ventricular arrhythmias
• Brugada pattern
• Pre-excitation pattern
• Long QTc
• Short QTc
• Arrhythmogenic right ventricular cardiomyopathy (ARVC)
• Presence of dysfunctional cardiac implantable electronic device (CIED)
• Including permanent pacemakers (PPMs) or implantable cardioverter-defibrillators (ICD)

Adapted from Shen et al. [21] and Brignole et al. [16]

Clinical Pearl
QT prolongation (>450 ms in men, >460 ms in women) is associated with increased risk for arrhythmogenic syncope, specifically from Torsades de pointes (TdP). Long QT can be hereditary or acquired – latter largely due to use of numerous classes of medications (namely anti-arrhythmics, antipsychotics, anti-infectives, and anti-depressives). Incidence of TdP with medication-induced long QT is not well-defined, but likely low. Threshold for discontinuing QT-prolonging medications and increased risk of TdP is ≥500 ms, extrapolating from studies performed with the anti-arrhythmic, dofetilide [23].

Further Evaluation

- Additional testing may be considered if:
  - No diagnosis reached with routine evaluation
  - Syncope recurs after initial diagnosis/treatment
  - High-risk features identified

Laboratory Studies

- Start with basic chemistry panel, complete blood cell count to assess for metabolic abnormalities, anemia, or infection
- If clinically indicated, cardiac biomarkers, pro-brain natriuretic peptide (proBNP), d-dimer, coagulation studies, liver function tests, and targeted culture studies can be performed

Continuous Electrocardiographic monitoring (Fig. 26.4)

- Inpatient telemetry:
  - Diagnostic yield reported as <3% and sensitivity/specificity 73%/86%, but may be justifiable to employ in high-risk patients [16, 24, 25].
- External ambulatory monitors:
  - Holter monitors:
    - Continuous ECG monitors, typically for 24-72 hours.
      - Arrhythmias, syncopal episodes unlikely to recur during monitoring period
      - Holter monitors only identify arrhythmias in 2% of patients with unexplained syncope [26].
      - One study reported diagnostic yield of 15% for arrhythmias, but only 1/51 patients reported concurrent symptoms [27].
    - Holter's may be useful if symptoms occurring near-daily to exonerate arrhythmia as underlying cause.
  - External loop recorders (ELR):
    - Used for longer timeframes (up to a month), with improved diagnostic yield over Holter monitors
    - Reported diagnostic yields (25-88%), but include rates of arrhythmias correlating with symptoms; asymptomatic arrhythmias; and reported symptoms associated with normal ECG [28, 29].
    - Reasonable to use for symptoms occurring at a weekly frequency

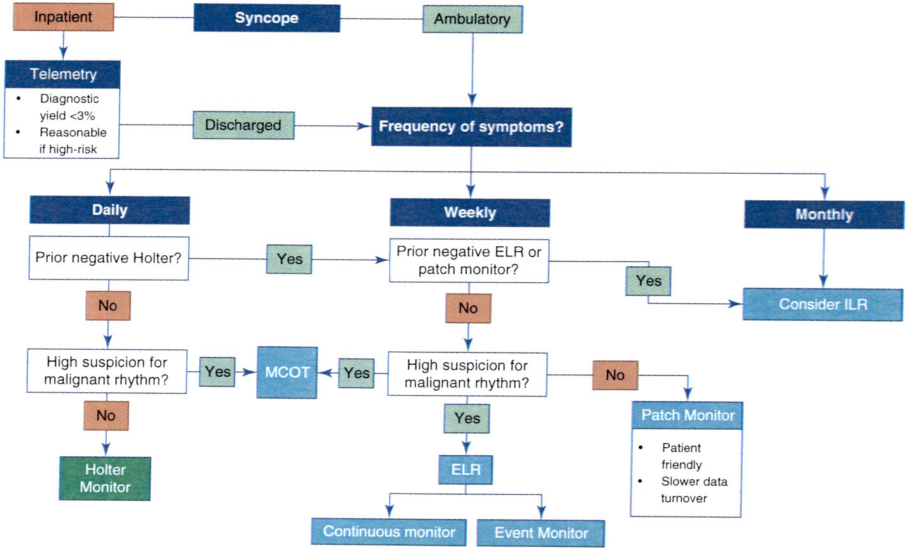

Figure 26.4 Choosing rhythm monitoring modality. Inpatient telemetry monitoring is of lower diagnostic yield, but potentially worthwhile in patients at high risk for arrhythmia. In the ambulatory setting, frequency of symptoms largely dictates optimal modality of monitoring. Prior negative study with any given monitor and degree of suspicion for malignant arrhythmia (and urgency of obtaining study results) also influence monitor choice. ELR external loop recorder, ILR implantable loop recorder, MCOT mobile cardiac outpatient telemetry

- Mobile cardiac outpatient telemetry (MCOT) systems:
  - Continuous ECG monitors similar in size to ELRs linked via cellular (as opposed to analog for ELRs and Holter's) technology to centralized monitoring units, staffed 24 hours/day by trained technicians
  - Do not require patient activation to transmit events (in contrast to Holter and ELR); occurs in real-time
  - Particularly useful when high-risk arrhythmias are suspected.
  - Diagnostic yield similar to, if not better than, that of ELRs [30, 31].
- External patch monitors (i.e., Zio XT patch):
  - Being used more frequently for ambulatory ECG monitoring
  - Smaller and convenient for patients
  - Allow for continuous ECG recording over a 2-week period, during which time the diagnostic yield has been reported to be roughly 74% [32].
  - No real-time transmission of data to ordering clinician

Clinical Pearl
Holter monitors and ELRs are capable of transmitting recorded ECG data remotely, but require the patient to trigger transfer (over an analog phone). MCOTS do not require patient activation and can relay information in real-time over cellular technology. This is particularly useful if malignant arrhythmias are suspected and/or detected, allowing for timely therapeutic intervention and response. Patch monitors such as the Zio XT patch do not possess this functionality and results can take weeks to return.

- Implantable loop recorders (ILR):
  - Subcutaneously implanted, leadless devices, allowing long-term (up to 2-3 years) rhythm monitoring
  - More invasive and expensive than external monitors, but useful in patients with recurrent but infrequent episodes of syncope.
  - Diagnostic yield in patients with syncope of unclear etiology range from 83-88% [33, 34].

Imaging Studies

- Echocardiography:
  - Very low diagnostic utility in the absence of history, exam, or ECG findings suggestive of underlying cardiac disease.
  - Should not be used routinely in evaluation of syncope, but can provide useful information when structural heart disease is suspected [21].
- Cardiac computed tomography (CT) and magnetic resonance imaging (MRI):
  - May be useful in very specific disease states, but should not be routinely pursued

Clinical Pearl
The diagnostic yield of echocardiogram has been estimated to be only about 3% and the cost per diagnosis made of echocardiography is over $34,000 [34, 35].

Tilt Table Testing

- Can be considered in individuals with suspected, but unproven, reflex syncope
  - Reported sensitivity and specificity ranges from 26-80% and 90%, respectively [36].

- Can be positive in cases of reflex, unexplained, and proven cardiac syncope [37]
  - Limited ability to distinguish between syncopal etiologies
  - Can identify individuals with high susceptibility to orthostatic stress [16].

Ischemic Evaluation

- Exercise stress testing:
  - Exertional syncope can be risky given association with dangerous underlying causes (severe AS, severe MS, or HCM with LVOT obstruction, sympathetically stimulated ventricular arrhythmias, and rarely heart block) [21].
  - Can provide useful information, but must be done with extreme caution in an appropriately equipped environment
- Coronary angiography:
  - Reasonable to pursue ± percutaneous coronary intervention (PCI) if patients present with symptoms of acute coronary syndrome or ischemia-induced arrhythmia, but adds no value with respect to syncope [38].

Management of Syncope

Risk Stratification and Patient Triage

- Risk stratification and triage should be initial goal of assessment using history, physical, and ECG (Fig. 26.2)

Treatment

- For orthostatic and reflex syncope, primary goal to improve symptoms and avoid complications from falls, other injuries
  - Non-pharmacologic interventions should be tried first [21, 39].
    - Increased oral intake of fluids and salt (in absence of medical contraindications)
    - Lower extremity compression garments and abdominal binders to prevent venous pooling
    - Avoid vasoplegic medications
    - Use of counter-pressure maneuvers and adaptive behaviors (changing positions more slowly)
    - Increased exercise and physical therapy
  - Pharmacologic therapies:
    - Fludrocortisone and midodrine used in treatment of orthostatic and reflex syncope. Both effectively increased BP and reduced symptoms [40–42].
      - Both carry significant adverse effects
- Additional condition-specific therapies:
  - Orthostatic syncope:
    - Droxidopa (pro-drug of norepinephrine) can be used as well to address autonomic insufficiency with potential benefits in functional status, although can cause supine hypertension as well [43].
    - Consider pyridostigmine as third line agent [44].
  - Reflex syncope:
    - Beta blockers and selective serotonin reuptake inhibitors (SSRIs) may benefit certain populations [21].
    - Pacemaker placement indicated for patients with cardioinhibitory syncope and CSS, especially for patients with prolonged spontaneous sinus pauses

and recurrent symptoms refractory to non-invasive therapies [45].

- Cardiogenic syncope: Treatments be tailored to specific diagnoses

- Driving after syncope:
  - Driving following syncopal event – particularly one without significant prodrome, obvious avoidable trigger, and treatable cause – poses significant risk to self and others
  - State laws frequently impose driving restrictions in this circumstance
    - Can interfere with personal, family, occupational obligations
  - Clinicians should be aware of local policies and engage in conversation with patients incorporating state-specific, occupational-specific, and individual factors [21].

Key Learning Points

- Syncope is a common and costly problem. It is often conflated with non-syncopal causes of transient loss of consciousness, for which diagnostic and management strategies are completely different.
- Transient cerebral hypoperfusion leads to syncope. Mechanistically, this is caused by some permutation of decreased cardiac output and vascular tone.
- Routine work-up of syncope should include a complete and thorough history (utilizing the patient and collateral report), physical exam, and electrocardiogram. The evaluation should focus on identifying high-risk features and patients, who require more aggressive and timely management.
- Inpatient telemetry in the hospital has very low diagnostic value. Ambulatory rhythm monitoring is much

more effective. Optimal monitor choice depends on frequency of symptoms, suspicion for malignant etiology of syncope, and urgency, with which study results are needed.

- Treatment of syncope depends heavily on the underlying cause. When possible, non-pharmacologic interventions should be tried first, then pharmacologic therapies, followed by invasive measures (such as pacemaker implantation). Clinicians should also recognize and address pre-emptively the matter of driving restrictions following syncope given the potentially enormous personal, societal, legal, and occupational ramifications.

References

1. Sun BC, Emond JA, Camargo CA. Direct medical costs of syncope-related hospitalizations in the United States. Am J Cardiol. 2005;95(5):668–71.
2. Schnipper JL, Kapoor WN. Diagnostic evaluation and management of patients with syncope. Med Clin N Am. 2001;85(2):423–56.
3. Soteriades, Elpidoforos S et al. Incidence and prognosis of syncope.N Engl J Med. 2002;347(12):878–85. https://doi.org/10.1056/NEJMoa012407.
4. Kapoor WN. Syncope. N Engl J Med. 2000;343(25):1856–62.
5. Morillo CA, et al. Vagal and sympathetic mechanisms in patients with orthostatic vasovagal syncope. Circulation. 1997;96(8):2509–13.
6. Thomson HL, Karen W, Michael F. Baroreflex sensitivity in patients with vasovagal syncope. Circulation. 1997;95(2):395–400.
7. Saadjian AY, Lévy S, Franceschi F, Zouher I, Paganelli F, Guieu RP. Role of endogenous adenosine as a modulator of syncope induced during tilt testing. Circulation. 2002;106(5):569–74.
8. Nallamothu BK, Mehta RH, Saint S. Syncope in acute aortic dissection: diagnostic, prognostic, and clinical implications. ACC Curr J Rev. 2003;12(2):17.

9. Georgeson S, Linzer M, Griffith JL, Weld L, Selker HP. Acute cardiac ischemia in patients with syncope. J Gen Intern Med. 1992;7(4):379–86.
10. Mitrani RD, Hendel RC. The appropriateness of an ischemia evaluation for syncope. Circ Cardiovasc Imaging. 2013;6(3):358–9.
11. Zimetbaum, Peter J, and Mark E Josephson. Use of the electrocardiogram in acute myocardial infarction. N Engl J Med. 2003;348(10):933–40. https://doi.org/10.1056/NEJMra022700.
12. Shukla, Gunjan J, and Peter J Zimetbaum. Cardiology patient page. Syncope. Circulation. 2006;113(16):e715–7. https://doi.org/10.1161/CIRCULATIONAHA.105.602250
13. Arthur W, Kaye GC. The pathophysiology of common causes of syncope. Postgrad Med J. 2000;76(902):750–3.
14. Albassam OT, Redelmeier RJ, Shadowitz S, Husain AM, Simel D, Etchells EE. Did this patient have cardiac syncope?: the rational clinical examination systematic review. JAMA. 2019;321(24):2448.
15. Zimetbaum PJ, Josephson ME. Practical clinical electrophysiology: Philadelphia, Pennsylvania. Lippincott Williams & Wilkins; 2009.
16. Brignole M, et al. 2018 ESC guidelines for the diagnosis and management of syncope. Eur Heart J. 2018;39(21):1883–948.
17. Saccilotto RT, Nickel CH, Bucher HC, Steyerberg EW, Bingisser R, Koller MT. San Francisco Syncope Rule to predict short-term serious outcomes: a systematic review. CMAJ. 2011;183(15):E1116–26.
18. Thiruganasambandamoorthy V, et al. Development of the Canadian Syncope Risk Score to predict serious adverse events after emergency department assessment of syncope. CMAJ. 2016;188(12):E289–98.
19. Freeman R, et al. Consensus statement on the definition of orthostatic hypotension, neurally mediated syncope and the postural tachycardia syndrome. Clin Auton Res. 2011;21(2):69–72.
20. Schaffer JT, Keim SM, Hunter BR, Kirschner JM, De Lorenzo RA. Do orthostatic vital signs have utility in the evaluation of syncope? J Emerg Med. 2018;55(6):780–7.
21. Shen W-K, et al. 2017 ACC/AHA/HRS guideline for the evaluation and management of patients with syncope: a report of the American College of Cardiology/American Heart Association

Task Force on Clinical Practice Guidelines and the Heart Rhythm Society. Circulation. 2017;136(5)
22. Wieling W, et al. At the heart of the arterial baroreflex: a physiological basis for a new classification of carotid sinus hypersensitivity. J Intern Med. 2013;273(4):345–58.
23. Al-Khatib SM, LaPointe NMA, Kramer JM, Califf RM. What clinicians should know about the QT interval. JAMA. Apr. 2003;289(16):2120–7.
24. Chiu DT, Shapiro NI, Sun BC, Mottley JL, Grossman SA. Are echocardiography, telemetry, ambulatory electrocardiography monitoring, and cardiac enzymes in emergency department patients presenting with syncope useful tests? A preliminary investigation. J Emerg Med. 2014;47(1):113–8.
25. Benezet-Mazuecos J, et al. Utility of in-hospital cardiac remote telemetry in patients with unexplained syncope. Europace. 2007;9(12):1196–201.
26. Gibson TC, Heitzman MR. Diagnostic efficacy of 24-hour electrocardiographic monitoring for syncope. Am J Cardiol. 1984;53(8):1013–7.
27. Bass EB, et al. The duration of Holter monitoring in patients with syncope: is 24 hours enough? Arch Intern Med. 1990;150(5):1073–8.
28. Gula LJ, Krahn AD, Massel D, Skanes A, Yee R, Klein GJ. External loop recorders: determinants of diagnostic yield in patients with syncope. Am Heart J. 2004;147(4):644–8.
29. Linzer M, Pritchett ELC, Pontinen M, McCarthy E, Divine GW. Incremental diagnostic yield of loop electrocardiographic recorders in unexplained syncope. Am J Cardiol. 1990;66(2):214–9.
30. Joshi AK, et al. First experience with a Mobile Cardiac Outpatient Telemetry (MCOT) system for the diagnosis and management of cardiac arrhythmia. Am J Cardiol. 2005;95(7):878–81.
31. Zimetbaum P, Goldman A. Ambulatory arrhythmia monitoring: choosing the right device. Circulation. 2010;122(16):1629–36.
32. Reed MJ, et al. Diagnostic yield of an ambulatory patch monitor in patients with unexplained syncope after initial evaluation in the emergency department: the PATCH-ED study. Emerg Med J. 2018;35(8):477–85.
33. Krahn AD, Klein GJ, Skanes AC, Yee R. Use of the implantable loop recorder in evaluation of patients with unexplained syncope. J Cardiovasc Electrophysiol. 2003;14(s9):S70–3.

34. Krahn AD, Klein GJ, Yee R, Mandab V. The high cost of syncope: cost implications of a new insertable loop recorder in the investigation of recurrent syncope. Am Heart J. 1999;137(5):870–7.
35. Recchia D, Barzilai B. Echocardiography in the evaluation of patients with syncope. J Gen Intern Med. 1995;10(12):649–55.
36. Flevari P, et al. Recurrent vasovagal syncope: comparison between clomipramine and nitroglycerin as drug challenges during head-up tilt testing. Eur Heart J. 2009;30(18):2249–53.
37. Brignole M, et al. Role of autonomic reflexes in syncope associated with paroxysmal atrial fibrillation. J Am Coll Cardiol. 1993;22(4):1123–9.
38. Anderson LL, Dai D, Miller AL, Roe MT, Messenger JC, Wang TY. Percutaneous coronary intervention for older adults who present with syncope and coronary artery disease? Insights from the National Cardiovascular Data Registry. Am Heart J. 2016;176:1–9.
39. Lanier JB, Mote MB, Clay EC. Evaluation and management of orthostatic hypotension. AFP. 2011;84(5):527–36.
40. Low PA, Gilden JL, Freeman R, Sheng K-N, McElligott MA. Efficacy of midodrine vs placebo in neurogenic orthostatic hypotension: a randomized, double-blind multicenter study. JAMA. 1997;277(13):1046–51.
41. Sheldon R, et al. Fludrocortisone for the prevention of vasovagal syncope: a randomized, placebo-controlled trial. J Am Coll Cardiol. 2016;68(1):1–9.
42. Wright RA, et al. A double-blind, dose-response study of midodrine in neurogenic orthostatic hypotension. Neurology. 1998;51(1):120–4.
43. Biaggioni, Italo et al. Integrated analysis of droxidopa trials for neurogenic orthostatic hypotension. BMC Neurol. 2017;17(1)90. https://doi.org/10.1186/s12883-017-0867-5
44. Singer W, et al. Pyridostigmine treatment trial in neurogenic orthostatic hypotension. Arch Neurol. 2006;63(4):513–8.
45. Varosy PD, Chen LY, Miller AL, Noseworthy PA, Slotwiner DJ, Thiruganasambandamoorthy V. Pacing as a treatment for reflex-mediated (vasovagal, situational, or carotid sinus hypersensitivity) syncope: a systematic review for the 2017 ACC/AHA/HRS guideline for the evaluation and management of patients with syncope: a report of the American College of Cardiology/American Heart Association Task Force on Clinical Practice Guidelines and the Heart Rhythm Society. J Am Coll Cardiol. 2017;70(5):664–79.

Chapter 27
Dyspnea

Susan McIlvaine and Eli V. Gelfand

Abbreviations

ACS	Acute coronary syndrome
AV	Arteriovenous
BNP	Brain natriuretic peptide
CHF	Congestive heart failure
COPD	Chronic obstructive pulmonary disease
CXR	Chest X-ray
DKA	Diabetic ketoacidosis
GERD	Gastroesophageal reflux disease
JVP	Jugular venous pressure
LE	Lower extremity
LV	Left ventricle
OSA	Obstructive sleep apnea
PE	Pulmonary embolism

S. McIlvaine (✉)
Department of Cardiology, Beth Israel Deaconess Medical Center, Boston, MA, USA
e-mail: smcilvai@bidmc.harvard.edu

E. V. Gelfand
Department of Cardiology, Beth Israel Deaconess Medical Center, Harvard Medical School, Boston, MA, USA
e-mail: egelfand@bidmc.harvard.edu

B. J. Wells et al. (eds.), *Handbook of Inpatient Cardiology*,
https://doi.org/10.1007/978-3-030-47868-1_27

PEFR	Peak expiratory flow rate
PND	Paroxysmal nocturnal dyspnea
RV	Right ventricle

Definition and Epidemiology

- Dyspnea is a subjective experience of breathing discomfort that consists of qualitatively distinct sensations that vary in intensity [1]
- Dyspnea is a subjective entity – can be experienced by patients who have compromise of their cardiac or respiratory status that prompts a physiologic change, or by patients who do not have any objective evidence of physiologic compromise
  - ∗*Clinical Pearl*: Dyspnea is a *symptom*, so providers should distinguish from *signs* like tachypnea, wheezing, cyanosis, lung hyperinflation, use of accessory respiratory muscles, and intercostal retractions [1]
- In patients > age 65 who present with dyspnea and signs of respiratory distress (increased respiratory rate, decreased oxygenation, acidosis), the top five diagnoses are decompensated congestive heart failure (CHF), pneumonia, chronic obstructive pulmonary disease (COPD), pulmonary embolism (PE), and asthma [2]
- Dyspnea is more closely associated with mortality (cardiac or all-cause) than angina in patients referred for stress testing [3]

Pathophysiology

- The sensation of dyspnea can be linked to specific cardiopulmonary physiologic mechanisms, but can also be affected by conscious thought, anxiety, cultural background, etc. (see Fig. 27.1). For example, the sense of air hunger may originate in the brainstem, the sense of chest tightness may be secondary to stimulation of vagal irritant receptors, and dyspnea in the setting of PE may be related to stimulation of pressure receptors in the pulmonary vasculature [4]

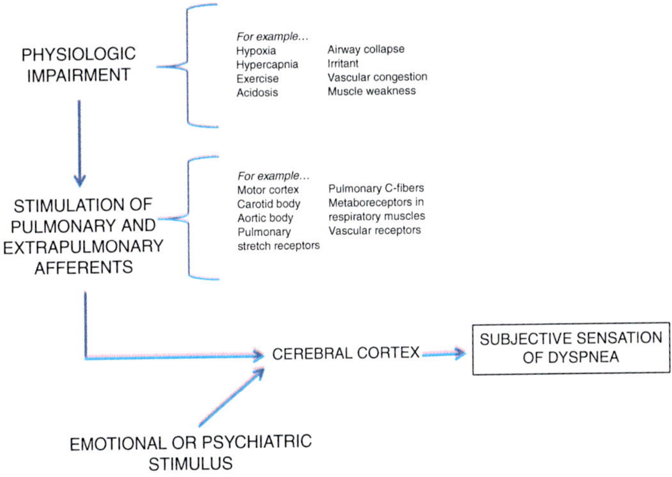

FIGURE 27.1 Physiology of Dyspnea. Dyspnea is a complicated subjective symptom that is caused by input from many different afferent receptors and emotional inputs

- Dyspnea can occur with or without an underlying issue with gas exchange and/or an impaired pump, which highlights the contribution of supratentorial factors
- The respiratory motor system has both automatic (brainstem) and voluntary (cortical) sources of input

History

- The language patients use to describe their dyspnea can often give clues as to the underlying etiology (see Table 27.1).
  - ∗*Clinical Pearl*: Ethnic and social differences exist with respect to the descriptors that patients use to characterize their symptoms. For example, one study showed that African American and white patients with asthma used significantly different descriptors when bronchoconstriction was induced – African American patients used primarily upper airway word descriptors (e.g.: *tight throat, voice tight*), whereas Caucasian patients used

Table 27.1 Patient descriptors of dyspnea. How patients describe their dyspnea may provide a clue as to the underlying etiology. However cultural differences exist in how patients describe their dyspnea [5–8]

Dyspnea descriptor	Potential underlying etiology
Tightness E.g.: *"My chest feels tight"*	Bronchoconstriction
Need or urge to breathe E.g.: *"I feel hunger for more air"*	Increased central drive (i.e., stimulation of brainstem respiratory neurons by exercise, hypoxia, hypercapnia, metabolic acidosis) Limited tidal volume
Suffocating sensation E.g.: *"I feel that I am suffocating/smothering"*	LV failure
Increased work or effort of breathing E.g.: *"My breathing requires effort"*	Difficulty with respiratory pump, i.e., muscle weakness, increased airway resistance
Depth and frequency of breathing E.g.: *"My breathing is shallow"* or *"I feel that I am breathing more"*	Increased exertion Hyperinflation due to obstructive lung disease Hyperventilation syndrome

lower airway or chest wall descriptors (*out of air, hurts to breathe*) [9]. Furthermore, non-English-speaking patients may describe their symptoms in a way that does not translate perfectly into the descriptors typical of English speakers. Non-native English speakers have often been excluded from studies that examine the language of dyspnea.

- If a patient reports difficulty with exertion, explore whether something other than dyspnea (i.e., chest pain, leg pain, leg weakness, joint pain) is limiting their exertion

- Ask about prior intubation, as these patients are at higher risk for severe disease
- More than one physiologic process can be contributing to a patient's symptoms, which helps contribute to diagnostic uncertainty
- Historical elements to clarify:
  - *Chronicity* (acute, subacute, chronic, acute on chronic): this may be the most useful initial clinical branchpoint, as the differential diagnosis for acute dyspnea is limited (see Table 27.2)
  - *Intermittent vs. persistent/progressive*: intermittent symptoms are likely due to a reversible cause (bronchoconstriction, CHF, pleural effusion, PE) as opposed to a chronic condition [5].
  - *Exertional vs. at rest*: If dyspnea is not worsened with exertion, it is unlikely to be due to cardiopulmonary disease. If feasible, consider ambulating the patient in the hallway to see how exertion affects their symptoms and vital signs.
  - *Nocturnal* dyspnea may indicate asthma, CHF, GERD, OSA, or nasal obstruction.
  - *Orthopnea* (worse with lying flat) may indicate CHF, ascites, diaphragmatic dysfunction.

TABLE 27.2 Causes of acute dyspnea. The differential for acute dyspnea is somewhat limited, and acute dyspnea is typically secondary to a cardiac or pulmonary cause

Causes of acute dyspnea		
Pulmonary	**Cardiac**	**Other**
Pneumonia Pulmonary Embolism Bronchospasm Pneumothorax Upper airway obstruction (aspiration, mucous plug)	Acute heart failure with pulmonary edema (can be due to various causes) Myocardial Ischemia Tamponade Arrhythmia	Anaphylaxis Angioedema Poisoning Psychogenic

- *Platypnea* (worse when upright) may indicate cirrhosis (hepatopulmonary syndrome), pulmonary AV malformations, interatrial shunting.

Diagnostic Approach

- Initial steps involve the evaluation of the acuity and severity of the dyspnea (i.e., is the patient hypoxemic? Is there impending respiratory failure?), and whether there is an urgent or emergent need for clinical intervention, such as mask ventilation or tracheal intubation. The physical exam can provide some clues (see Table 27.3).
- The differential for *acute severe* dyspnea is relatively narrow. Such symptoms are typically (though not always) due to an underlying pulmonary or cardiac etiology.
- Underlying pathology causes dyspnea via:
- 1. increase in the respiratory drive, via hypoxia, increased dead space, hypercapnia, metabolic acidosis
- 2. mechanical constraint, muscle weakness, or airway obstruction
- 3. psychologic processes

Some causes of dyspnea fall into more than one of these categories (see Table 27.4).

- Diagnostic tests to help distinguish the cause of dyspnea:
  - *BNP* or NT-proBNP may be helpful in identifying heart failure as the cause/contributor, especially in those patients in whom physical exam for signs of volume overload is difficult. Familiarity with the local assays and normal ranges is critical for interpretation. Prior BNP/NT-proBNP values in a particular patient with a history of heart failure may be useful when combined with other clinical parameters to suggest volume overload over prior "baseline."

    **Clinical Pearl*: BNP < 100 has a negative predictive value of >90% for acute heart failure, and > 500 has a positive predictive value of >90% [10]. BNP may

TABLE 27.3 Physical exam findings. Attention to certain features of the physical exam can provide clues as to the underlying etiology (or etiologies) of dyspnea

Physical exam findings	Possible underlying etiology
Pursed lip breathing, accessory muscle use	COPD
Retractions	Airway obstruction: asthma, COPD, foreign body aspiration
Cough with deep breaths	Asthma, interstitial lung disease
Diffusely poor air movement	Emphysema, bronchoconstriction
Wheezing	Obstruction below trachea (asthma, anaphylaxis, mainstem bronchus foreign body, acute CHF)
Crackles	Interalveolar fluid: pneumonia, CHF, or pulmonary fibrosis
Localized decreased breath sounds	Pneumonia, pleural effusion, diaphragmatic paralysis, airway obstruction, pneumothorax
RV heave	Pulmonary hypertension
Systolic murmur	Aortic stenosis or mitral regurgitation
S3 or S4	Left or right ventricular dysfunction
Loud P2	Pulmonary hypertension
Distant heart sounds	Pericardial effusion, COPD
Elevated JVP	R- or L-sided heart failure, pericardial tamponade
Clubbing	COPD, bronchiectasis, other intrinsic lung pathology
Symmetric LE edema	CHF
Asymmetric LE edema	Deep venous thrombosis/PE

Table 27.4 Dyspnea differential diagnosis and mechanism of dyspnea. Chemoreceptor stimulation is caused by hypoxemia, increased dead space, hypercapnia, and metabolic acidosis. Pulmonary receptor stimulation is caused by irritants, and stimulation of mechanical and vascular lung afferent receptors [6]

	Increased respiratory drive		Increased work of breathing			
	Chemoreceptor Stimulation	**Pulmonary Receptor Stimulation**	**Muscle Weakness**	**Decreased chest wall compliance**	**Airflow obstruction**	**Behavioral**
CNS/Neuro						
Stroke	x		x			
Spinal cord injury			x			
Cardiac						
ACS	x					x
PE	x	x				
CHF	x	x				
Arrhythmia	x					x
Tamponade	x					

Pulm				
Asthma	x	x		x
COPD	x	x		x
Pneumonia	x			
Pleural effusion		x		
Aspiration		x		x
Pneumothorax	x	x		
Pulmonary hypertension	x	x		
GI				
Ascites			x	
Renal				
Renal failure	x			

(continued)

TABLE 27.4 (continued)

	Increased respiratory drive		Increased work of breathing			
	Chemoreceptor Stimulation	**Pulmonary Receptor Stimulation**	**Muscle Weakness**	**Decreased chest wall compliance**	**Airflow obstruction**	**Behavioral**
Endocrine						
DKA	x					
Thyroid disorder	x					
Heme						
Anemia	x					
Rheum						
Myasthenia gravis	x		x			
Guillain-Barre			x			
Other						

Chest wall deformity/ trauma				x		
Altitude	x					
Anxiety						x
Acute chest syndrome	x	x				
Toxic ingestion or inhalation	x	x				
Angioedema		x			x	
Obesity	x			x		

be falsely low/normal in patients with flash pulmonary edema and in the obese [11]. Other factors causing distention of the cardiac chambers such as fluid overload from renal failure or pulmonary hypertension can also elevate BNP.

- *D-Dimer*: sensitivity is much greater than specificity. Check a d-dimer only in patients with a low pretest probability for PE (according to modified Wells criteria, PERC rule) [12].
- *Hemoglobin/Hematocrit*: anemia of any cause can contribute to dyspnea. Polycythemia can indicate chronic hypoxemia.
- *Procalcitonin* can be used as a biomarker for a bacterial infection such as pneumonia. In dyspneic patients judged to be at high risk for heart failure, sensitivity of procalcitonin to rule out pneumonia is high. In dyspneic patients judged to be at low risk for heart failure, elevated procalcitonin is highly specific for pneumonia [10].
- *Elevated Troponin*: can indicate ACS, but can also be elevated with PE, sepsis, CHF, pericarditis, myocarditis, renal failure, and in other situations where there is myocardial oxygen supply-demand mismatch.
- *ECG*: useful to evaluate for ACS, pericardial effusion, or right heart strain (possibly indicating PE).
- *Transthoracic echocardiography*: helps identify valvular disease, reduced ejection fraction, RV strain in the setting of PE or pulmonary hypertension. Doppler analysis of mitral inflow pattern is more accurate in diagnosing heart failure than BNP, especially in patients with flash pulmonary edema [11]. Even if systolic function is normal, consider diastolic dysfunction as a cause of exertional dyspnea, as this diagnosis is easy to miss. *Focused ultrasound* at the bedside can be useful to detect pulmonary edema, tamponade, pneumothorax, pleural effusion, and cardiac wall motion abnormalities. Assessment of IVC compressibility can be a more reliable estimate of right atrial pressure or volume status than visual

inspection of JVP in patients in whom assessment of volume status is challenging [13]. As technology advances, bedside ultrasound is becoming a tool that will prove to be feasible for the internist to use to improve diagnostic accuracy.

- *Lung Ultrasound* showing B-lines is more sensitive than CXR in diagnosing acute cardiogenic pulmonary edema [7].
- *Chest radiography*: useful in evaluating for pulmonary edema, pneumonia, pneumothorax, and signs of COPD. However, ~20% of the patients admitted with acute decompensated heart failure have a nondiagnostic CXR [14].
- *Peak flow*: can help distinguish cardiac from pulmonary causes of dyspnea. Peak expiratory flow rate is generally higher in patients with a cardiac cause of dyspnea. PEFR less than 25% of normal or 200 L/minute can indicate the presence of hypercapnia.
- *Chest CT*: should not be used as a screening test, but CTA is standard for evaluation for PE. In patients with a low clinical probability of PE (according to Wells score) and a normal D-Dimer, CTA does not need to be performed to rule out PE [12].
- *V/Q Scan*: cannot be used in patients with an abnormal chest X-ray or known lung disease
- *JAMA Rational Clinical Exam: Does this Dyspneic Patient in the Emergency Department Have Congestive Heart Failure?* [15]

  Features that best *increased* the probability of heart failure: past history of heart failure, PND, S3 gallop, CXR with pulmonary venous congestion, ECG with AFib

  Features that best *decreased* the probability of heart failure: ABSENCE of – prior history of heart failure, DOE, rales, CXR with cardiomegaly, any ECG abnormality

  Most useful test: low (<1000 pg/mL) BNP (negative LR = 0.11)

Key Learning Points

- Dyspnea is a subjective experience of breathing discomfort that consists of qualitatively distinct sensations that vary in intensity [1]. It can be experienced by patients who have compromise of their cardiac or respiratory status that prompts a physiologic change, or by patients who do not have any objective evidence of physiologic compromise
- The pathophysiology of dyspnea is complex, and dyspnea can often be multifactorial
- Underlying pathology causes dyspnea via: (1) increase in the respiratory drive, via hypoxia, increased dead space, hypercapnia, metabolic acidosis; (2) mechanical constraint, muscle weakness, or airway obstruction; and/or (3) psychologic processes.
- The descriptors patients use to describe their dyspnea can give clues as to its underlying etiology, but language and cultural differences exist that may limit the extent to which providers can rely on these descriptors to map to a specific etiology
- The differential for *acute severe* dyspnea is relatively narrow. Such symptoms are typically (though not always) due to an underlying pulmonary or cardiac etiology

References

1. Parshall MB, Schwartzstein RM, Adams L, et al. An official American Thoracic Society statement: update on the mechanisms, assessment, and management of dyspnea. Am J Respir Crit Care Med. 2012;185(4):435–52. https://doi.org/10.1164/rccm.201111-2042ST.
2. Ray P, Birolleau S, Lefort Y, et al. Acute respiratory failure in the elderly: etiology, emergency diagnosis and prognosis. Crit Care. 2006;10(3):R82. https://doi.org/10.1186/cc4926.

3. Abidov A, Rozanski A, Hachamovitch R, et al. Prognostic significance of dyspnea in patients referred for cardiac stress testing. N Engl J Med. 2005;353(18):1889–98. https://doi.org/10.1056/NEJMoa042741.
4. Manning HL, Schwartzstein RM. Pathophysiology of dyspnea. N Engl J Med. 1995;333(23):1547–53. https://doi.org/10.1056/NEJM199512073332307.
5. Broaddus V, Mason R. Murray and Nadel's Textbook of Respiratory Medicine: 2-Volume Set. 6th ed. Saunders: an imprint of Elsevier Incorporated; 2016.
6. Chang AS, Munson J, Gifford AH, Mahler DA. Prospective use of descriptors of dyspnea to diagnose common respiratory diseases. Chest. 2015;148(4):895–902. https://doi.org/10.1378/chest.15-0308.
7. Elliott MW, Adams L, Cockcroft A, MacRae KD, Murphy K, Guz A. The language of breathlessness. Use of verbal descriptors by patients with cardiopulmonary disease. Am Rev Respir Dis. 1991;144(4):826–32. https://doi.org/10.1164/ajrccm/144.4.826.
8. Mahler DA, Harver A, Lentine T, Scott JA, Beck K, Schwartzstein RM. Descriptors of breathlessness in cardiorespiratory diseases. Am J Respir Crit Care Med. 1996;154(5):1357–63. https://doi.org/10.1164/ajrccm.154.5.8912748.
9. Hardie GE, Janson S, Gold WM, Carrieri-Kohlman V, Boushey HA. Ethnic differences: word descriptors used by African-American and white asthma patients during induced bronchoconstriction. Chest. 2000;117(4):935–43. https://doi.org/10.1378/chest.117.4.935.
10. Mueller C, Scholer A, Laule-Kilian K, et al. Use of B-type natriuretic peptide in the evaluation and management of acute dyspnea. N Engl J Med. 2004;350(7):647–54. https://doi.org/10.1056/NEJMoa031681.
11. Logeart D, Saudubray C, Beyne P, et al. Comparative value of Doppler echocardiography and B-type natriuretic peptide assay in the etiologic diagnosis of acute dyspnea. J Am Coll Cardiol. 2002;40(10):1794–800.
12. van Belle A, Buller HR, Huisman MV, et al. Effectiveness of managing suspected pulmonary embolism using an algorithm combining clinical probability, D-dimer testing, and computed tomography. JAMA. 2006;295(2):172–9. https://doi.org/10.1001/jama.295.2.172.
13. Saha NM, Barbat JJ, Fedson S, Anderson A, Rich JD, Spencer KT. Outpatient use of focused cardiac ultrasound to assess the

inferior vena cava in patients with heart failure. Am J Cardiol. 2015;116(8):1224–8. https://doi.org/10.1016/j.amjcard.2015.07.040.
14. Collins SP, Lindsell CJ, Storrow AB, Abraham WT. Prevalence of negative chest radiography results in the emergency department patient with decompensated heart failure. Ann Emerg Med. 2006;47(1):13–8. https://doi.org/10.1016/j.annemergmed.2005.04.003.
15. Wang CS, FitzGerald JM, Schulzer M, Mak E, Ayas NT. Does this dyspneic patient in the emergency department have congestive heart failure? JAMA. 2005;294(15):1944–56. https://doi.org/10.1001/jama.294.15.1944.

Chapter 28
Perioperative Cardiac Risk Assessment

Mark K. Tuttle and Joseph P. Kannam

Abbreviations

CABG	Coronary artery bypass graft
CVA	Cerebrovascular accident
MET	Metabolic equivalent
LVEF	Left ventricular ejection fraction
LMCA	Left main coronary artery
MACE	Major adverse cardiac event
MI	Myocardial infarction
NTG	Nitroglycerin
PTCA	Percutaneous transluminal coronary angioplasty
TIA	Transient ischemic attack
VF	Ventricular fibrillation

M. K. Tuttle (✉) · J. P. Kannam
Division of Cardiology, Beth Israel Deaconess Medical Center/
Harvard Medical School, Boston, MA, USA
e-mail: mtuttle1@bidmc.harvard.edu

B. J. Wells et al. (eds.), *Handbook of Inpatient Cardiology*,
https://doi.org/10.1007/978-3-030-47868-1_28

Risk Assessment [Table 28.1]

Goldman Revised Cardiac Index (for Noncardiac Surgery) [2]

High-risk procedure [Table 28.3]
Peritoneal, thoracic, suprainguinal vascular
History of ischemic heart disease
MI, (+) stress test, angina, using NTG, Pathologic Q
History of CABG or PTCA or stent does not count
History of heart failure
History of cerebrovascular disease (TIA or CVA)
Diabetes mellitus treated with insulin
Serum creatinine >2.0

Selected Clinical Predictors of Risk [3]

- *Heart failure*: Particularly if currently decompensated
- *Aortic stenosis*: Perioperative mortality of 13% (compared with 1.6% without AS) in RCRI cohort
  - With modern anesthetic approaches, moderate-severe AS: 2.1% 3-day mortality (compared with 1.0% in propensity-matched patients without AS) [4]

Table 28.1 Goldman risk factors and complication rate

Risk factors	Complication rate
No risk factors	0.4%
1 risk factor	0.9%
2 risk factors	6.6%
3+ risk factors	11.0%

Major cardiac complications: MI, VF, cardiac arrest, complete heart block, pulmonary edema

- *Severe pulmonary hypertension*: 4–26% mortality
- *Coronary artery disease*: 2.9% 30-day postoperative mortality
- *Functional capacity* [Tables 28.2 and 28.3]
  - Less than 4 METs: >5% complication rate
  - 4–10 METs: 1–5% complication rate
  - Greater than 10 METs: <1% complication rate

Table 28.2 Duke Activity Status Index [5]

Activity	METs
Walk indoors	1
Eating, dressing, bathing	2
Dusting, washing dishes	3
Climb 1 flight of stairs	4
Vacuuming, sweeping	5
Playing golf, doubles tennis	6
Scrubbing floors, lifting furniture	7
Swimming, singles tennis	>10

Table 28.3 Selected types of operations and associated risk [6] (because there are so many different types of operations, a surgical risk calculator should likely be used.)

High risk (MACE ≥ 5%)	Intermediate risk (MACE 1–5%)	Low risk (MACE < 1%)
Emergency major operations, particularly in the elderly Aortic, major vascular, and peripheral vascular surgery Extensive operations with large volume shifts/ and or blood loss	Intraperitoneal and intrathoracic Carotid endarterectomy Head and neck surgery Orthopedic surgery Prostate surgery	Endoscopic procedures Superficial biopsy Cataract surgery Breast surgery

> **Clinical Pearl**
> Perioperative mortality is more often due to underlying medical conditions than surgical error or anesthesia.

Approach to the Patient Undergoing Noncardiac Surgery

Definitions of Surgical Urgency [3]

- *Urgent/Emergent*: Life or limb is threatened if not in the operating room between 6 and 24 hours.
- *Time-sensitive*: A delay of 1–6 weeks would negatively affect outcome.
- *Elective*: Procedure could be delayed for up to 1 year.

Management Algorithm [3]

- *Urgent/Emergent surgery?* Proceed to surgery.
- *Very low risk surgery?* Proceed to surgery.

1. *Time-sensitive or elective procedure?* If optimization is needed, delay surgery.
   (a) *Acute coronary syndrome:* Delay surgery and manage per AHA guidelines
   (b) Calculate risk of major adverse cardiac event (MACE, defined as death, MI, or revascularization)
   Low risk (<1% MACE): Proceed to surgery
   Elevated risk (>1% MACE)
      1. Good functional capacity (>4 METs): Proceed to surgery.
      2. Poor functional capacity (< 4 METS)
   (c) If valvular intervention is indicated on the basis of symptoms and severity of lesion, this should be performed before elective surgery (Class I, evidence C)

Clinical Pearl
Climbing one flight of stairs requires 4 METs.

Pre-operative Optimization

Indications for Pre-Operative Diagnostics

- Indications for ECG [3]
  - Never needed in patients undergoing low-risk surgery
  - Known CAD, arrhythmia, PAD, CVD, structural heart disease (IIa, Evidence B)
  - Can be considered in asymptomatic patients with no cardiac history (IIb, Evidence B)
- Indications for TTE [3]
  - Dyspnea of unknown origin (Class IIa, Evidence C)
  - History of heart failure and change in clinical status since last TTE (Class IIa, Evidence C)
  - History of heart failure and > 1 year since last TTE (Class IIb, Evidence C)
  - History of at least moderate stenosis or regurgitation and > 1 year since last TTE or change in clinical status (Class I, Evidence C)
- Indications for stress testing [3]
  - With elevated surgical risk (>1% MACE) and unknown functional capacity, it may be reasonable to perform exercise testing to assess functional capacity if it will change management (Class IIb, Evidence B)
  - With elevated surgical risk and poor functional capacity, it may be reasonable to perform exercise testing OR pharmacological stress with cardiac imaging if it will change management (Level IIb, Evidence C)

    No studies compare dobutamine stress echo with nuclear imaging and are considered equivalent
  - Impact on management [3]

Moderate to large areas of myocardial ischemia means increased risk of MI and/or death.
A normal study has a very high negative predictive value.
The presence of an old MI identified on rest imaging is of little predictive value.
The benefit of revascularization is unclear in this setting and is controversial. The CARP trial (see below "Relevant Studies") showed no benefit of pre-op revascularization prior to vascular surgery.

- Indications for cardiac catheterization
  - Preoperative intervention is rarely necessary simply to lower the risk of surgery unless such intervention is indicated irrespective of the preoperative context [9].
  - Situations in which we consider pre-operative cardiac catheterization:

    Active ischemia
    Large territory of ischemia on stress testing (e.g. "large reversible perfusion defect" on nuclear imaging.)
    Newly depressed ejection fraction

Clinical Pearl
Routine pre-operative cardiac catheterization and revascularization do not decrease mortality or peri-operative MI.

Pre-Operative Medications

- Beta blockers [3]
  - Beta blockers should be continued for patients who have been on them chronically (Class I, Evidence B)
  - Beta blockers in naive patients can be considered if intermediate-high risk of ischemia on stress test (Class IIb, Evidence C)

- In patients with 3+ RCRI risk factors, it may be reasonable to begin beta blocker (Class IIb, Evidence B)
- In patients with a compelling long-term indication for beta blocker but no other RCRI risk factors, initiating beta blockers in the perioperative setting is of uncertain benefit (Class IIb, Evidence B)

- Statins [3]
  - Continue in patients already taking (Class I, Evidence B)
  - Initiate in patients undergoing vascular surgery (Class IIa, Evidence B)
  - Initiate in patients when otherwise indicated (Class IIb, Evidence C)

- ACE inhibitors [3]
  - Continue in patients already taking (Class IIa, Evidence B)

    Increases intraoperative hypotension but reduces postoperative hypertension. Unclear impact on MACE.
- Antiplatelet agents [3]
  - Within 4–6 weeks after stenting (BMS or DES), DAPT should be continued (Class I, Evidence C)
  - With no coronary stent, aspirin should still be continued where possible (Class IIb, Evidence B)
- Pulmonary hypertension [3]
  - Chronic pulmonary vascular therapy (e.g. PDE5 inhibitors) should be continued (Class I, Evidence C)
  - Pre-op evaluation by a pulmonary hypertension specialist is beneficial (Class IIa, Evidence C)

Relevant Studies

CARP Trial: Coronary Artery Revascularization Prophylaxis (CARP) Trial [7]

- *Sites*: 18 VA medical centers (VA Co-op study) in 1997–1998 (98% male patients)

- *Inclusion criteria*: Elective vascular operation of AAA or PAD of legs
  - Cardiology consultant felt patient was high risk
  - Underwent angiography
  - Included if stenosis >70%
- *Exclusion criteria*:
  - LMCA stenosis >50%
  - LVEF <20%
  - Severe AS
  - Emergent operation, severe coexisting illness, recent revascularization
  - Coronary anatomy not suitable for revascularization
- *Intervention*: Then, randomized to revascularization (CABG/PCI) vs. conservative management
- *Outcomes* (revascularization vs. conservative management):
  - All-cause mortality at 2.7 years 22% vs. 23% (RR 0.98; 95% CI 0.70–1.37, $P = 0.92$)
  - Post-operative MI within 30 days (Positive enzymes): 11.6% vs. 14.3% ($P = 0.37$)

VISION Study: Vascular Events in Noncardiac Surgery Patients Cohort Evaluation [8]

- *Purpose*: To evaluate the value of post-operative TnT measurement
- *Inclusion criteria*: 45 years or older undergoing noncardiac surgery with general or regional anesthetic
  - Did not necessarily have to have CAD
- *Findings*: Post-op peak TnT predicts 30 day mortality
  - TnT ≤ 0.01 ng/mL: 1% 30-day mortality
  - TnT = 0.02 ng/mL: 4% 30-day mortality
  - TnT between 0.03–0.29 ng/mL: 9.3% 30-day mortality
  - TnT ≥ 3.0 ng/mL: 16.9% 30-day mortality

Key Learning Points

1. Preoperative intervention is rarely necessary simply to lower the risk of surgery unless such intervention is indicated irrespective of the preoperative context.
2. ECG and other cardiovascular diagnostics are not indicated prior to low-risk (<1% MACE) surgery.
3. With contemporary anesthesia, patients with asymptomatic moderate/severe aortic stenosis may generally undergo elective procedures.

Sources

1. Fleisher LA, Anderson GF. Perioperative risk: how can we study the influence of provider characteristics? Anesthesiology. 2002;96:1039–41.
2. Lee TH, Marcantonio ER, Mangione CM, et al. Derivation and prospective validation of a simple index for prediction of cardiac risk of major noncardiac surgery. Circulation. 1999;100:1043–9.
3. Fleisher LA, Fleischmann KE, Auerbach AD, et al. 2014 ACC/AHA guideline on perioperative cardiovascular evaluation and management of patients undergoing noncardiac surgery. J Am Coll Cardiol. 2014;64:e77–e137.
4. Agarwal S, Rajamanickam A, Bajaj N, Catacutan T, Griffin B, Svensson L, Anabtawi A, Tuzcu E, Kapadia S. Impact of aortic stenosis on postoperative outcomes after noncardiac surgeries. Chest. 2012;142:88A.
5. Hlatky MA, Boineau RE, Higginbotham MB, Lee KL, Mark DB, Califf RM, Cobb FR, Pryor DB. A brief self-administered questionnaire to determine functional capacity (the Duke Activity Status Index). Am J Cardiol. 1989;64:651–4.
6. Mukherjee D, Eagle KA. Perioperative cardiac assessment for noncardiac surgery: eight steps to the best possible outcome. Circulation. 2003;107:2771–4.
7. Moneta GL. Coronary-artery revascularization before elective major vascular surgery. Yearbook of Vascular Surgery. 2006;2006:81–2.

8. Vascular Events In Noncardiac Surgery Patients Cohort Evaluation (VISION) Study Investigators, Devereaux PJ, MTV C, et al. Association between postoperative troponin levels and 30-day mortality among patients undergoing noncardiac surgery. JAMA. 2012;307:2295–304.
9. Eagle KA, Berger PB, Calkins H, et al. ACC/AHA guideline update for perioperative cardiovascular evaluation for noncardiac surgery—executive summary. J Am Coll Cardiol. 2002;39:542–53.

Part III
Cardiac Diagnostic Imaging and Procedures

Chapter 29
Approach to ECG Interpretation

Geoffrey Southmayd and David Hirsh

Abbreviations

ACS	Acute coronary syndrome
AV node	Atrioventricular node
BPM	Beats per minute
ECG	Electrocardiogram
HR	Heart rate
LAA	Left atrial abnormality
LVH	Left ventricular hypertrophy
MI	Myocardial infarction
PE	Pulmonary embolism
RAE	Right atrial enlargement
RV	Right ventricle
RVH	Right ventricular hypertrophy
SA node	Sinoatrial node

G. Southmayd (✉) · D. Hirsh
Division of Cardiology, Emory University, Atlanta, GA, USA
e-mail: gsouthm@emory.edu; david.hirsh@emory.edu

B. J. Wells et al. (eds.), *Handbook of Inpatient Cardiology*,
https://doi.org/10.1007/978-3-030-47868-1_29

Electrocardiogram (ECG) BASICS

Electrical Conduction System

- Sinoatrial node (SA node) ➔ Atrioventricular node (AV node) ➔ His bundle ➔ Left and Right bundle branches ➔ Purkinje fibers ➔ Myocytes
- An action potential leads to myocyte depolarization, which spreads quickly among adjoining cells. Summation of the movement of this current through the myocardium over time produces the surface ECG tracing.

Introduction to the 12-Lead ECG (Standard Calibration)

- Limb leads: I, II, III, aVL, aVR, aVF. Measure electrical activity in the frontal plane.
- Precordial leads: $V_1 - V_6$. Measure electrical activity in the horizontal plane.
- Standard 12-lead ECG = 10 s
- Horizontal grid represents time: 1 mm small box = 0.04 s, 5 mm large box = 0.2 s
- Vertical grid represents voltage amplitude: 10 mm = 1 mV

The Normal ECG: (See Fig. 29.1)

- P wave: atrial depolarization
- QRS complex: ventricular depolarization
- T wave: ventricular repolarization

Standard Approach to ECG Assessment

Rate

- 300–150–100-75-60-50 rule (See Fig. 29.2)
- Tachycardia = rate > 100 bpm; Bradycardia = rate < 60 bpm; Accelerated = rate > expected (For non-sinus rhythms. AV

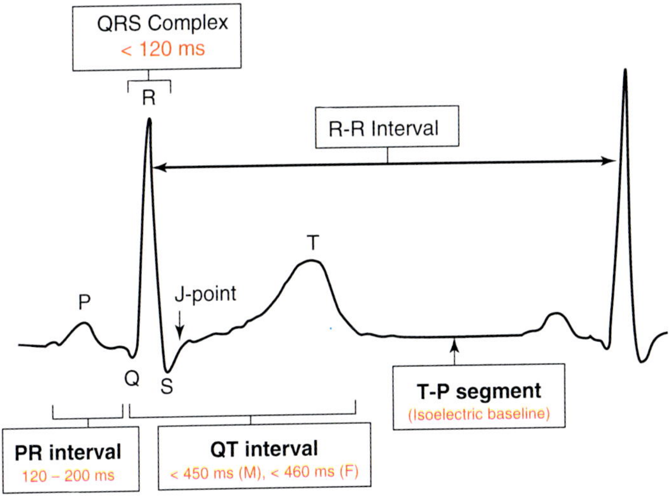

FIGURE 29.1 Normal ECG

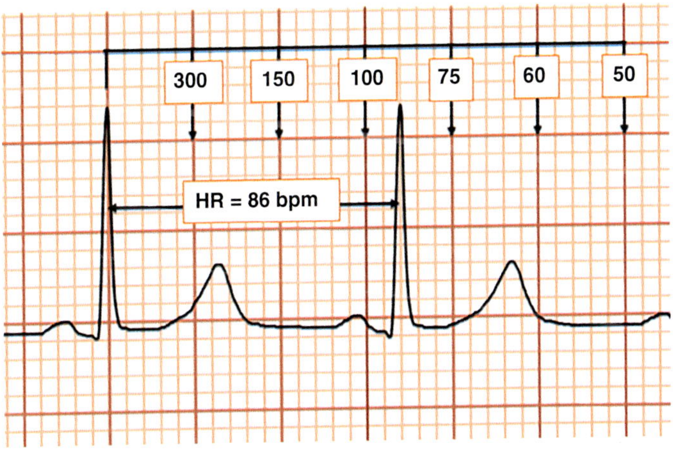

FIGURE 29.2 Heart rate assessment using ECG

node expected rate = 40–60 bpm, Ventricular expected rate = 20–40 bpm)

- For irregular rhythms: Heart rate (HR) = (Total # QRS complexes on 10-second ECG) × 6
- Atrial and ventricular rates may differ from one another (AV block, AV dissociation)

Rhythm

- Important considerations:
  - Is the rhythm regular or irregular?
  - Are P waves present? What is the P wave relationship with QRS?
  - Is the QRS complex wide or narrow?
  - Are there premature or dropped beats?
  - How did an arrhythmia begin or terminate?
- See Table 29.1 for common rhythm abnormalities.
- The reader is directed to the corresponding chapters elsewhere in the text for details on the diagnosis and management of various rhythm disturbances.

> **Clinical Pearl**
> A narrow complex tachycardia with ventricular rate near 150 bpm should be considered atrial flutter until proven otherwise. Look closely for flutter waves that may be buried in the tracing.

Axis

- Represents cumulative current vector at any point in time during cardiac cycle.
- Depolarization current *toward* the positive electrode will cause an *upward* deflection in the ECG tracing. Similarly, depolarization direction *away* from the positive electrode will cause a *downward* deflection, and depolarization *perpendicular* to the electrode will not cause any deflection (isoelectric).
- Approach to QRS axis determination (See Fig. 29.3):
  1. Examine QRS complex in leads I and aVF to determine vector quadrant.
  2. Find isoelectric limb lead. QRS axis is perpendicular to this lead in the selected quadrant.
  3. If no isoelectric lead is present, keep narrowing the scope of vectors by analyzing additional leads.

Table 29.1 ECG rhythm assessment

Rhythm	ECG	Distinguishing features
Normal sinus rhythm	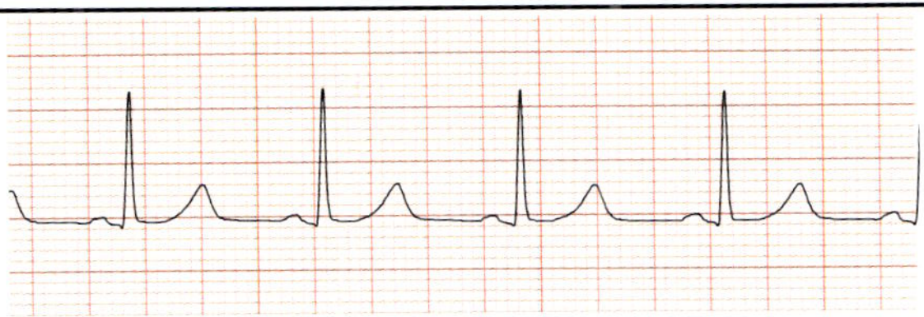	Normal P-QRS-T relationship
Sinus arrhythmia	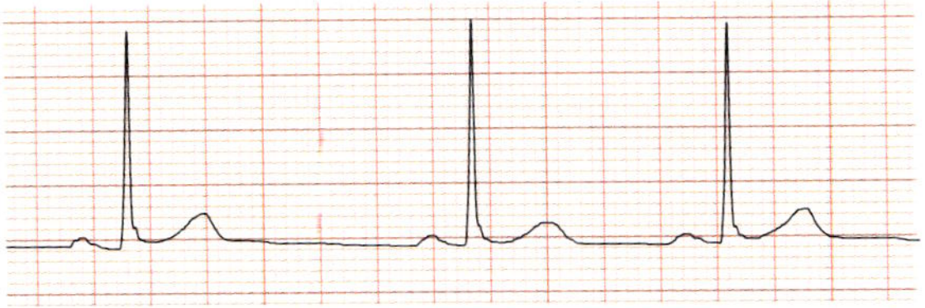	Respirophasic variation in PP interval by >10%, normal P-QRS-T relationship. Benign finding.
Ectopic Atrial Rhythm	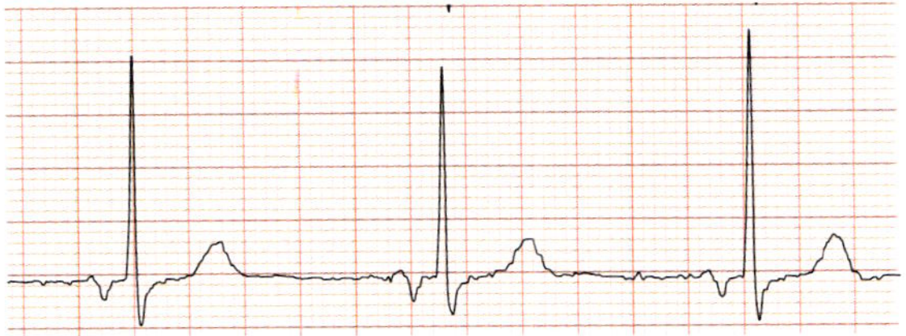	Abnormal P wave morphology and P wave axis.

(continued)

TABLE 29.1 (continued)

Rhythm	ECG	Distinguishing features
Atrial flutter	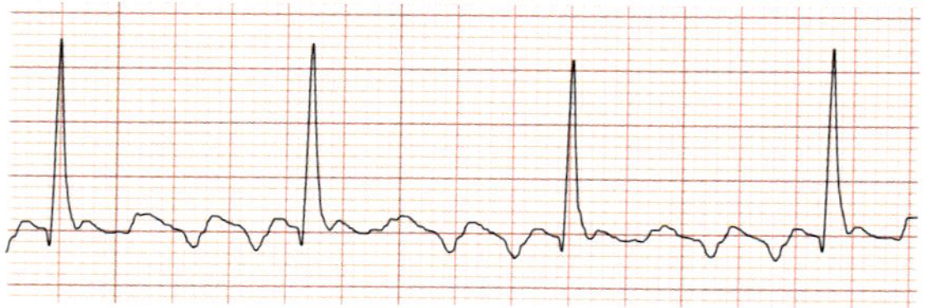	Sawtooth flutter waves with atrial rate 250–350. Ventricular rate near 150 bpm during 2:1 AV conduction.
Atrial fibrillation	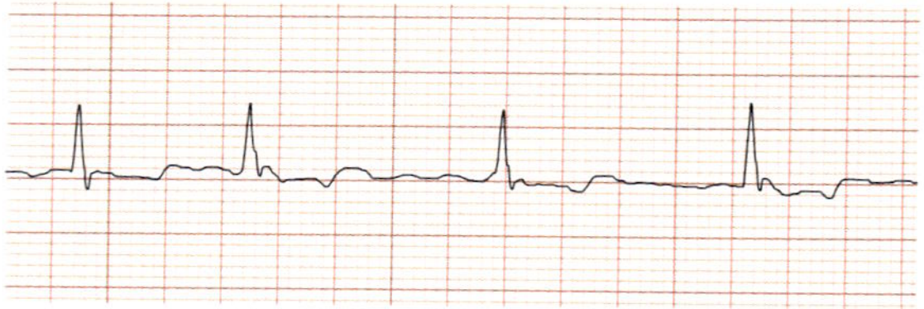	Irregularly irregular rhythm with absent P waves.
Supraventricular Tachycardia	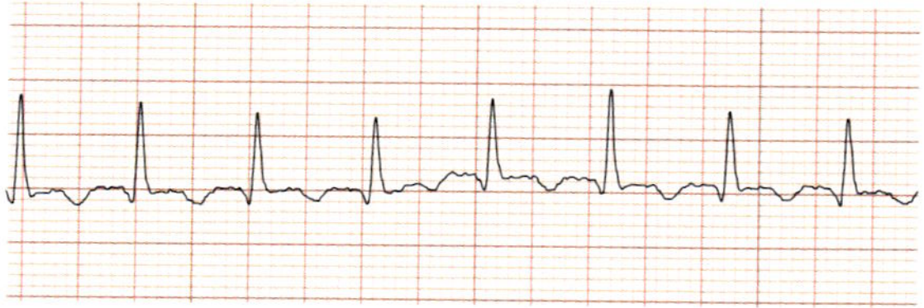	Regular, narrow complex tachycardia. P waves often buried within or shortly after QRS complex and may not be visible. In cases of aberrant conduction, can mimic VT.

Junctional rhythm	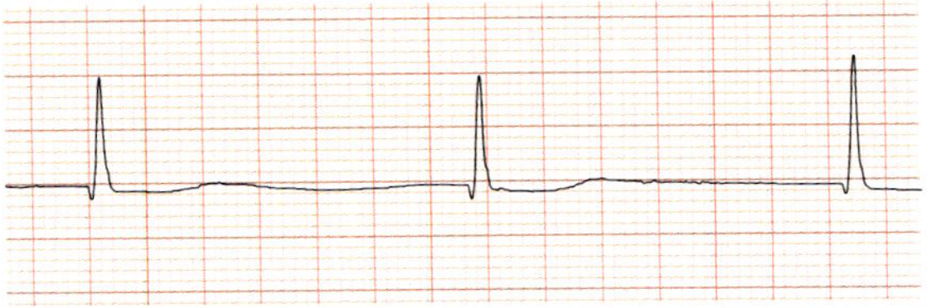	Regular rhythm, QRS narrow complex, or borderline wide. P waves often buried within or just after QRS (retrograde P waves). Rate > 60 bpm = Accelerated junctional rhythm. Rate > 100 = junctional tachycardia.
First degree AV block	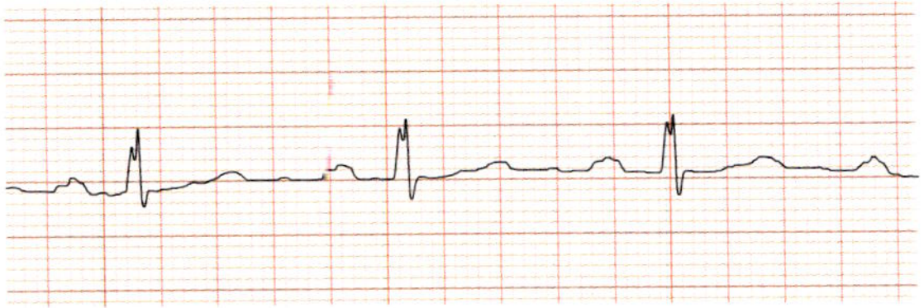	Prolonged PR interval > 200 ms
Mobitz Type I AV block (Wenckebach)	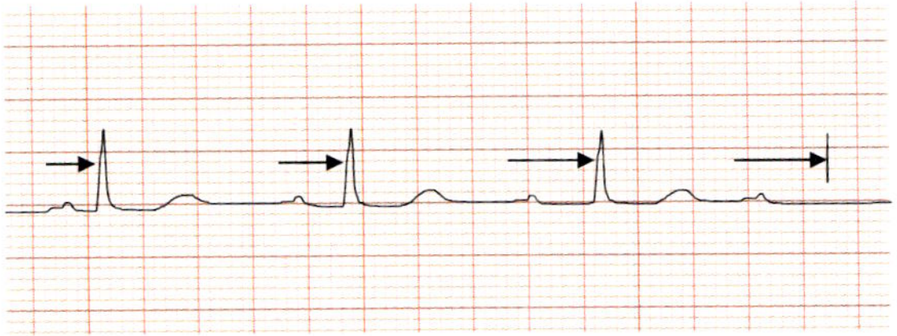	PR interval gradually prolongs until non-conducted impulse. Level of block generally at level of AV node, with narrow QRS. Most often benign.

(continued)

TABLE 29.1 (continued)

Rhythm	ECG	Distinguishing features
Mobitz II AV block	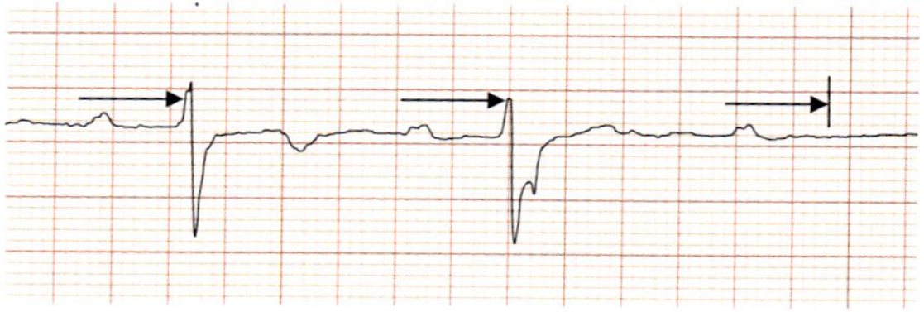	Constant PR intervals before non-conducted impulse. QRS may be narrow or wide. Level of block below AV node. Typically requires treatment.
Complete Heart Block	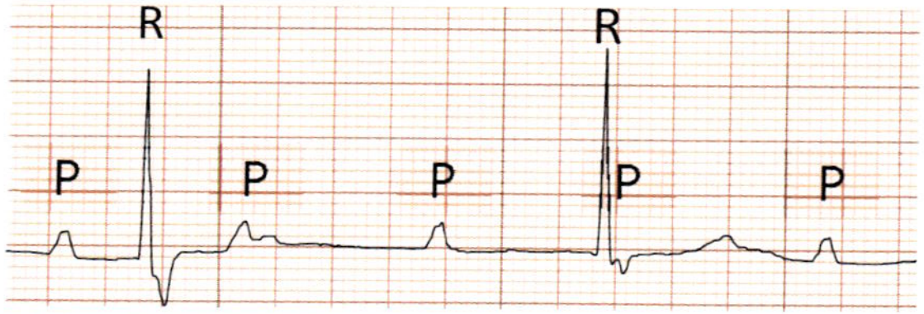	Independent atrial and ventricular rates (AV dissociation) with regular PP and RR intervals. QRS may be narrow or wide depending on the level of escape rhythm.

Monomorphic VT	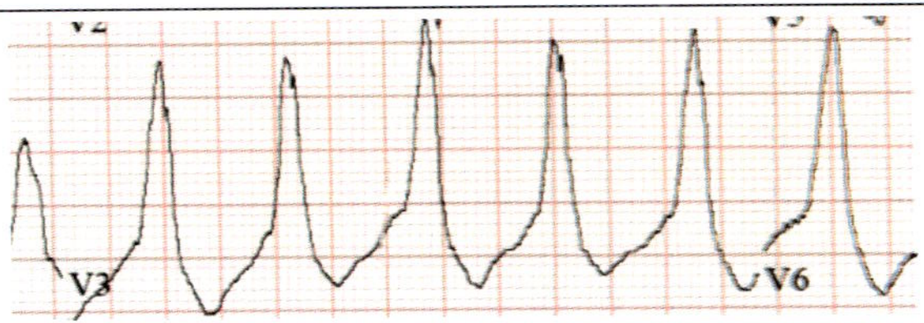	Regular wide complex tachycardia. AV dissociation is common. Should be distinguished from SVT with aberrancy.
Polymorphic VT	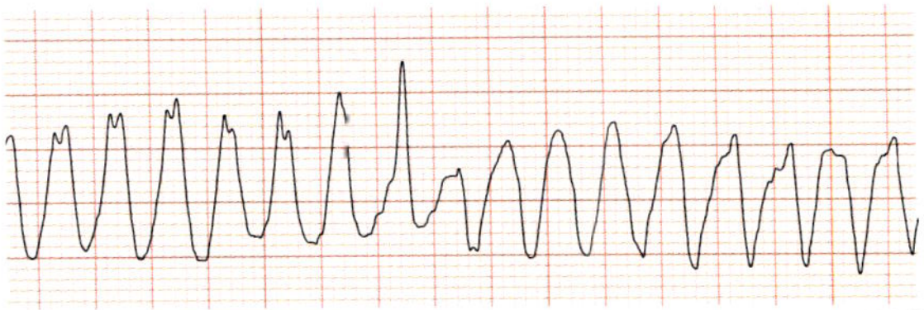	Undulating changes in QRS amplitude and polarity. Polymorphic VT in the setting of long QT = *Torsades de Pointes*

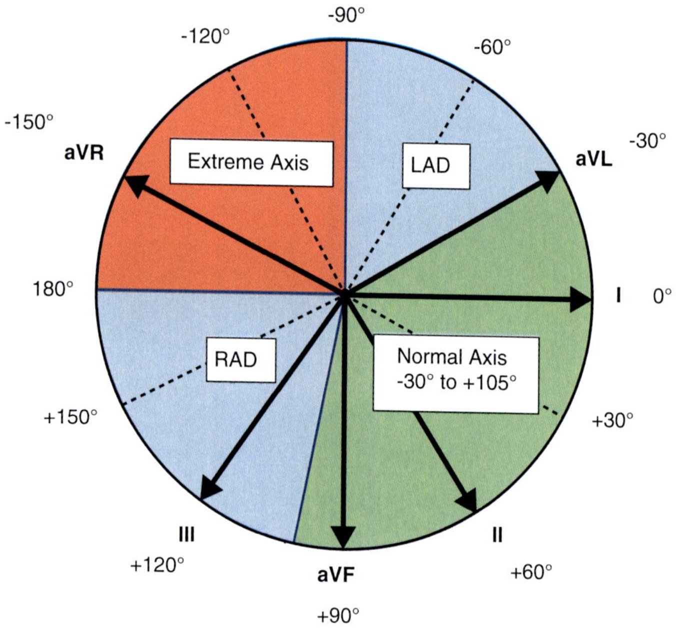

FIGURE 29.3 Axis

- Normal QRS axis = –30° to 105°
- Left axis deviation (–30° to –90°): Causes include LAFB, LBBB, LVH, ostium primum ASD, inferior MI, horizontal heart (pregnancy, ascites)
- Right axis deviation (105° to 180°): Causes include LPFB, RBBB, RVH, ostium secundum ASD, vertical heart, chronic lung disease, pulmonary embolism, lateral MI, dextrocardia
- Extreme axis deviation (180° to –90°): Causes include ventricular rhythm, limb lead reversal, inferolateral MI
- Normal P wave axis = 0–75°
- Normal T wave axis = 0–60°

Clinical Pearl
If QRS is positive in leads I and II, then the QRS vector is located between –30° and 90° and QRS axis is normal.

Intervals: (See Fig. 29.1)

- PR interval: normal 120–200 ms
- QRS duration: normal <120 ms
- QT interval:
  - Normal QTc < 450 ms (male) or < 460 ms (female)
  - Use the single lead with the longest QT interval
  - If the T and U waves are superimposed, measure the QT in leads which do not have an obvious U wave and/or draw a tangent from the steepest part of the T wave to the TP segment
  - Widened QRS (> 120 ms): consider using the J-T interval (QT interval-QRS duration)
  - QT interval must be adjusted for HR. Bazett's formula has been used classically: Corrected QT $(QTc) = \frac{QT}{\sqrt{RR\,interval}}$. Currently, other linear regression formulae are recommended.
  - When estimating QTc on ECG, in general, the QT interval should be < ½ RR interval [1]

Chamber Enlargement: (See Fig. 29.4)

- Right atrial enlargement (RAE): P wave ≥ 2.5 mm in lead II, or ≥ 1.5 mm in V_1/V_2
- Left atrial abnormality (LAA): Terminal portion of P wave in V_1 ≥ 0.04 sec duration and ≥ 1 mm deep; P wave duration ≥0.12 sec in leads II, III, or aVF.

Hypertrophy

- Left ventricular hypertrophy (LVH) [2]:
  - Criteria:

    S (V_1) + R (V_5 or V_6) ≥ 35 mm (Sokolow Lyon)

    R (aVL) + S (V_3) ≥ 28 mm (male) or ≥ 20 mm (female) (Cornell criteria)

    R (aVL) ≥ 11 mm

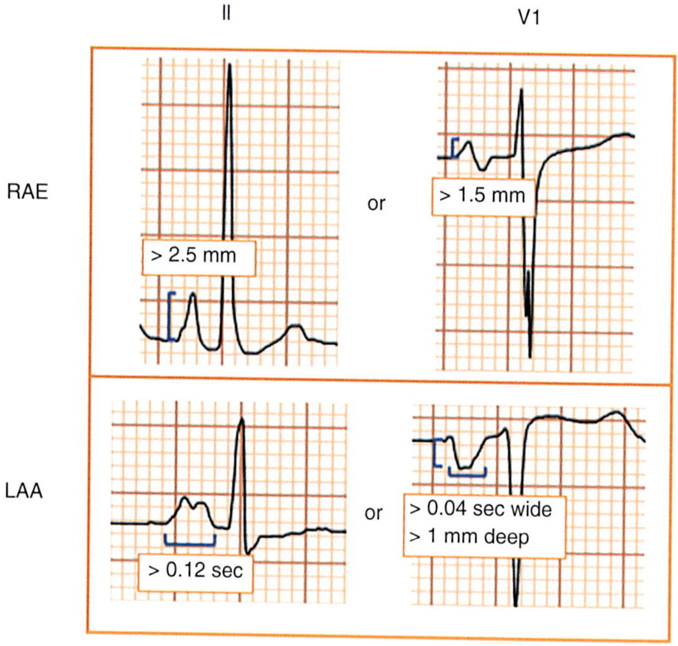

FIGURE 29.4 Chamber enlargement

- Supporting features on ECG: LAA, repolarization abnormality, Q waves in anterior precordial leads (pseudo-infarct pattern)

• Right ventricular hypertrophy (RVH):
  - Criteria less well defined. Look for R/S ratio > 1 in V_1, R/S ratio < 1 in V_6, R (V_1) ≥ 7 mm, or R (V_1) + S (V_5 or V_6) ≥ 10.5 mm
  - Supporting features: Right axis deviation, right ventricle (RV) strain pattern (ST depression and T wave inversion in V_1-V_3), incomplete/complete right bundle branch block, RAE

Clinical Pearl
The differential diagnosis for tall R waves in V_1 (R > S) includes: Right bundle branch block, RV hypertrophy or strain pattern, Posterior MI, WPW syndrome, Dextrocardia, and Muscular dystrophy

ST Segment and T Wave Changes

- ST segment: Represents time between ventricular depolarization and repolarization. Usually isoelectric. Depression or elevation >1 mm is considered abnormal.
- ST depression:
  - Subendocardial ischemia: flat or down-sloping ST depressions ± T wave abnormalities.
  - Posterior acute MI: Can be difficult to recognize. Look for tall R waves with ST depressions and upright T waves in V_1, V_2 (Inverse of changes seen in anterior MI).
  - LVH with repolarization abnormality: ST-T wave changes opposite to the direction of major QRS deflection. Typically mild ST depressions in I, V_5, V_6 and mild ST elevations in anterior precordial leads.
  - Other causes: Bundle branch blocks, drug/electrolyte effects.
- ST elevation:
  - Early repolarization: upwardly concave ST elevation with elevated take-off of the ST-segment, large upright T waves, and no reciprocal ST depressions, typically in precordial leads.
  - Myocardial injury: upwardly convex ST elevation ("tombstone" pattern) often with reciprocal ST depressions, T wave abnormality, QT prolongation.
  - Acute Pericarditis: diffuse ST elevation without reciprocal ST depressions, PR segment depressions.
  - Other causes: Coronary vasospasm, ventricular aneurysm, takotsubo cardiomyopathy.

Clinical Pearl
You cannot localize ischemic ST depressions on ECG to a particular region of the myocardium. This is in contrast to ST elevations from myocardial injury, which we can use to predict the culprit vessel in ACS.

- T wave inversion: consider myocardial ischemia/infarct, repolarization abnormality in LVH/RVH (strain pattern), bundle branch block, metabolic abnormality, or normal variant in V_1-V_4 in children (Juvenile T waves)
- Tall T waves: early acute MI, hyperkalemia

Conduction Abnormalities: (See Fig. 29.5)

- Right bundle branch block (RBBB) [3]:
  - rSR pattern in V_1, V_2; Wide, slurred S wave in I, V_5, V_6
  - T wave inversion +/– ST depression in V_1, V_2
  - Complete (QRS $\geq$ 120 ms) or incomplete (QRS 100–120 ms)
  - Does not interfere with diagnosis of acute MI or hypertrophy
- Left bundle branch block (LBBB) [3]:
  - QS or rS complex in V_1, V_2; Broad monophasic R waves in I, V_5, V_6
  - Secondary ST-T wave changes in direction opposite to major QRS deflection
  - QRS > 120 ms
  - LBBB interferes with ability to diagnose acute MI and LVH. Use Sgarbossa criteria to assess for ischemia, and echo to assess for LVH.
- Left anterior fascicular block (LAFB):
  - qR complex in I, aVL; rS complex in III, aVF
  - Left axis deviation for diagnosis (−45 to −90 deg)
  - QRS narrow or borderline wide
- Left posterior fascicular block (LPFB):

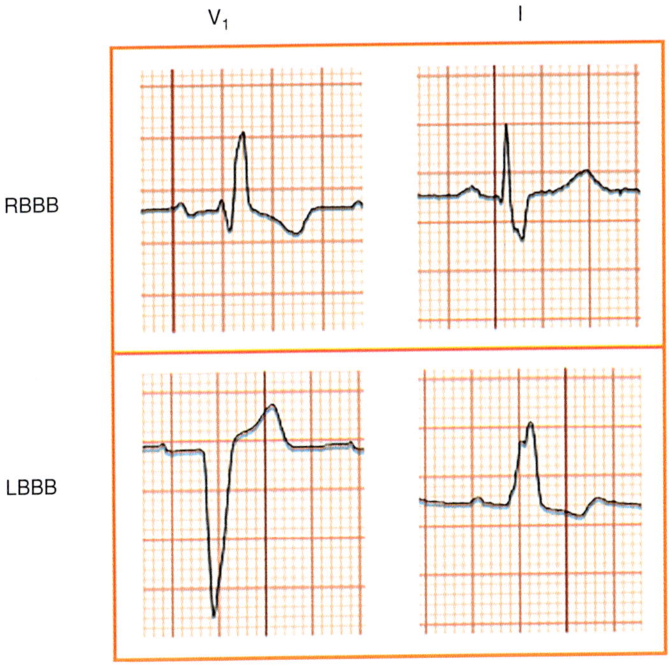

FIGURE 29.5 Bundle branch blocks

  - rS complex in I, aVL; qR complex in III, aVF
  - Right axis deviation (100 to 180 deg)
  - QRS narrow or borderline wide
- Bifascicular block = RBBB + LAFB/LPFB
- Trifascicular block = first degree AV block + RBBB + LAFB/LPFB

Clinical Pearl
In patients with RBBB, you should use only the first 60 ms of QRS complex for axis assessment, since the latter half of the QRS complex represents primarily RV depolarization.

Q Waves: Significant when ≥30-40 ms wide in 2 contiguous leads.

Low-Voltage ECG: QRS amplitude (R + S) < 5 mm in limb leads, < 10 mm in precordial leads

Clinical ECG Patterns

Electrolytes

- Hyperkalemia: Peaked T waves ➔ QRS widening, PR prolongation ➔ Sine wave pattern
- Hypokalemia: T wave flattening, prominent U waves, sagging ST depressions. prolonged QT.
- Hypercalcemia: QT shortening – limited to ST-segment
- Hypocalcemia: QT prolongation – limited to ST-segment

Drugs

- Digoxin:
  - Common effects: Scooping ST depressions (*Digitalis effect*), mild PR prolongation. Findings do not imply toxicity.
  - Toxicity: Numerous possible arrhythmias. High suspicion for toxicity if atrial tachycardia with variable AV block, or bidirectional VT.
- Tricyclic antidepressant toxicity: QRS widening, QT prolongation.
- Common QT prolonging meds: Antiarrhythmics, antipsychotics, TCA, macrolides, fluoroquinolones, methadone, ondansetron.
  - Full list can be found at https://www.crediblemeds.org (AZCERT, Inc.)

Systemic/Metabolic Abnormalities

- Acute Pulmonary Embolism (PE): RAD, RBBB (incomplete or complete), T wave inversions in anterior precordial leads, S1Q3T3 pattern. Most common ECG finding in acute PE = sinus tachycardia
- Pericardial Tamponade: Tachycardia, electrical alternans, ± low voltage
- Hypothermia: bradycardia, prolongation of PR/QRS/QT intervals, J point elevation ("Osborn wave")
- Central Nervous System disorder: classically with large, deeply inverted T waves in precordial leads and marked QT prolongation.

Key Learning Point

1. The approach to ECG assessment should include a systematic evaluation of the rate, rhythm, axis, intervals, chamber enlargement, and any associated ST-T wave changes.
2. Rhythm interpretation requires careful evaluation of the P-QRS-T relationship. Remember to distinguish the atrial rate from the ventricular rate, as these may differ and provide clues to rhythm identification.
3. The beginning and end of a tachyarrhythmia provide the best clues to determine etiology. Pay attention to events that trigger or terminate the rhythm.
4. Maintain a high index of suspicion for atrial flutter for any narrow complex tachycardia with ventricular rates near 150 bpm.

References

1. Rautaharju PM, Surawicz B, Gettes LS, et al. AHA/ACCF/HRS recommendations for the standardization and interpretation of the electrocardiogram: part IV: the ST segment, T and U waves, and the QT interval: a scientific statement from the American

Heart Association Electrocardiography and Arrhythmias Committee, Council on Clinical Cardiology; the American College of Cardiology Foundation; and the Heart Rhythm Society. Endorsed by the International Society for Computerized Electrocardiology. J Am Coll Cardiol. 2009;53(11):982–91. https://doi.org/10.1016/j.jacc.2008.12.014.

2. Hancock EW, Deal BJ, Mirvis DM, Okin P, Kligfield P, Gettes LS. AHA/ACCF/HRS recommendations for the standardization and interpretation of the electrocardiogram, part V: electrocardiogram changes associated with cardiac chamber hypertrophy: a scientific statement from the American Heart Association electrocardiography and arrhythmias committee, council on clinical cardiology; the American College of Cardiology Foundation; and the Heart Rhythm Society. Circulation. 2009;119:e251–61.
3. Surawicz B, Childers R, Deal BJ, Gettes LS. AHA/ACCF/HRS recommendations for the standardization and interpretation of the electrocardiogram, part III: intraventricular conduction disturbances: a scientific statement from the American Heart Association electrocardiography and arrhythmias committee, council on clinical cardiology; the American College of Cardiology Foundation; and the Heart Rhythm Society. Circulation. 2009;119:e235–40.

Chapter 30
Basic Principles of Echocardiography

Bryan Kindya and Byron Robinson Williams III

Assessment of Left Ventricle (LV) Function

Systolic Assessment

- LV systolic function is quantified by the amount of blood ejected from the ventricle during systole. This is expressed as an absolute value (stroke volume) or as a percentage (ejection fraction) [1].
- Assessment of LV function is accomplished with five traditional views: (parasternal long axis (PLAX), parasternal short axis (PSAX), apical four chamber (A4C), apical two chamber (A2C), and subcostal) [Fig. 30.1].
- E-point septal separation can be used to quickly assess LV function as normal or abnormal [2]. To calculate this, measure the distance between the anterior mitral leaflet and the septum during early diastole.
- E-point septal separation greater than 7 mm is generally associated with a reduced ejection fraction [3]

B. Kindya (✉) · B. R. Williams III
Department of Medicine, Division of Cardiology, Emory University School of Medicine, Atlanta, GA, USA
e-mail: bkindya@emory.edu; brwilli@emory.edu

B. J. Wells et al. (eds.), *Handbook of Inpatient Cardiology*,
https://doi.org/10.1007/978-3-030-47868-1_30

Highlights and Clinical Pearls

- EF less than 50% defines systolic dysfunction and is diagnosed by echo. This aids in diagnosis of Heart Failure with Reduced Ejection Fraction.
- The severity of EF reduction helps guide medical therapy for heart failure treatment.

Assessment of Right Ventricular (RV) Function

Due to the RV's complex shape, it is difficult to assess size and function in the traditional cardiac windows [1].

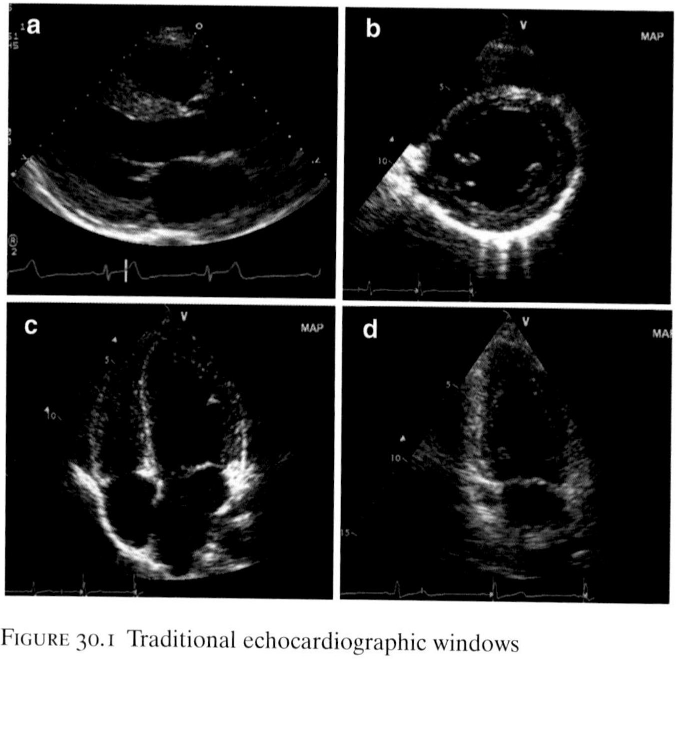

FIGURE 30.1 Traditional echocardiographic windows

RV Size

- RV size is best assessed in the subcostal or A4C view. To estimate RV size, compare it to the LV and estimate how much of the cardiac apex it comprises.
  - Normal – RV is smaller than the LV and makes up little to none of the cardiac apex.
  - Mildly enlarged – Smaller than the LV but contributes to the cardiac apex.
  - Moderately enlarged – Equal in size to the LV and makes up about half of the cardiac apex.
  - Severely enlarged – Bigger than the LV and makes up more than half of the cardiac apex.

Function

- RV dysfunction is classified as mild, moderate, or severe. Though this is often a subjective assessment, there are objective means to classify RV function. One is Tricuspid Annular Planar Systolic Excursion, or TAPSE [4]. In the A4C view, use M-mode to view the lateral RV wall at the level of the tricuspid annulus. Measure the distance the tricuspid annulus moves during systole. Normal movement is greater than 14 mm. Movement less than this indicates RV dysfunction.

McConnell's Sign

- McConnell's sign may indicate acute pulmonary embolism and should not be overlooked [5]. In the A4C view, hyperkinesis of the RV apex, akinesia of the mid lateral RV free wall, and septal flattening or bowing of the septum into the LV are seen. These findings signify acute RV pressure overload, commonly seen in large pulmonary embolism, and should prompt immediate consultation.

Highlights and Clinical Pearls

- Assess RV size in the subcostal or A4C view.
- RV dysfunction can be due to LV failure or intrinsic pulmonary pathology. RV dysfunction in the setting of a normal LV suggests pulmonary pathology.
- Acute RV dysfunction should raise concern for large pulmonary embolism.

Assessment of Valves

Valve disease is typically characterized by stenosis (narrowing, decreased forward flow) or regurgitation (insufficiency, increased backward flow).

Stenosis is defined by small valve area, high flow velocities, and high-pressure gradients.

Regurgitation is characterized by increased regurgitant volumes and large regurgitant orifice areas. Regurgitation is classified as acute or chronic. Acute regurgitation occurs due to rapid change in valve function, which may be caused by a ruptured papillary muscle, whereas chronic regurgitation occurs more slowly. Enlarged cardiac chambers can be seen in chronic regurgitation, as cardiac remodeling happens over time and is not usually seen in acute regurgitation.

Aortic Valve Disease

Aortic Stenosis (AS)

- AS can be due to congenital unicuspid or bicuspid valve, especially in patients younger than 70, or due to age-related calcification. Symptoms of severe disease include chest pain, dyspnea, and syncope.
- The severity of stenosis is measured in the A4C view with the left ventricular outflow tract brought into view by angulating the transducer anteriorly toward the patient's chest wall.

Table 30.1 Markers of severe valve stenosis

	Aortic valve	**Mitral valve**	**Tricuspid valve**
Mean pressure gradient (mm Hg)	40	10	5
Valve area (cm^2)	1.0	1.0	1.0
Peak flow velocity (m/s)	4.0	–	–
Pressure half time (ms)	–	150	190
Other findings	–	Pulmonary artery pressure above 50 mm Hg	–

- Severe disease is defined by:
  - Maximum flow velocity ≥ 4 m/s
  - Mean pressure gradient ≥40 mm Hg
  - Calculated aortic valve area of ≤1.0 cm^2 [Table 30.1] [6] [7].
- Low flow – low gradient AS should be suspected when the calculated aortic valve area is less than 1 cm^2 but mean pressure gradient is less than 40 mm Hg [6]. This finding should prompt cardiology consultation.
- Severe, symptomatic AS requires cardiology consultation for procedural intervention.

Aortic Regurgitation (AR)

- AR is typically caused by aortic disease (dilation, dissection) or primary leaflet disease (endocarditis, etc.). Chronic AR leads to a LV volume overload and subsequent LV dilation followed by a reduction in EF [Fig. 30.2].
- Severe disease is defined by:
  - Regurgitant volume ≥ 60 mL/beat
  - Regurgitant fraction ≥50%

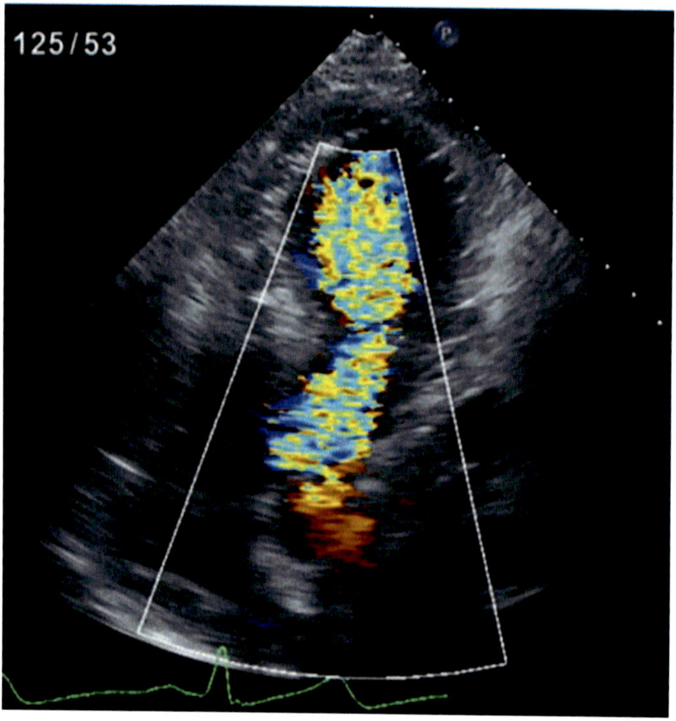

FIGURE 30.2 Severe aortic regurgitation with diastolic backflow into the left ventricle

- Effective regurgitant orifice area $\geq 0.3\ \text{cm}^2$
- Diastolic flow reversal (backward flow) in the abdominal aorta suggests severe disease [Table 30.2] [6, 8]

- Severe disease requires cardiology consultation.

Highlights and Clinical Pearls

- AS is characterized by high gradients, high velocities, and low valve areas. Severe or symptomatic disease requires cardiology consult.

- AR is characterized by high regurgitant volumes and large orifice areas. Acute severe regurgitation usually warrants emergent or urgent intervention. Chronic, severe regurgitation requires monitoring by a cardiologist.

Mitral Disease

The mitral valve is seen in the PLAX, PSAX, and A4C, but objective measurement is best accomplished in the A4C view.

Mitral Stenosis (MS)

- MS is usually caused by rheumatic disease, but can also be caused by mitral annular calcification. MS causes atrial arrhythmias, pulmonary hypertension, LV diastolic dysfunction, and left atrial enlargement.
- Severe disease requires cardiology consultation and is defined by:
  - Mitral valve area ≤ 1.0 cm^2
  - Mean diastolic gradient above 10 mm Hg
  - Pressure half time of ≥150 ms [Table 30.1] [6] [7].

Table 30.2 Markers of severe valve regurgitation

	Aortic valve	**Mitral valve**
Regurgitant volume (mL)	60	60
Regurgitant fraction (%)	50	50
Effective regurgitant orifice area (cm^2)	0.3	0.4
Other findings	Abdominal aortic diastolic flow reversal	Pulmonic vein systolic flow reversal

Mitral Regurgitation (MR)

- MR is characterized by its underlying etiology. Degenerative MR refers to diseases of the leaflet apparatus itself. Functional MR refers to remodeling of the valve, usually due to LV dysfunction and/or dilation. MR causes atrial dilation, arrhythmias, pulmonary hypertension, and dilated cardiomyopathy. Subjective assessment of MR severity can be accomplished in the A4C view using color Doppler across the mitral valve.
  - Mild MR – small, central, often brief jets
  - Moderate MR – variable in size, longer in duration than mild
  - Severe MR – Holosystolic, often more than 50% of the LA is filled by regurgitation [Fig. 30.3] [6].
- Severe disease is defined by:
  - Regurgitant volume ≥ 60 mL/beat
  - Regurgitant fraction ≥50%
  - Effective regurgitant orifice area ≥ 0.4 cm^2 [Table 30.2] [6, 8]
- Severe disease requires cardiology consultation to determine if valve repair/replacement is indicated.

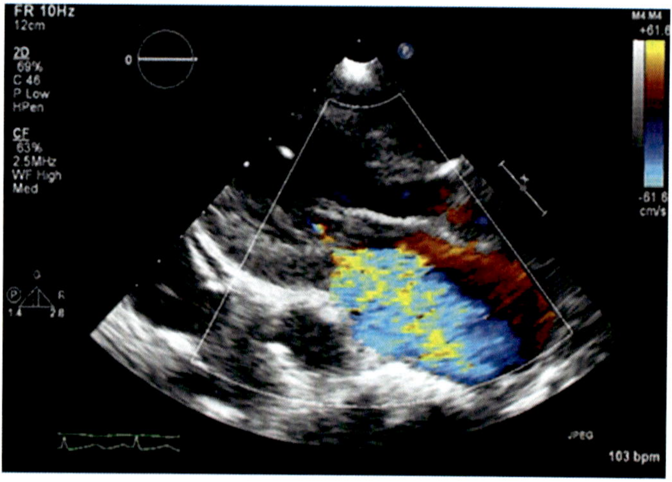

FIGURE 30.3 Severe mitral regurgitation

Tricuspid Disease

Tricuspid Stenosis (TS)

- TS is rare and seen in rheumatic disease or other clinical conditions such as carcinoid syndrome. TS always requires cardiology consultation [Table 30.1].

Tricuspid Regurgitation (TR)

- TR occurs secondary to RV disease, pulmonary hypertension, or primary leaflet pathology. It leads to RA and RV volume overload and dilatation. Assess in the A4C view with color doppler across the tricuspid valve.
  - Mild TR – Narrow jet
  - Moderate TR – Intermediate-sized jet
  - Severe TR – Large jet encompassing more than half the RA
  - Systolic reversal of flow in the hepatic veins suggests severe TR
- Severe disease requires cardiology consultation.

Pulmonic Disease

Pulmonic Stenosis (PS)

- PS is rare and usually seen in congenital heart disease (Tetralogy of Fallot, Noonan's syndrome). Evaluation of the pulmonic valve requires special windows and requires cardiology evaluation.

Pulmonic Regurgitation (PR)

- PR is usually benign. If there is concern for severe or symptomatic disease, a cardiology referral for specialized imaging is indicated.

Great Vessel Assessment

Aorta

- Assessment of the aorta is important when evaluating for aneurysm or dissection. In the PLAX view, angulate the probe toward the patient's right shoulder to bring the proximal aorta into view. Measure during end diastole [1].

Ascending Aortic Aneurysms

- Aneurysms are caused by hypertension or genetic disorders (bicuspid valve, Marfan syndrome). Ascending aorta diameters >3.5 cm are considered dilated and require serial echocardiography and cardiology consultation. Indications for repair include diameter > 5.5 cm (5.0 cm in Marfan syndrome), or growth greater than 0.5 cm/year.

Aortic Dissection

- TTE is not a sensitive test for dissection. Assessment of aortic dissection involves PLAX for the proximal aorta, the suprasternal notch window for the aortic notch, and the proximal descending aorta via the subcostal window. A dissection flap may be visualized in the aorta [Fig. 30.4]. Other indicators of dissection include differences in color flow across the dissection flap or a dilated aorta. Assessment for AR in the PLAX or A4C view is important in patients going for surgery to determine if concurrent aortic valve intervention is indicated.

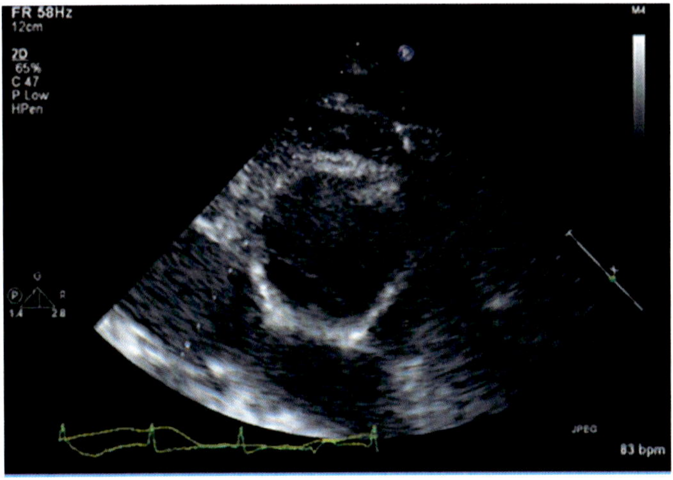

FIGURE 30.4 Aortic dissection with dissection flap present

Highlights and Clinical Pearls

- Aortic aneurysms weaken wall integrity and are at risk of rupture. Serial monitoring is necessary, and indications for repair are based on size.
- Dissection can be acute or chronic. Ascending aortic dissection requires surgical repair, and assessment of aortic valve disease is essential before surgery.

Inferior Vena Cava (IVC)

IVC assessment assists in the evaluation of a variety of cardiac conditions including heart failure and cardiac tamponade. Assess the IVC in the subcostal view with the transducer positioned longitudinally. Then, angulate the probe side to side to bring the IVC into view. Ensure IVC is being viewed and not the descending aorta by angulating the probe toward the patient's head to view the junctions of the hepatic vein and IVC, and the IVC and RA. Estimate the RA pressure based on diameter of the IVC and its collapsibility when the patient “sniffs” [9].

- IVC size >2.1 cm and IVC collapsibility <50% = 10–20 mm Hg
- IVC size >2.1 cm and IVC collapsibility >50% = 5–10 mm Hg
- IVC size <2.1 cm and IVC collapsibility >50% = 0–5 mm Hg

Highlights and Clinical Pearls

- A dilated IVC that does not collapse >50% with “sniff” suggests elevated RA pressures. This may be seen in decompensated heart failure, pericardial tamponade, TS, and severe TR.

Pericardial Disease

Pericardial Effusion

- Effusions occur due to various etiologies (malignancy, viral pericarditis, autoimmune, trauma).
- Assess for pericardial effusion in all five standard views, as it may present in any location in the pericardium and may not be visible in all views.

Tamponade Assessment

- Cardiac tamponade occurs when the pressure in the pericardial space exceeds that of the chambers of the heart, causing impaired filling and collapse. Echo findings suggesting tamponade include sustained systolic collapse of the RA, diastolic collapse of the RV [Fig. 30.5], and a

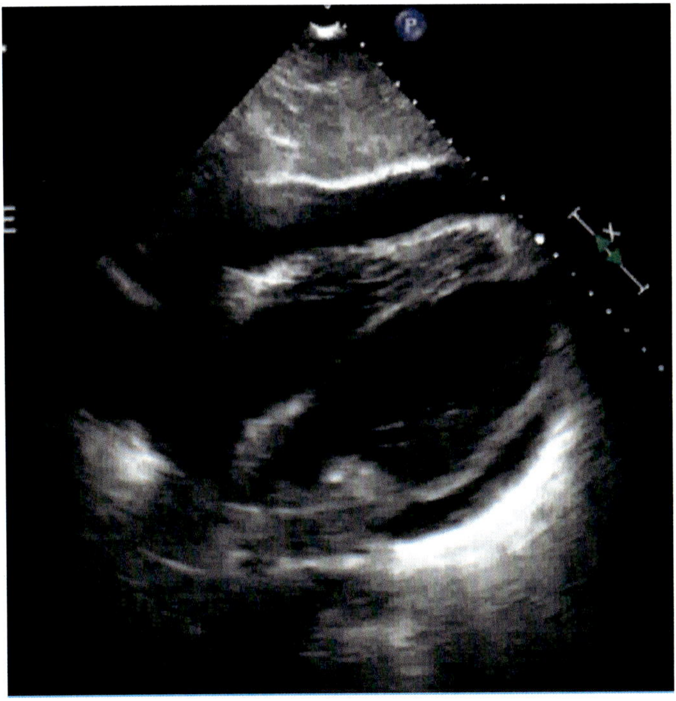

FIGURE 30.5 Cardiac tamponade with diastolic collapse of the right ventricle

dilated IVC with respiratory variation less than 50% [1]. In normal physiology, inspiration causes a drop in thoracic pressure, increased RV filling, and decreased LV filling. In tamponade, this finding is accentuated. Assess in the A4C view by measuring Doppler inflow across the mitral valve. Greater than 25% variation in peak flow velocity between inspiration and expiration across the mitral valve suggests tamponade physiology. Concern for tamponade should prompt emergent cardiology consultation to determine further management.

Key Learning Points

1. Complete assessment of ventricular function requires visualization of the heart in all views. Obtaining these views requires practical experience and practice, and skill doing so varies from person to person.
2. Assessment of valve regurgitation and stenosis use both qualitative and quantitative parameters. Severe disease, especially when acute, requires cardiac consultation.
3. Acute aortic dissection is a medical emergency with high mortality when not detected. Despite this, transthoracic echocardiography has low sensitivity and is not an accurate diagnostic test to assess for dissection. Once dissection has been diagnosed, echocardiography is useful for aortic valve assessment to determine if valve repair is indicated at the time of surgery.
4. Cardiac tamponade is a medical emergency. Abnormal collapse of any cardiac chamber (atrial, ventricular, left sided, or right sided) indicates tamponade physiology and warrants urgent consultation.
5. Inferior vena cava assessment can play an important role in volume assessment and can be used to estimate cardiac filling pressures.

References

1. Otto CM, Pearlman AS. Textbook of clinical echocardiography, vol. xiv. Philadelphia: W.B. Saunders; 1995. p. 404.
2. Massie BM, Schiller NB, Ratshin RA, Parmley WW. Mitral-septal separation: new echocardiographic index of left ventricular function. Am J Cardiol. 1977;39(7):1008–16.
3. McKaigney CJ, Krantz MJ, La Rocque CL, Hurst ND, Buchanan MS, Kendall JL. E-point septal separation: a bedside tool for emergency physician assessment of left ventricular ejection fraction. Am J Emerg Med. 2014;32(6):493–7.

4. Kaul S, Tei C, Hopkins JM, Shah PM. Assessment of right ventricular function using two-dimensional echocardiography. Am Heart J. 1984;107(3):526–31.
5. McConnell MV, Solomon SD, Rayan ME, Come PC, Goldhaber SZ, Lee RT. Regional right ventricular dysfunction detected by echocardiography in acute pulmonary embolism. Am J Cardiol. 1996;78(4):469–73.
6. Nishimura RA, Otto CM, Bonow RO, Carabello BA, Erwin JP 3rd, Guyton RA, et al. 2014 AHA/ACC guideline for the Management of Patients with Valvular Heart Disease: executive summary: a report of the American College of Cardiology/American Heart Association task force on practice guidelines. Circulation. 2014;129(23):2440–92.
7. Baumgartner H, Hung J, Bermejo J, Chambers JB, Evangelista A, Griffin BP, et al. Echocardiographic assessment of valve stenosis: EAE/ASE recommendations for clinical practice. J Am Soc Echocardiogr. 2009;22(1):1–23; quiz 101-2.
8. Zoghbi WA, Adams D, Bonow RO, Enriquez-Sarano M, Foster E, Grayburn PA, et al. Recommendations for noninvasive evaluation of native valvular regurgitation: a report from the American Society of Echocardiography developed in collaboration with the Society for Cardiovascular Magnetic Resonance. J Am Soc Echocardiogr. 2017;30(4):303–71.
9. Porter TR, Shillcutt SK, Adams MS, Desjardins G, Glas KE, Olson JJ, et al. Guidelines for the use of echocardiography as a monitor for therapeutic intervention in adults: a report from the American Society of Echocardiography. J Am Soc Echocardiogr. 2015;28(1):40–56.

Chapter 31
Stress Testing, Nuclear Imaging, CT Angiography, and Cardiac MRI

Talal Khalid Al-Otaibi and Thomas H. Hauser

Abbreviation

ABI	Ankle–brachial pressure index
ARVC	Arrhythmogenic Right Ventricular Cardiomyopathy
AVB	Atrioventricular block
CAC	Coronary Artery Calcium Score
CAD	Coronary artery disease
CCT	Cardiac CT
CCTA	Coronary CT angiography
DTS	Duke Treadmill Prognostic Score
ECG	Electrocardiogram
EGE	Early gadolinium enhancement
EIBBB	Exercise-induced BBB
EMB	Endomyocardial biopsy
FFRCT	Fractional flow reserve CT
HHR	Heart Rate Recovery

T. K. Al-Otaibi (✉) · T. H. Hauser
Department of Medicine, Cardiovascular Institute, Beth Israel Deaconess Medical Center, Boston, MA, USA
e-mail: talotaib@bidmc.harvard.edu

B. J. Wells et al. (eds.), *Handbook of Inpatient Cardiology*,
https://doi.org/10.1007/978-3-030-47868-1_31

HR	Heart rate
ICA	Intracoronary angiogram
LBBB	Left bundle branch block
LGE	Late gadolinium enhancement
LVEF	Left ventricular ejection fraction
LVH	Left ventricular hypertrophy
MET	Metabolic Equivalent of Task
MI	Myocardial infarction
PAD	Peripheral Arterial Disease
Pt	Patient
Qp/Qs	Pulmonary-to-systemic shunt ratio
RV	Right ventricular
SBP	Systolic blood pressure
SE	Stress Echocardiography
SSFP	Steady-state free precession
V-paced	Ventricular paced rhythm
WMA	Wall motion abnormality
WPW	Wolff-Parkinson-White syndrome

Stress Test

Stress testing is performed using either standardized exercise protocols or a pharmacological agent.

Exercise Stress Test

Generally preferred if able to exercise. Modalities include treadmill (most common), stationary cycle, or arm ergometry. The goal peak HR is 85% age predicted maximal HR to ensure adequacy of exercise.

Pharmacologic Stress Test

- Use if unable to exercise or unable to achieve goal HR.
- Must be paired with nuclear imaging or echo.
- Similar sensitivity and specificity to exercise stress with imaging but without the hemodynamic and symptomatic information.

- Preferred in LBBB or V-paced due to false positive exercise imaging (artefactual septal perfusion defect).
- Types of pharmacological stress:
  - *Coronary vasodilator:* causes coronary arteriolar vasodilation, diseased vessels do not dilate while normal vessels have increased flow, causing coronary flow heterogeneity. Agents available are adenosine, dipyridamole (increases circulating adenosine), or regadenoson (selective A2A receptor agonist). Side effects: flushing, AVB, and bronchospasm. Contraindications: allergy, theophylline within 36 h, uncontrolled asthma, significant AVB, caffeine within 12 to 24h. Caution in those with seizure disorders.
  - *Chronotropes/inotropes:* dobutamine, which is more physiologic but can induce ischemia and be arrhythmogenic.

Indications/Contraindications: See Table 31.1

Table 31.1 Summary of indications and contraindications to exercise stress testing

Indication	Contraindication
Coronary Artery Disease	*Absolute*
Asymptomatic Pt with chest pain and intermediate likelihood of obstructive CAD, management of Pt with stable CAD, following myocardial infarction, limited usefulness in Pt post PCI.	Acute myocardial infarction (within 2 days). High-risk unstable angina. Uncontrolled arrhythmia with hemodynamic compromise.
Peripheral Arterial Disease	
Assessment of questionable PAD, functional assessment in known PAD, evaluation of post-surgical or endovascular revascularization procedures.	Active endocarditis. Symptomatic severe aortic stenosis. Decompensated heart failure
Valvular Heart Disease	Acute pulmonary embolism
Assessing functional capacity in patients with valvular heart disease.	Acute myocarditis or pericarditis

(continued)

TABLE 31.1 (continued)

Indication	Contraindication
Hypertrophic Cardiomyopathy	*Relative*
Risk stratification and functional assessment.	Known left main coronary artery stenosis
Heart Rhythm Disorders	Hypertrophic cardiomyopathy with a severe resting gradient
Evaluation of Pt with exercise-induced arrhythmias, evaluate with medical or ablative therapy.	Severe hypertension
Adult Congenital Heart Disease	High-grade AV block
Functional assessment of Pt with congenital heart disease associated with pulmonary hypertension.	

Assessment of Coronary Arterial Disease

- Sensitivity of 68% and specificity of 77%. Exercise test has a higher sensitivity with triple-vessel disease than in those with single-vessel disease.
- Exercise capacity is the most important prognostic variable; Pt able to perform >10 METs are in general at low risk for cardiovascular events.
- *Hemodynamic Response*:
  - *Maximum Heart rate*: an adequate study is defined by achieving 85% of the age-predicted maximum heart rate [HRmax = 220 – age, for Pt with coronary artery disease CAD on B-Blocker HRmax = 164 – (0.7× age)].
  - *Systolic Blood Pressure:* Exaggerated SBP Response >210 mmHg in men and > 190 mmHg in women indicative of the future development of hypertension in normotensive Pt. *Exercise-Induced Hypotension* SBP during exercise falling below resting systolic pressure is predictive of a poor prognosis typically due to severe multivessel CAD with left ventricular dysfunction, also seen in Pt with cardiomyopathy, left ventricular outflow tract obstruction, enhanced vagal tone, hypovolemia, antihypertensive medications, and arrhythmias.

- *Heart Rate Recovery HRR*: Normal recovery is defined as >12 beats/min after 1 min with post exercise cool down or > 18 beats/min after 1 min with immediate cessation of movement. HRR of 12 beats or less predicts an increased relative risk of sudden cardiac death and all-cause mortality independent of CAD severity.
- *Electrocardiographic Responses*:
  - ST-segment evaluated 80 ms after the J point.
  - ST depression does not localize ischemia, whereas ST-segment elevation localizes the vascular region; Lead V5 is the most sensitive.
  - *Downsloping* or *horizontal* ST depression (≥1 mm) is more predictive of CAD, whereas upsloping ST depression is less specific.
  - Presence of ventricular ectopy during exercise recovery is an indicator of worse prognosis.
  - Exercise-induced BBB EIBBB suggests CAD (especially at lower HR <125 bpm) or conduction disease. ST-segment changes before onset of the EIBBB are still interpretable.
- *Multivariable Score*:
  - Duke Treadmill Prognostic Score (DTS):
    DTS = Exercise time on Bruce protocol – (5 × ST deviation [mm]) – (4 × Angina index [0 for no chest pain, 1 for chest pain, 2 for chest pain that stops the test])
    (>10 low risk, 10 to −5 intermediate risk, <−5 high risk)
    Does not include clinical variables (age, HR, etc.)
  - Cleveland Clinic Prognostic Score. Includes most clinical and exercise prognostic variables.

Assessment of Peripheral Arterial Disease (PAD)

Evaluate functional limitations caused by PAD and the response to therapy. Post exercise ankle brachial index ABI: in Pt with PAD will show a decrease in ABI (greater than a 5% drop in post exercise ABI from resting levels) and a prolonged recovery time.

Exercise Stress Testing in Women: Exercise stress testing without imaging is less sensitive and specific in women, while still providing valuable information in evaluating symptomatic patients.

Clinical Pearl
Beta-blockers may be held for modalities that rely on chronotropic response, e.g., exercise or dobutamine stress. Whereas, beta-blockers should not be held in Pt with known CAD when attempting to assess the quality of medical management.

Stress Echocardiography SE

Evaluation of CAD: Typically performed with exercise or dobutamine stress. Echocardiography performed at peak stress to assess for stress-induced wall motion abnormalities. SE has sensitivity of 84% and specificity of 82% in detecting CAD.

- Negative SE test has a low risk of subsequent events (< 1% per year), whereas a positive study indicates increased risk of MI, revascularization, or death.
- For Pt undergoing major noncardiac surgery, a negative dobutamine SE is associated with a high negative predictive value of death and MI.

Viability Assessment: Viable myocardium is defined as an increase in wall thickening at low-dose dobutamine (5 μg/kg/min). Viable segments may show a biphasic response (improvement at low dose and then worsening at high dose) due to ischemia present with higher dose dobutamine. *Limitations:* Images need to be obtained as close to peak stress as possible to accurately assess ischemia; image quality limited in those with poor echo windows.

Nuclear Cardiology

Evaluation of CAD: Myocardial perfusion imaging typically performed using SPECT with Tc-99 m based tracers. PET is more expensive and less available, but may be more accurate. Reversible defects (abnormal perfusion with stress and normal at rest) are consistent with ischemia, while fixed defects are consistent with infarction. SPECT has a sensitivity of 88% and a specificity of 76% in detecting CAD.

- Normal myocardial perfusion implies an excellent prognosis with <1% mortality or MI rate at 1 year. Abnormal perfusion implies high risk, with increasing risk with severity and extent of perfusion defects.
- For Pt undergoing major noncardiac surgery, normal myocardial perfusion is associated with a high negative predictive value of death and MI.

Myocardial viability: Often assessed with metabolic PET imaging using FDG, with mismatched PET defects (normal FDG uptake with abnormal perfusion) indicating viability. Resting Tl-201 and Tc-99 m SPECT are also used, with preserved perfusion indicating viability.

LV function: LV function routinely assessed with SPECT and PET imaging. MUGA can assess LV and RV function, but rarely used in current practice.

Limitations: Attenuation (breast, diaphragmatic), LBBB if performed with exercise (vasodilator preferred), rarely balanced ischemia, radiation exposure.

Clinical Pearl

Important signs of the presence of left main or multivessel CAD are transient ischemic dilation TID of the left ventricle, reversible right ventricular uptake, and/or a decline in the LVEF after stress.

Cardiac CT (CCT)

Indications/Contraindications/Safety: See Table 31.2

Coronary CT angiography (CCTA) vs. functional testing led to more radiation, coronary angiography, and revascularization, but no difference in clinical outcomes [(PROMISE *NEJM* 2015; 372:1291)].

Table 31.2 Summary of indications, contraindications, and safety considerations for Cardiac CT

Indication	**Contraindication**[a]	**Safety**
Chest pain Acute or chronic low-intermediate risk chest pain syndromes with equivocal stress test. Coronary artery anomalies. Graft patency. *Cardiac Masses* *Congenital heart disease* *Pericardial disease* Constrictive pericarditis, mass, surgical complication. *Aortic* Dissection, aneurysm, prior surgery or EVS. *Pulmonary embolism* *Pre-interventional planning* Surgical, TAVR, TMVR, EP ablation procedures, LAA closure device *Intracardiac thrombus*	Renal insufficiency, (GFR <30 ml/min) Contrast allergy (pretreat with steroid and diphenhydramine. Hx of anaphylaxis is an absolute contraindication.) Recent IV contrast (should avoid contrast CT for 24 h) Hyperthyroidism (iodine may precipitate thyrotoxicosis). Irregular heart rhythm due to suboptimal ECG gating. Inability to breath-hold >10 sec (respiratory motion artifact)	Radiation exposure Contrast induced nephropathy Risk factors: Renal insufficiency, DM, volume of contrast

[a]Are considered relative contraindication, and risk-benefit should be evaluated

CCT has a high NPV and may be used as a method to exclude CAD among patients of low/intermediate risk presenting with acute chest pain to the emergency department, which leads to more rapid triage/discharge times. An approach including cardiac CT leads to identification of more coronary atherosclerosis and higher frequency of invasive testing and revascularization, with more contrast and radiation.

Physiologic Evaluation of Coronary Artery Disease

Fractional flow reserve (FFR) can be estimated from the CT images without the need for a coronary vasodilator to determine the hemodynamic significance of a coronary stenosis. When applied to coronary stenosis of intermediate severity, FFRCT may correctly identify hemodynamically significant lesions to better determine the need for invasive angiography and revascularization.

Coronary Artery Calcium (CAC) Score

CAC is sensitive (91%) but not specific (49%) for detecting obstructive CAD with high NPV. CAC assessment is useful for risk stratification and is reasonable in asymptomatic patients with intermediate risk (10–20% 10-y Framingham risk) to determine the need for statin therapy. Radiation exposure for CAC is lower than for CCTA.

Cardiac MRI CMR

MRI provides high spatial resolution images; quantitative assessment of ventricular function; myocardial viability; quantification of intra- and extracardiac shunts; measurements of valvular velocities and gradients; and contrast-enhanced angiography without the use of ionizing radiation. See Table 31.3 for common applications of CMR.

Clinical Pearl
Avoid gadolinium when there is impaired renal function (eGFR <30) to avoid nephrogenic systemic fibrosis.

TABLE 31.3 Common clinical application of cardiac MRI

CMR clinical application:
Coronary artery disease
Myocardial infarction: Assess ventricular function, late gadolinium enhancement LGE for myocardial infarction and infarct size, complications of MI. ***Assessment of myocardial viability:*** Presence and extent of LGE involvement (< 50% transmurality cutoff) typically used to determine probability of contractile recovery. Dobutamine-induced systolic wall thickening of >2 mm or improved wall motion also predicts recovery. ***Myocardial ischemia:*** Stress CMR imaging can be performed using vasodilator agents to assess myocardial perfusion or with dobutamine to assess for inducible wall motion abnormalities. Normal stress CMR predicts an annualized cardiac event rate of less than 1%.
Cardiomyopathy
Hypertrophic Cardiomyopathy: Gold standard for determination of LVH and LV mass. Max wall thickness (>30 mm) is specific for predicting SCD. Detects the presence of LGE, systolic anterior motion (SAM) of the mitral valve, and apical aneurysms. ***Arrhythmogenic Right Ventricular Cardiomyopathy ARVC:*** Assessment of RV size and function, myocardial fibrofatty infiltration, localized aneurysms. CMR has been shown to have a sensitivity of 96% and a specificity of 78% in detecting ARVC. ***Myocarditis:*** Using the modified Lake Louise criteria, CMR assessment of T2-weighted imaging for myocardial edema, early gadolinium enhancement (EGE) for regional hyperemia and capillary leak, and LGE imaging for myocardial fibrosis (usually subepicardial and/or mid-myocardial). T2 mapping showed the most benefit in patients with chronic symptoms.

TABLE 31.3 (continued)

Cardiac Sarcoidosis: Assesses ventricular function, LGE for scar/fibrosis (usually patchy involvement). Presence of LGE has been associated with major arrhythmias, guide endomyocardial biopsy (EMB) (if septal LGE noted). Higher sensitivity in identifying cardiac sarcoidosis than the modified Japanese Ministry of Health guidelines.
Cardiac Amyloidosis: Assessment of LV systolic function, presence of concentric increase in LV wall thickness, diffuse EGE and/or LGE of the LV (may involve the RV).
Other cardiomyopathies: *Iron Overload Cardiomyopathy*, preserved systolic LV function in most cases, T2$*$ technique for quantifying myocardial iron deposition (myocardial T2$*$ $<$ 10 ms highest risk of heart failure within 1 year). *Left Ventricular Noncompaction,* measuring diastolic noncompacted-to-compacted thickness ratio of >2.3 has been used to diagnose LV noncompaction.

Valvular heart disease

In aortic valve disease, CMR can measure the aortic valve orifice by direct planimetry of the valve orifice. CMR phase-contrast imaging is used to measure blood and to quantify regurgitant valvular lesions.

Pericardial disease

Assessment of pericardial thickness, LGE imaging to assess for active inflammation or pericardial fibrosis. Real-time imaging during free breathing for the detection of cardiac constriction. Myocardial tagged (CSPAMM) imaging may be useful to identify any regional tethering caused by adhesions. CMR can help in differentiating constrictive pericarditis from restrictive cardiomyopathy.

Congenital heart disease

Atrial septal defect: Presence of an atrial septal defect, assess suitability for transcatheter ASD closure, quantify right heart size and function, measure pulmonary-to-systemic shunt ratio (Qp/Qs).

(continued)

TABLE 31.3 (continued)

Ventricular septal defect: Presence of a ventricular septal defect, quantify ventricular size and function, measure pulmonary-to-systemic shunt ratio (Qp/Qs), LGE imaging may help to determine if a VSD developed as a complication of MI. ***Coarctation of the Aorta:*** Assess the aortic anatomy, the degree of obstruction, and aortic valvular dysfunction. Phase-contrast imaging can estimate pressure gradient across the coarctation. Detection of collateral formation ***Tetralogy of Fallot:*** Identifying pulmonary blood flow. Quantitation of the severity of infundibular or pulmonary stenosis, assessment of RV function, presence of an anomalous coronary artery. Post-surgical RV outflow aneurysm evaluation, pulmonary regurgitation, biventricular size and function, and residual shunt.

Key Learning Points

- Multiple imaging options exist for the evaluation of cardiac disease. It is important to be aware of the wide array of choices available.
- Stress testing, whether exercise or pharmacologic, provides a functional evaluation of ischemia.
- The addition of imaging (either echo or nuclear) increases the diagnostic accuracy of stress testing for the detection of CAD, particularly in women.
- CCT provides an anatomic evaluation of CAD and is particularly useful in the exclusion of disease in low-risk patients.
- Cardiac MRI has broad capabilities that are important across many specific cardiac disorders.

References

1. Johnson NP, Goldberger JJ. Prognostic value of late heart rate recovery after treadmill exercise. Am J Cardiol. 2012;110:45–9.
2. Weiss SA, Blumenthal RS, Sharrett AR, et al. Exercise blood pressure and future cardiovascular death in asymptomatic individuals. Circulation. 2010;121:2109–16.

3. Stein R, Nguyen P, Abella J, et al. Prevalence and prognostic significance of exercise-induced right bundle branch block. Am J Cardiol. 2010;105:677–80.
4. Marine JE, Shetty V, Chow GV, et al. Prevalence and prognostic significance of exercise induced nonsustained ventricular tachycardia in asymptomatic volunteers: BLSA (Baltimore longitudinal study of aging). J Am CollCardiol. 2013;62:595–600.
5. Gibbons RJ, Balady GJ, Bricker JT, et al. ACC/AHA 2002 guideline update for exercise testing: summary article: a report of the American College of Cardiology/American Heart Association task force on practice guidelines (committee to update the 1997 exercise testing guidelines). Circulation. 2002;106:1883–92.
6. Morise AP, Jalisi F. Evaluation of pretest and exercise test scores to assess all-cause mortality in unselected patients presenting for exercise testing with symptoms of suspected coronary artery disease. J Am Coll Cardiol. 2003;42:842–50.
7. Mieres JH, Gulati M, Bairey Merz N, et al. Role of noninvasive testing in the clinical evaluation of women with suspected ischemic heart disease: a consensus statement from the American Heart Association. Circulation. 2014;130:350–79.
8. Kiviniemi AM, Lepojarvi S, Kentta TV, et al. Exercise capacity and heart rate responses to exercise as predictors of short-term outcome among patients with stable coronary artery disease. Am J Cardiol. 2015;116:1495–501.
9. Fleisher LA, Fleischmann KE, Auerbach AD, et al. 2014 ACC/AHA guideline on perioperative cardiovascular evaluation and management of patients undergoing noncardiac surgery: a report of the American College of Cardiology/American Heart Association task force on practice guidelines. J Am Coll Cardiol. 2014;64:e77–e137.
10. Anderson JL, Halperin JL, Albert NM, et al. Management of patients with peripheral artery disease (compilation of 2005 and 2011 ACCF/AHA guideline recommendations): a report of the American College of Cardiology Foundation/American Heart Association task force on practice guidelines. Circulation. 2013;127:1425–43.
11. Marwick TH, Case C, Sawada S, et al. Prediction of mortality by exercise echocardiography: a strategy for combination with Duke treadmill score. Circulation. 2001;103:2566–71.
12. Cornel JH, Bax JJ, Ehendy A, et al. Biphasic response to dobutamine predicts improvement of global left ventricular dysfunction after surgical revascularization in patients with stable coronary

artery disease : implications of time course of recovery on diagnostic accuracy. J Am Coll Cardiol. 1998;31:1002–10.
13. Holly TA, Abbott BG, Al-Mallah M, et al. ASNC imaging guidelines for nuclear cardiology procedures: single photon-emission computed tomography. J Nucl Cardiol. 2010;17:941–73.
14. Dilsizian V. SPECT and PET myocardial perfusion imaging: tracers and techniques. In: Dilsizian V, Narula J, Braunwald E, editors. Atlas of nuclear cardiology. 4th ed. New York: Springer; 2013. p. 55–94.
15. Schindler TH, Schelbert HR, Quercioli A, Dilsizian V. Cardiac PET imaging for the detection and monitoring of coronary artery disease and microvascular health. JACC Cardiovasc Imaging. 2010;3:623–40.
16. Amsterdam EA, Wenger NK, Brindis RG, et al. 2014 AHA/ACC guideline for the management of patients with non-ST-elevation acute coronary syndromes: a report of the American College of Cardiology/American Heart Association task force on practice guidelines. Circulation. 2014;130:e344–426.
17. Wolk MJ, Bailey SR, Doherty JU, et al. ACCF/AHA/ASE/ASNC/HFSA/ HRS/SCAI/SCCT/SCMR/ STS 2013 multimodality appropriate use criteria for the detection and risk assessment of stable ischemic heart disease. A report of the American College of Cardiology Foundation Appropriate Use Criteria Task Force, American Heart Association, American Society of Echocardiography, American Society of Nuclear Cardiology, Heart Failure Society of America, Heart Rhythm Society, Society for Cardiovascular Angiography and Interventions, Society of Cardiovascular Computed Tomography, Society for Cardiovascular Magnetic Resonance, and Society of Thoracic Surgeons. J Am Coll Cardiol. 2014;63:380–406.
18. Patel MR, White RD, Abbara S, et al. 2013 ACCF/ACR/ASE/ASNC/SCCT/SCMR appropriate utilization of cardiovascular imaging in heart failure. A joint report of the American College of Radiology Appropriateness Criteria Committee and the American College of Cardiology Foundation appropriate use criteria task force. J Am Coll Cardiol. 2013;61:2207–31.
19. Soman P, Udelson JE. Assessment of myocardial viability by nuclear imaging in coronary heart disease. UptoDate.
20. Fleisher LA, Fleischmann KE, Auerbach AD, et al. 2014 ACC/AHA guideline on perioperative cardiovascular evaluation and management of patients undergoing noncardiac surgery: executive summary. A report of the American College of Cardiology/

American Heart Association task force on practice guidelines. Circulation. 2014;130:2215–45.
21. Abbara S, Arbab-Zadeh A, Callister TQ, et al. SCCT guidelines for performance of coronary computed tomographic angiography: a report of the Society of Cardiovascular Computed Tomography Guidelines Committee. J Cardiovasc Comput Tomogr. 2009;3:190–204.
22. El-Hajjar M, Bashir I, Khan M, et al. Incidence of contrast-induced nephropathy in patients with chronic renal insufficiency undergoing multidetector computed tomographic angiography treated with preventive measures. Am J Cardiol. 2008;102:353–6.
23. Nasir K, Bittencourt MS, Blaha MJ, et al. Implications of coronary artery calcium testing among statin candidates according to American College of Cardiology/American Heart Association cholesterol management guidelines: MESA (multi-ethnic study of atherosclerosis). J Am Coll Cardiol. 2015;66:1657–68.
24. Criqui MH, Denenberg JO, Ix JH, et al. Calcium density of coronary artery plaque and risk of incident cardiovascular events. JAMA. 2014;311:271–8.
25. Nasir K, Clouse M. Role of nonenhanced multidetector CT coronary artery calcium testing in asymptomatic and symptomatic individuals. Radiology. 2012;264:637–49.
26. Wolk MJ, Bailey SR, Doherty JU, et al. ACCF/AHA/ASE/ASNC/HFSA/HRS/SCAI/SCCT/SCMR/ STS 2013 multimodality appropriate use criteria for the detection and risk assessment of stable ischemic heart disease: a report of the American College of Cardiology Foundation Appropriate Use Criteria Task Force, American Heart Association, American Society of Echocardiography, American Society of Nuclear Cardiology, Heart Failure Society of America, Heart Rhythm Society, Society for Cardiovascular Angiography and Interventions, Society of Cardiovascular Computed Tomography, Society for Cardiovascular Magnetic Resonance, and Society of Thoracic Surgeons. J Am Coll Cardiol. 2014;63:380–406.
27. Miller JM, Rochitte CE, Dewey M, et al. Diagnostic performance of coronary angiography by 64-row CT. N Engl J Med. 2008;359:2324–36.
28. Neglia D, Rovai D, Caselli C, et al. Detection of significant coronary artery disease by noninvasive anatomical and functional imaging. Circ Cardiovasc Imaging. 2015;8:e002179.

29. Min JK, Dunning A, Lin FY, et al. Rationale and design of the CONFIRM (coronary CT angiography evaluation for clinical outcomes: an international multicenter) registry. J Cardiovasc Comput Tomogr. 2011;5:84–92.
30. Dwivedi G, Cocker M, Yam Y, et al. Predictive value of cardiac computed tomography and the impact of renal function on all-cause mortality (from coronary CT angiography evaluation for clinical outcomes). Am J Cardiol. 2013;111:1563–9.
31. Hulten E, Villines TC, Cheezum MK, et al. Calcium score, coronary artery disease extent and severity, and clinical outcomes among low Framingham risk patients with low vs high lifetime risk: results from the CONFIRM registry. J Nucl Cardiol. 2014;21:29–37. quiz 38-29
32. Goldstein MA, Roy SK, Hebsur S, et al. Relationship between routine multi-detector cardiac computed tomographic angiography prior to reoperative cardiac surgery, length of stay, and hospital charges. Int J Cardiovasc Imaging. 2013;29:709–17.
33. Meijboom WB, Van Mieghem CA, van Pelt N, et al. Comprehensive assessment of coronary artery stenoses: computed tomography coronary angiography versus conventional coronary angiography and correlation with fractional flow reserve in patients with stable angina. J Am Coll Cardiol. 2008;52:636–43.
34. Hoffmann U, Bamberg F, Chae CU, et al. Coronary computed tomography angiography for early triage of patients with acute chest pain: the ROMICAT (rule out myocardial infarction using computer assisted tomography) trial. J Am Coll Cardiol. 2009;53:1642–50.
35. Hoffmann U, Truong QA, Schoenfeld DA, et al. Coronary CT angiography versus standard evaluation in acute chest pain. N Engl J Med. 2012;367:299–308.
36. Douglas PS, Hoffmann U, Patel MR, et al. Outcomes of anatomical versus functional testing for coronary artery disease. N Engl J Med. 2015;372:1291–300.
37. Newby D, Williams M, Hunter A, et al. CT coronary angiography in patients with suspected angina due to coronary heart disease (SCOT-HEART): an open-label, parallel-group, multicenter trial. Lancet. 2015;385:2383–91.
38. Min JK, Leipsic J, Pencina MJ, et al. Diagnostic accuracy of fractional flow reserve from anatomic CT angiography. JAMA. 2012;308:1237–45.
39. Douglas PS, Pontone G, Hlatky MA, et al. Clinical outcomes of fractional flow reserve by computed tomographic angiography-

guided diagnostic strategies vs. usual care in patients with suspected coronary artery disease: the prospective longitudinal trial of FFR(CT): outcome and resource impacts study. Eur Heart J. 2015;36:3359–67.

40. Hlatky MA, De Bruyne B, Pontone G, et al. Quality-of-life and economic outcomes of assessing fractional flow reserve with computed tomography angiography: PLATFORM. J Am Coll Cardiol. 2015;66:2315–23.
41. Blanke P, Naoum C, Webb J, et al. Multimodality imaging in the context of transcatheter mitral valve replacement: establishing consensus among modalities and disciplines. JACC Cardiovasc Imaging. 2015;8:1191–208.
42. Achenbach S, Delgado V, Hausleiter J, et al. SCCT expert consensus document on computed tomography imaging before transcatheter aortic valve implantation (TAVI)/transcatheter aortic valve replacement (TAVR). J Cardiovas Comput Tomogr. 2012;6:366–80.
43. Njeim M, Desjardins B, Bogun F. Multimodality imaging for guiding EP ablation procedures. JACC Cardiovasc Imaging. 2016;9:873–86.
44. Saw J, Lopes JP, Reisman M, et al. Cardiac computed tomography angiography for left atrial appendage closure. Can J Cardiol. 2016;32(1033):e1031–9.
45. Choi BH, Ko SM, Hwang HK, et al. Detection of left atrial thrombus in patients with mitral stenosis and atrial fibrillation: retrospective comparison of two-phase computed tomography, transoesophageal echocardiography and surgical findings. Eur Radiol. 2013;23:2944–53.
46. Heydari B, Juan YH, Liu H, et al. Stress perfusion cardiac magnetic resonance imaging effectively risk stratifies diabetic patients with suspected myocardial ischemia. Circ Cardiovasc Imaging. 2016;9:e004136.
47. Pasupathy S, Air T, Dreyer RP, et al. Systematic review of patients presenting with suspected myocardial infarction and nonobstructive coronary arteries. Circulation. 2015;131:861–70.
48. Fihn SD, Gardin JM, Abrams J, et al. 2012 ACCF/AHA/ACP/AATS/PCNA/SCAI/STS guideline for the diagnosis and management of patients with stable ischemic heart disease: executive summary: a report of the American College of Cardiology Foundation/American Heart Association task force on practice guidelines, and the American College of Physicians, American Association for Thoracic Surgery, Preventive Cardiovascular

Nurses Association, Society for Cardiovascular Angiography and Interventions, and Society of Thoracic Surgeons. Circulation. 2012;126:3097–137.

49. Mordini FE, Haddad T, Hsu LY, et al. Diagnostic accuracy of stress perfusion CMR in comparison with quantitative coronary angiography: fully quantitative, semiquantitative, and qualitative assessment. JACC Cardiovasc Imaging. 2014;7:14–22.
50. Chan RH, Maron BJ, Olivotto I, et al. Prognostic value of quantitative contrast-enhanced cardiovascular magnetic resonance for the evaluation of sudden death risk in patients with hypertrophic cardiomyopathy. Circulation. 2014;130:484–95.
51. te Riele AS, Tandri H, Bluemke DA. Arrhythmogenic right ventricular cardiomyopathy (ARVC): cardiovascular magnetic resonance update. J Cardiovasc Magn Reson. 2014;16:50.
52. Radunski UK, Lund GK, Stehning C, et al. CMR in patients with severe myocarditis: diagnostic value of quantitative tissue markers including extracellular volume imaging. JACC Cardiovasc Imaging. 2014;7:667–75.
53. Murtagh G, Laffin LJ, Beshai JF, et al. Prognosis of myocardial damage in sarcoidosis patients with preserved left ventricular ejection fraction: risk stratification using cardiovascular magnetic resonance. Circ Cardiovasc Imaging. 2016;9:e003738.
54. Gati S, Rajani R, Carr-White GS, Chambers JB. Adult left ventricular noncompaction: reappraisal of current diagnostic imaging modalities. JACC Cardiovasc Imaging. 2014;7:1266–75.
55. Cawley PJ, Hamilton-Craig C, Owens DS, et al. Prospective comparison of valve regurgitation quantitation by cardiac magnetic resonance imaging and transthoracic echocardiography. Circ Cardiovasc Imaging. 2013;6:48–57.
56. Myerson SG, d'Arcy J, Mohiaddin R, et al. Aortic regurgitation quantification using cardiovascular magnetic resonance: association with clinical outcome. Circulation. 2012;126:1452–60.

Chapter 32
Left and Right Heart Catheterization

Mistyann-Blue Miller and Duane Pinto

Cardiac Catheterization

General Principles

- Cardiac catheterization includes a combination of diagnostic coronary angiography, percutaneous coronary intervention (PCI), left ventricular and aortic angiography, right heart catheterization, hemodynamic pressure measurements, blood oximetry, evaluation and treatment of valvular heart disease, or diagnostic and therapeutic removal of pericardial fluid.
- Left heart catheterization (LHC) involves invasive percutaneous techniques that require arterial access, i.e., coronary angiography and/or left ventricular angiography.
- Right heart catheterization (RHC) involves the hemodynamic assessment of right-sided (venous) cardiac chambers and pulmonary arterial vasculature using balloon-tipped catheters to measure pressure and obtain blood oximetry samples.

M.-B. Miller (✉) · D. Pinto
Department of Interventional Cardiology, Beth Israel Deaconess Medical Center/Harvard Medical School, Boston, MA, USA
e-mail: mmille16@bidmc.harvard.edu

B. J. Wells et al. (eds.), *Handbook of Inpatient Cardiology*,
https://doi.org/10.1007/978-3-030-47868-1_32

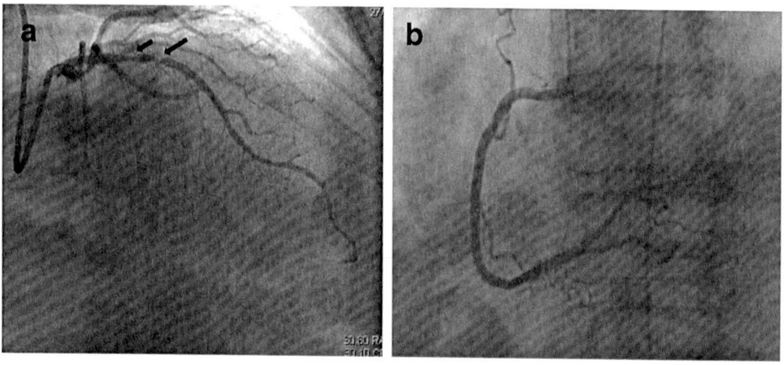

Figure 32.1 Diagnostic coronary angiograms depicting an RAO cranial projection of the left main coronary artery (**a**) and LAO cranial projection of the right coronary artery (**b**). Note the serial stenotic lesions (*arrows*) of the mid-left anterior descending artery

- Cardiac catheterization should be performed as a confirmatory or diagnostic complement to noninvasive testing.
- Small catheters of various sizes and shapes are used for invasive hemodynamic measurements and for injection of radiopaque contrast that allows visualization of coronary arteries and cardiac chambers under fluoroscopic X-ray imaging (Fig. 32.1).

LHC and Coronary Angiography

- Coronary angiography is the mainstay of diagnostic and therapeutic cardiac catheterization laboratory procedures.
- Coronary angiography should be performed to identify the presence, extent, and severity of coronary artery disease.
- Indications for cardiac catheterization are listed in Table 32.1. A complete list of indications can be reviewed in the ACC/AHA guidelines [1–4].
- Adjunctive procedures to coronary angiography include functional and physiologic assessment of stenotic coronary lesions using fractional flow reserve (FFR) or instanta-

TABLE 32.1 Indication for Coronary Angiography
Acute coronary syndrome
Preoperative valve surgery for patients older than 35 years of age
When the presence of clinically relevant coronary artery disease remains unclear despite noninvasive testing and imaging
Differentiation between ischemic versus non-ischemic cardiomyopathy
Cardiogenic shock
When clinical history and noninvasive testing suggest high likelihood of significant ischemic heart disease

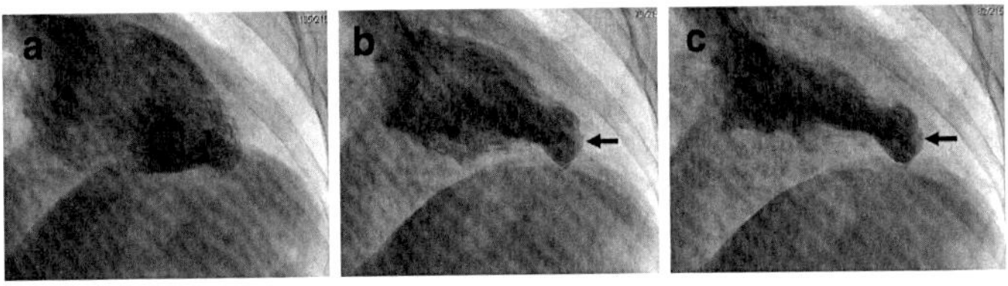

FIGURE 32.2 Left ventriculography demonstrating an apical LV aneurysm (*arrows*) in (**a**) diastole, (**b**) mid-systole, (**c**) end-systole

neous wave-free ratio (IFR); assessment of coronary lumen compromise, calcium density, or plaque characteristics using intravascular ultrasound (IVUS) or optical coherence tomography (OCT); or measurement of myocardial and coronary blood flow.

- Left ventricular (LV) angiography (i.e., left ventriculography) is helpful in the assessment of LV systolic function, regional wall motion abnormalities, VSD and mitral regurgitation (Fig. 32.2).

Periprocedural Considerations for Cardiac Catheterization

Informed Consent and Contraindications

- Informed consent, full history and physical exam, medication reconciliation, and review of basic labs (i.e., CBC, BMP, coagulations studies) are obtained prior to any elective cardiac catheterization procedure.
- The only absolute contraindication to cardiac catheterization is the refusal of a competent patient (or healthcare proxy if the patient does not have decision-making capacity) to undergo the procedure.
- Relative contraindications should be reviewed in Table 32.2.

Preparation of the Patient

- The patient should be NPO at least 6 hours prior to the procedure, except in the case of urgent or emergent indications.

Clinical Pearl

- Patients with documented contrast (or iodine) allergies should be premedicated with steroids and diphenhydramine. Protocols for pre-medication may vary among institutions, but in general the patient should receive 50 mg Prednisone PO (or 100 mg Hydrocortisone IV) 12 hours prior to the procedure and an additional dose immediately before the procedure. Intravenous methylprednisolone can also be used. Premedication also includes the use of H2 blockers – either cimetidine, ranitidine, or famotidine – and diphenhydramine 25 mg or 50 mg IV given once.
- Shellfish allergy does not warrant premedication with steroids, diphenhydramine, or H2-blockers.

Table 32.2 Relative Contraindications to Cardiac Catheterization

Severe hypokalemia
Severe anemia
Active blood loss
Acute stroke
Severe coagulopathy
Significant acute kidney injury (AKI) or acute renal failure
Digoxin toxicity
Untreated infection

- Patients should receive pre- and post-procedure hydration with normal saline unless patients are volume overloaded.
- Sodium bicarbonate has not been proven to be superior to normal saline in the prevention of contrast-induced nephropathy in patients with renal insufficiency [3].
- Metformin should be discontinued the morning of the procedure and should not be restarted until renal function has remained stable 48 hours post-procedure.
- Systemic anticoagulation should be held for elective catheterization procedures requiring arterial access.
- Direct oral anticoagulants should be held for 2–4 doses prior to the procedure.
- Heparin for acute coronary syndrome, DVT, or atrial fibrillation, can be held 1–4 hours prior to the scheduled catheterization.
- For mechanical heart valves, systemic anticoagulation should be continued as close to the procedure as reasonably accepted and may require discussions with the physician operator.
- INR goals for femoral artery and radial artery access should be <1.8 and 2.2, respectively.
- Procedures that involve only venous access (i.e., RHC) do not require cessation of anticoagulation and can safely be performed with an INR ≤ 3.

Vascular Access

- Routine vascular access sites for cardiac catheterization procedures include femoral and transradial arterial access.
- Transradial access has become increasingly prevalent for routine, urgent, and emergent procedures with fewer vascular complications [5]. Time to ambulation is also significantly reduced with transradial access.
- The common femoral vessels are used for procedures that require large-bore access, including placement of mechanical circulatory support devices (e.g. Impella, intra-aortic balloon pump), or structural interventions including balloon aortic valvuloplasty, transcatheter aortic valve replacement (TAVR), or percutaneous mitral valve interventions.
- Alternative vascular access sites include the distal radial artery (via anatomical snuffbox), ulnar artery, brachial artery, axillary artery, or subclavian artery.

Post-procedure Care

- Common femoral artery hemostasis is achieved with either manual compression or with the use of active or passive vascular closure devices (VCD).
- Patients should remain flat without bending of the ipsilateral leg typically 2–4 hours after hemostasis is achieved with manual compression and 1–2 hours with VCDs.
- Longer bedrest times are required for larger sheath sizes (6Fr and larger).
- Femoral artery occlusion may occur with the use of VCDs, but the incidence is low [6].
- Radial artery hemostasis is achieved with the use of a compression band that provides hemostasis while still allowing radial artery patency, which reduces the risk of radial artery occlusion [7].
- After most routine catheterization procedures without vascular complications, anticoagulation can generally be restarted 4–6 hours after documented hemostasis. Protocols may vary by institution.

Pharmacotherapy During Cardiac Catheterization

- Antiplatelet and anticoagulants are required for any percutaneous coronary, peripheral, or structural intervention.

> **Clinical Pearl**
> Patients with unexplained anemia should be evaluated for sources of bleeding, bleeding diatheses, or coagulopathy prior to referring for cardiac catheterization procedure.

- Unfractionated heparin (UFH) is the most commonly used anticoagulant in cardiac catheterization procedures. UFH is administered in weight-based boluses and its therapeutic effects are monitored by measuring the activated clotting time (ACT).
- Diagnostic transradial procedures also require the use of heparin to reduce the risk of radial artery occlusion.
- Low molecular weight heparin (LMWH) is less frequently used, but can be administered subcutaneously or intravenously.
- Other anticoagulants or antiplatelets used during cardiac catheterization may include GP IIb/IIIa inhibitors (tirofiban, eptifibatide, abciximab) and direct thrombin inhibitors (argatroban and bivalirudin).
- Moderate sedation (conscious sedation) is the desired level of sedation for most cardiac catheterization procedures. This induces a depressed consciousness that still permits the patient to respond to verbal commands without respiratory or cardiovascular compromise. This is most commonly achieved with an intravenous short-acting benzodiazepine (e.g., midazolam) and an opiate, typically fentanyl [7].

Right Heart Catheterization

- RHC can be performed via the internal jugular vein, femoral vein, subclavian vein, or antecubital vein.
- Indications for RHC can be reviewed in Table 32.3.
- A balloon-tipped PA catheter is advanced through the right atrium, right ventricle, pulmonary artery (PA), and pulmonary capillary bed where pressure measurements are recorded in each chamber.
- Pulmonary capillary wedge pressure is used as a surrogate for left atrial pressure.
- Cardiac output (CO) is calculated using the Fick equation (Fig. 32.3) or using the thermodilution (TD) technique.
- The Fick principle is based on the concept that uptake or release of oxygen in blood by an organ is the product of the arteriovenous concentration difference of oxygen and the blood flow to that organ.

Table 32.3 Indications for Right Heart Catheterization

Assessment of pulmonary hypertension and response to therapy: Epoprostenol, nitric oxide
Assessment of volume status when clinically ambiguous
Differentiation of cardiogenic shock from other forms of shock
Leave-in swan-Ganz catheters for continuous hemodynamic monitoring and tailored inotrope or diuretic therapy
Evaluate for constrictive or restrictive pathophysiology
Intracardiac shunt assessment
Assessment of RV failure
Determine severity of valvular disease

$$\frac{\text{O}_2\text{ Consumption (VO2) mL/min}}{\text{AVO}_2\text{ Difference x 10}}$$

- *O_2 consumption is typically calculated as 3mL O2/kg*
- *A VO_2 = The arteriovenous oxygen difference calculated from arterial - mixed venous (PA) O2 content, where O2 content= saturation x 1.36 x hemoglobin.*

Figure 32.3 Fick equation for calculating cardiac output

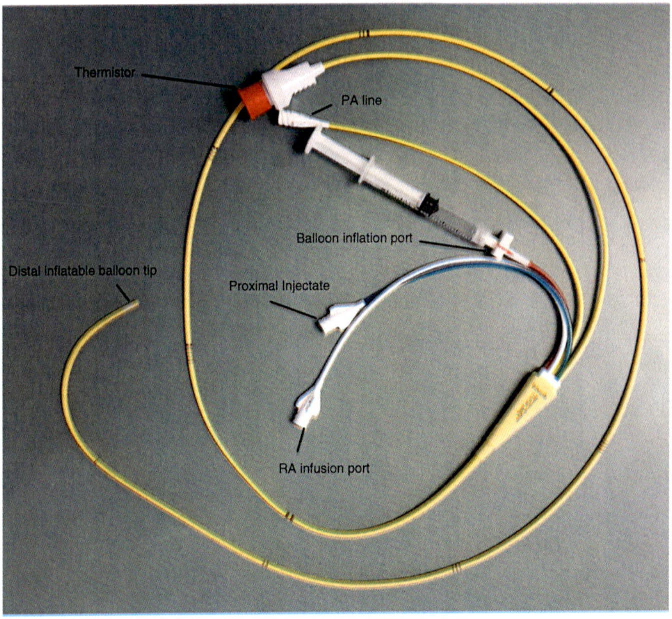

FIGURE 32.4 Swan Ganz catheter with thermistor port

- The Fick method is the most widely used technique to calculate CO in the catheterization lab.
- The thermodilution technique is performed using a balloon-tipped PA catheter with a distal thermistor (Fig. 32.4). Cold (4 ° C) or room temperature normal saline is injected into the right atrium which mixes with and cools the blood. Change in temperature of the indicator (mixed saline and blood) is calculated and plotted over time. The area under this curve is the cardiac output.
- Accuracy of the thermodilution technique decreases with lower CO and severe tricuspid regurgitation.
- Patients with primary pulmonary arterial hypertension may undergo invasive hemodynamic response testing in the catheterization lab with intravenous pulmonary vasodilators (e.g., epoprostenol or inhaled nitric oxide).
- Protocols for vasodilator response testing vary among institutions.

Combined RHC and LHC Hemodynamic Assessments

- Invasive assessment of any valve disease is performed when noninvasive assessment remains ambiguous.
- Most valvular assessments require combined left and right heart catheterization techniques.
- The assessment of valvular stenosis involves invasive measurement of right heart pressures, cardiac output, and transvalvular gradients which are then used to calculate valve area.
- Mitral and aortic insufficiency are assessed angiographically with power injection of contrast into the left ventricle and aortic root, respectively.
- Severity of regurgitation is graded from 0 (no regurgitation) to 4+ (severe, wide-open regurgitation).
- Pulmonic and tricuspid insufficiency are assessed using PA catheters and similar angiographic techniques described above.

Complications of Cardiac Catheterization

- Due to relatively low complication rates, percutaneous catheterization procedures are safe for the majority of patients.
- The risk of any adverse event is less than 1%. The risk of mortality is about 0.08% while the risk of stroke or periprocedural MI are 0.2% and 0.5%, respectively [7].
- Bleeding, vascular injury, acute kidney injury, allergic reactions, arrhythmias, and heart failure occur at risks <1%.
- Arterial access site hematomas are the most common post-procedural complications.
- If a hematoma is detected, immediately apply manual pressure and notify the physician or staff involved in the initial procedure.

- Duplex ultrasound studies may be needed to evaluate the presence of a pseudoaneurysm. These can be treated with ultrasound-guided compression or direct injection of thrombin.

Clinical Pearl

If a patient becomes hypotensive and tachycardic post-cardiac catheterization, particularly with femoral arterial access, retroperitoneal hematomas should be suspected and these patients should undergo urgent CT or ultrasound of the abdomen, pelvis, and groin, in addition to serial CBCs and cessation of systemic anticoagulation. With high index suspicion or an unstable patient, immediate angiography is often preferred over diagnostic imaging to allow for more prompt identification and initiation of catheter-based treatment.

Key Learning Points

1. The decision to proceed with cardiac catheterization is based on a risk-benefit model and should be performed as a confirmatory or diagnostic complement to noninvasive testing.
2. Informed consent is obtained prior to any elective cardiac catheterization procedure. This is paired with a full history and physical, medication reconciliation, and review of basic labs including CBC, BMP, and coagulation studies.
3. Premedication with steroids, diphenhydramine, and H_2 blockers is required for patients with documented contrast or iodine allergy.
4. Shellfish allergy does not warrant premedication with steroids, diphenhydramine, or H2-blockers.
5. In patients who become hypotensive and tachycardic post-cardiac catheterization, retroperitoneal hematomas should be highly suspected.

References

1. Nishimura RA, Otto CM, Bonow RO, et al. 2014 AHA/ACC guideline for the management of patients with valvular heart disease: a report of the American College of Cardiology/American Heart Association task force on practice guidelines. J Am Coll Cardiol. 2014;63:e57.
2. Fihn SD, Blankenship JC, Alexander KP, et al. 2014 ACC/AHA/AATS/PCNA/SCAI/STS focused update of the guideline for the diagnosis and management of patients with stable ischemic heart disease: a report of the American College of Cardiology/American Heart Association task force on practice guidelines, and the American Association for Thoracic Surgery, Preventive Cardiovascular Nurses Association, Society for Cardiovascular Angiography and Interventions, and Society of Thoracic Surgeons. J Am Coll Cardiol. 2014;64:1929–49.
3. Levine GN, O'Gara PT, Bates ER, et al. 2015 ACC/AHA/SCAI focused update on primary percutaneous coronary intervention for patients with ST-elevation myocardial infarction: an update of the 2011 ACCF/AHA/SCAI guideline for percutaneous coronary intervention and the 2013 ACCF/AHA guideline for the management of ST-elevation myocardial infarction. J Am Coll Cardiol. 2016;67:1235–50.
4. Fleisher LA, Fleischmann KE, Auerbach AD, et al. 2014 ACC/AHA guideline on perioperative cardiovascular evaluation and management of patients undergoing noncardiac surgery: a report of the American College of Cardiology/American Heart Association task force on practice guidelines. J Am Coll Cardiol. 2014;64:e77–137.
5. Jolly SS, Yusuf S, Cairns J, et al. Radial versus femoral access for coronary angiography and intervention in patients with acute coronary syndromes (RIVAL): a randomised, parallel group, multicentre trial. Lancet. 2011;377:1409–20.
6. Dauerman HL, Applegate RJ, Cohen DJ. Vascular closure devices: The second decade. J Am Coll Cardiol. 2007;50:1617–26.
7. Kern MJ, Sorajja P, Lim M. The cardiac catheterization handbook. 6th ed. Philadelphia: Elsevier; 2016.

Index

B. J. Wells et al. (eds.), *Handbook of Inpatient Cardiology*,
https://doi.org/10.1007/978-3-030-47868-1

B

C

9783030478674